D1267153

Integration of
Pharmacokinetics,
Pharmacodynamics,
and Toxicokinetics
in Rational
Drug Development

Integration of
Pharmacokinetics, Pharmacodynamics, and Toxicokinetics
in Rational Drug Development

Edited by

Avraham Yacobi
American Cyanamid Company
Pearl River, New York

Jerome P. Skelly
Food and Drug Administration
Washington, D.C.

Vinod P. Shah
Food and Drug Administration
Rockville, Maryland

and

Leslie Z. Benet
University of California, San Francisco
San Francisco, California

Published in cooperation with the
American Association of Pharmaceutical Scientists

Plenum Press • New York and London

Library of Congress Cataloging-in-Publication Data

Integration of pharmacokinetics, pharmacodynamics, and toxicokinetics
in rational drug development / edited by Avraham Yacobi ... [et
al.].
        p.   cm.
      "Sponsored by the American Association of Pharmaceutical
Scientists, the U.S. Food and Drug Administration, and the American
Society for Clinical Pharmacology and Therapeutics"--T.p. verso.
      "Published in cooperation with the American Association of
Pharmaceutical Scientists."
      Includes bibliographical references and indexes.
      ISBN 0-306-44356-2
      1. Drugs--Research--Methodology--Congresses. 2. Pharmacokinetics-
-Congresses. 3. Drugs--Physiological effect--Congresses. 4. Drugs-
-Toxicology--Congresses.   I. Yacobi, Avraham.   II. American
Association of Pharmaceutical Scientists.   III. United States. Food
and Drug Administration.   IV. American Society for Clinical
Pharmacology and Therapeutics.
      [DNLM: 1. Drug Evaluation--congresses. 2. Drug Screening-
-congresses. 3. Drugs, Investigational--congresses.
4. Pharmacokinetics--congresses.   QV 771 I602]
RM301.25.I58 1993
615'.1'072--dc20
DNLM/DLC
for Library of Congress   92-48285
                                                              CIP

This limited facsimile edition has been issued
for the purpose of keeping this title available
to the scientific community.

Invited papers presented at a conference entitled "The Integration of Pharmacokinetic,
Pharmacodynamic, and Toxicokinetic Principles in Rational Drug Development," held
April 24–26, 1991, in Arlington, Virginia, sponsored by the American Association of
Pharmaceutical Scientists, the U.S. Food and Drug Administration, and the American
Society for Clinical Pharmacology and Therapeutics

ISBN 0-306-44356-2

© 1993 Plenum Press, New York
A Division of Plenum Publishing Corporation
233 Spring Street, New York, N.Y. 10013

Printed in the United States of America

PREFACE

This volume contains the invited papers presented at the conference entitled "The Integration of Pharmacokinetic, Pharmacodynamic and Toxicokinetic Principles in Rational Drug Development" held in April, 1991. The conference was sponsored by the American Association of Pharmaceutical Scientists, the U.S. Food and Drug Administration and the American Society for Clinical Pharmacology and Therapeutics. The conference was organized with three objectives:

To identify the roles and interrelationships between pharmacokinetics, pharmacodynamics and toxicokinetics in the drug development process.

To evolve strategies for the effective application of the principles of pharmacokinetics, pharmacodynamics and toxicokinetics in drug development, including early clinical trials.

To prepare a report on the use of pharmacokinetics and pharmacodynamics in rational drug development as a basis for the development of future regulatory guidelines.

The report from this conference, a copy of which can be found on pages 249-262 of this volume, was published in mid 1992 in four leading journals of special interest to the more than 600 scientists who attended the conference. However, a great deal of information on the use of pharmacokinetics, pharmacodynamics and toxicokinetics in drug development was presented by the 25 academic, governmental and industrial scientists who made formal presentations at this unique meeting. It was strongly felt by the Editors, that this wealth of useful information would be of benefit to those in the pharmaceutical industry as well as to those in the regulatory agencies who are most concerned with the use of pharmacokinetics, pharmacodynamics and toxicokinetics in drug development. Therefore, the authors were requested to prepare formal documents of their presentations. However, it was also felt by the Editors that the volume should be more than a "conference proceedings". Thus the 25 individual chapters have been edited, prepared in a common print type face, with references updated as necessary, and supplemented with a complete subject index, which should make the book quite useful to those interested in particular topics.

The Editors greatly appreciate the efforts of Ms. Amy Miller of the AAPS staff who has spent innumerable hours and great efforts in assuring that this volume represents a first-class contribution to the drug development literature. We also appreciate the efforts of Ms. Leah

v

Dible of the Department of Pharmacy at the University of California, San Francisco in assisting the Editors in reference updates and index preparation.

The Editors anticipate that the conference summary report and this volume will only be the first of the publications which emanate from the 1991 workshop as we develop and hone our skills in the use of pharmacokinetics, pharmacodynamics and toxicokinetics in rational drug development.

CONTRIBUTORS

Antal, Edward J., Ph.D. Director, Clinical Pharmacokinetics, The Upjohn Company, Kalamazoo, Michigan.

Batra, Vijay K., Ph.D. Associate Director of Pharmacokinetics, Drug Metabolism and Pharmacokinetics Division, Schering Plough Research Institute, Bloomfield, New Jersey.

Benet, Leslie Z., Ph.D., Pharm.D.(Hon.) Professor and Chairman, Department of Pharmacy, School of Pharmacy, University of California, San Francisco, California.

Branch, Robert A., M.D. Professor of Medicine and Pharmacology, Director, Center for Clinical Pharmacology, University of Pittsburgh Medical Center, Pittsburgh, Pennsylvania.

Brater, D. Craig, M.D. John B. Hickman Professor of Medicine, Chairman, Department of Medicine, Director, Clinical Pharmacology Division, Professor of Medicine and Pharmacology, Indiana University, Indianapolis, Indiana.

Chen, Conrad, Ph.D. Pharmacologist, Pilot Drug Evaluation Staff, Center for Drug Evaluation and Research, Food and Drug Administration, Rockville, Maryland.

Collins, Jerry M., Ph.D. Director, Division of Clinical Pharmacology, Office of Research Resources, Center for Drug Evaluation and Research, Food and Drug Administration, Rockville, Maryland.

Coutinho, Claude B., Ph.D., M.D. Pharmacologist, Pilot Drug Evaluation Staff, Center for Drug Evaluation and Research, Food and Drug Administration, Rockville, Maryland.

Danhof, Meindert, Ph.D. Division of Pharmacology, Center for Biopharmaceutical Sciences, Leiden University, Leiden, The Netherlands.

Desjardins, Robert E., M.D. Vice President for Clinical Research, Medical Research Division, American Cyanamid Company, Pearl River, New York.

Faulkner, Robert D., Ph.D. Group Leader, Clinical Pharmacokinetics/Pharmacodynamics, American Cyanamid Company, Medical Research Division, Pearl River, New York.

Fitzgerald, Glenna G., M.D. Supervisory Pharmacologist, Division of Neuropharmacological Drug Products, Center for Drug Evaluation and Research, Food and Drug Administration, Rockville, Maryland.

Furst, Daniel E., M.D. Clinical Professor of Rheumatology, University of Medicine and Dentistry of New Jersey, R. W. Johnson Medical School, New Brunswick, New Jersey; (presently) Director of Clinical Research Programs, Virginia Mason Medical Center, Seattle, Washington.

Grasela, Thaddeus H., Jr., Pharm.D. Associate Professor of Pharmacy and Social and Preventive Medicine, Schools of Pharmacy and Medicine, University of Buffalo, Buffalo, New York.

Green, M. David, Ph.D. Supervisory Pharmacologist, Division of Antiviral Drug Products, Office of Drug Evaluation II, Center for Drug Evaluation and Research, Food and Drug Administration, Kensington, Maryland.

Greenblatt, David J., M.D. Professor of Pharmacology and Experimental Therapeutics, Psychiatry, and Medicine, Tufts University School of Medicine, Division of Clinical Pharmacology, New England Medical Center Hospital, Boston, Massachusetts.

Hoogerkamp, Arendien, M.Sc. Division of Pharmacology, Center for Bio-Pharmaceutical Sciences, Leiden University, Leiden, The Netherlands.

Jackson, Edwin K., Ph.D. Professor of Pharmacology and Medicine, Associate Director, Center for Clinical Pharmacology, University of Pittsburgh Medical Center, Pittsburgh, Pennsylvania.

Jean, Lucy, Ph.D., Pharmacologist, Pilot Drug Evaluation Staff, Center for Drug Evaluation and Research, Food and Drug Administration, Rockville, Maryland.

Leal, Mauricio, Ph.D. Group Leader, Non Clinical Pharmacokinetics, Medical Research Division, American Cyanamid Company, Pearl River, New York.

Levy, Gerhard, Pharm.D. Distinguished Professor of Pharmacy, Department of Pharmaceutics, School of Pharmacy, State University of New York at Buffalo, Amherst, New York.

Mandema, Jaap W., Ph.D. Departments of Laboratory Medicine and Pharmacy, Schools of Medicine and Pharmacy, University of California, San Francisco, California.

Miller, Lawrence G., M.D. Assistant Professor of Psychiatry and Pharmacology, Division of Clinical Pharmacology, Departments of Pharmacology and Psychiatry, Tufts University School of Medicine and New England Medical Center, Boston, Massachusetts.

Mukherjee, Asoke, Ph.D. Pharmacologist, Pilot Drug Evaluation Division, Center for Drug Evaluation and Research, Food and Drug Administration, Rockville, Maryland.

Nicolau, Gabriela, Ph.D. Department Head, Drug Metabolism/Disposition, American Cyanamid Company, Medical Research Division, Pearl River, New York.

O'Reilly, Robert A., M.D. Chairman, Department of Medicine, Santa Clara

Valley Medical Center, San Jose, California; Professor of Medicine, Stanford University Medical Center, Stanford, California; Clinical Professor of Medicine, School of Medicine, University of California, San Francisco, California.

Peck, Carl C., M.D. Director, Center for Drug Evaluation and Research, Food and Drug Administration, Rockville, Maryland.

Pool, William R., Ph.D. Executive Director, Pharmaceutical Development, American Cyanamid Company, Medical Research Division, Pearl River, New York.

Roden, Dan M., M.D. Director of Clinical Pharmacology, Professor of Medicine and Pharmacology, School of Medicine, Clinical Pharmacology, Vanderbilt University, Nashville, Tennessee.

Rozman, Karl K., M.D. Professor of Pharmacology and Toxicology. University of Kansas Medical Center, Kansas City, Kansas; Head, Section of Environmental Toxicology, Gesellschaft fur Strahlen - Unh Umweltforschung Munchen, Institut fur Toxikologie, Neuherberg, Germany.

Sanathanan, Lilly P., Ph.D. Director, Research and Methodology Planning Staff, Center for Drug Evaluation and Research, Food and Drug Administration, Rockville Maryland; (presently) Vice President, Bio Statistics and Clinical Data Systems, Institute for Biological Research and Development, Inc., Blue Bell, Pennsylvania.

Schentag, Jerome J., Pharm.D. Professor of Pharmaceutics and Pharmacy, State

University of New York at Buffalo, and Director, The Clinical Pharmacokinetics Lab, Millard Fillmore Hospital, Buffalo, New York.

Schwartz, Sorell L., Ph.D. Professor, Division of Clinical Pharmacology, Department of Pharmacology, Georgetown University Medical Center, Washington, District of Columbia.

Shah, Anita, Ph.D. Assistant Director, Clinical Pharmacology, Miles, Inc., West Haven, Connecticut.

Shah, Vinod P., Ph.D. Acting Deputy Associate Director for Science, Office of Generic Drugs, Center for Drug Evaluation and Research, Food and Drug Administration. Rockville, Maryland.

Sheiner, Lewis B., M.D. Professor of Laboratory Medicine, Pharmacy, and Medicine. Schools of Medicine and Pharmacy, University of California, San Francisco, California.

Skelly, Jerome P., Ph.D. Deputy Director, Office of Research Resources, Center for Drug Evaluation and Research, Food and Drug Administration, Washington, District of Columbia.

Stanski, Donald R., M.D. Professor and Chairman, Department of Anesthesia, Stanford University School of Medicine, Stanford, California.

Tonelli, Alfred P., Ph.D. Department Head, Bioanalytical Research, American Cyanamid Company, Medical Research Division, Pearl River, New York.

Verotta, Davide, Ph.D. Assistant Professor, Department of Pharmacy, University of California, San Francisco, California.

Weissinger, Judi, Ph.D. Assistant Director for Toxicology, Office of Drug Evaluation II, Center for Drug Evaluation and Research, Food and Drug Administration, Rockville, Maryland; (presently) Director of Preclinical Compliance, Glaxo Inc., Research Triangle Park, North Carolina.

Wellstein, Anton, M.D., Ph.D. Associate Professor, Division of Clinical Pharmacology, Departments of Pharmacology and Medicine, Georgetown University Medical Center, Washington, District of Columbia.

Woosley, Raymond L., M.D., Ph.D. Chairman, Department of Pharmacology, Director, Clinical Pharmacology Center, Professor of Pharmacology and Medicine, Georgetown University Medical Center, Washington, District of Columbia.

Yacobi, Avraham, Ph.D. Director, Pharmacodynamics Research, American Cyanamid Company, Medical Research Division, Pearl River, New York.

Yasuda, Sally Usdin, Pharm.D., M.S. Instructor, Division of Clinical Pharmacology, Department of Pharmacology, Georgetown University Medical Center, Washington, District of Columbia.

CONTENTS

SECTION

III

METHODOLOGY FOR PRECLINICAL PHARMACODYNAMIC STUDIES

SECTION

IV

PRECLINICAL & CLINICAL PHARMACOKINETICS

SECTION

V

CLINICAL PHARMACODYNAMICS

SECTION
VI

APPLICATION OF PHARMACODYNAMICS & PHARMACOKINETICS IN THE DRUG DEVELOPMENT PROCESS

SECTION
VII

SUMMARY REPORT

INTRODUCTION

In 1962 Congress passed the Kefauver Harris Amendments to the Pure Food and Drug Act. Drugs approved by the Food and Drug Administration from 1938 to that date had been approved only on the basis of safety, i.e., 'lack of toxicity.' To be sure, the toxicity data required in NDA submissions were considerably more onerous in 1960, than in the late 30's and early 40's. But the amended law now provided that drugs henceforth approved would require proof of efficacy as well. Moreover, those drugs approved between 1938 and October 10, 1962, would be reviewed to determine whether or not they were efficacious. Those that were judged to meet the efficacy provision, were additionally required to demonstrate that they were "bioavailable". Generic versions were required, among labeling and other considerations, to establish that they were bioequivalent to the bioavailable product.

The argument of the late 60's and early 70's was over whether the new sciences of biopharmaceutics and pharmacokinetics could be employed to demonstrate product bioequivalence, or whether generic firms would have to also conduct clinical studies. Such studies were neither economically feasible nor scientifically advisable. They would require many patients, and for many drugs, differences on the order of 50 to 100% could not be detected clinically. The Agency, with academic support, opted for in vivo human bioavailability and bioequivalence studies.

Over time, thousands of such studies were conducted. But determinations of drug bioavailability/bioequivalence provide for a very limited use of the pharmacokinetic information obtained. Gradually pharmacokinetics (the study of the time course of drug and metabolite concentrations and amounts in biological fluids, tissues, and excreta) came to be routinely employed in the design of dosage regimen and drug interaction studies. Today it is especially useful in the design of dosage regimens in subpopulations which differ markedly in their physiological responses. Nevertheless, while these studies have been conducted in humans to great advantage, similar employment has not been utilized in animal toxicity studies. Toxicokinetics, which encompasses the kinetics of absorption, distribution, metabolism, and elimination of large doses of drugs in the body and the safety evaluation and assessment of adverse reactions caused by excessive drug dosage, has yet to reach its full potential. It is interesting that even at this point in time, 20 years after the discovery of the importance of drug blood levels, our animal toxicity data is still largely dose based, even when the dose may not have been completely absorbed. Pharmacodynamics, which provides an assessment on how drugs exert their therapeutic and toxic effect on the body by describing the relationship of drug concentration to drug effect, is still an infant science. Yet we are aware that for many drugs the pharmacokinetic and pharmacodynamic effects appear to be unrelated.

The Editors, through this book, are resolved to make available all of the information presented at the AAPS/FDA/ASCPT workshop in April 1991, along with the summary document which was issued as a result. Our purpose is to take that first real public step toward the rational integration of pharmacokinetics, pharmacodynamics, and toxicokinetics. We hope that this step will encourage others to follow.

RATIONALE FOR THE EFFECTIVE USE OF PHARMACOKINETICS AND PHARMACODYNAMICS IN EARLY DRUG DEVELOPMENT

Carl C. Peck
Center for Drug Evaluation and Research
Food and Drug Administration
Rockville, MD 20857

MOTIVATIONS

Premarketing development of new drugs is time-consuming, costly, and does not always lead to optimal dosages. DiMasi and coworkers (1991) estimate that the mean development time of new drugs approved during the mid-80's was 11.8 years and the average direct cost was 117 million dollars. Despite such lengthy and costly premarketing research efforts, as of April 1991, 8.3% of 192 new drugs approved during the 1980's had undergone significant dosage changes in the approved drug labels (examples: midazolam, zidovudine, buprenorphine, alprazolam). These dosage changes were prompted by a recognition that modifications in recommended doses or dosing intervals would lead to even more efficacious or safer therapy in individual patients. Thus, if efficiency in premarketing drug development is measured by its duration, cost and optimality of dosages, it appears that the process is often inefficient.

The key objective of drug development is the formation of a scientific database that supports the effectiveness and safety profile of the dosage regimen(s) intended for marketing. An informal polling of experienced FDA reviewers has revealed some valuable clues to the inefficiency of some drug development programs. For example, while minimally two adequate and well controlled clinical trials are required for drug approval, many new drug applications (NDA's) contain results of numerous non-contributory clinical trials, e.g. trials that failed to add to the effectiveness or safety database. In many instances, failed trials represented costly Phase III clinical studies that were inadequate attempts to establish effective and safe dosage regimens. Hence, a fundamental flaw in many drug development programs has been the lack of early discovery of effective and safe dosage regimens that can be efficiently employed in the few pivotal clinical trials that are required for drug approval.

Regulatory scientists at FDA are keenly interested in the quality and efficiency of premarketing drug development programs, for their ability to review and approve NDA's in a

Integration of Pharmacokinetics, Pharmacodynamics, and Toxicokinetics in Rational Drug Development, Edited by A. Yacobi *et al.*, Plenum Press, New York, 1993

timely fashion is dependent upon receipt of compact and scientifically persuasive applications. Moreover, FDA relies upon informative NDA's to fulfill it's public health obligation to approve dosage regimens with accompanying labels that enable effective and safe treatment of individual patients.

Thus, premarketing drug development programs are often cluttered by multiple failed clinical trials that lead to excessive development times and costs or even suboptimal dosages, and are difficult for FDA to review and approve efficiently. Herein lies the potential contribution of pharmacokinetics (PK) and pharmacodynamics (PD) for improving the efficiency of drug development. By establishment of informative dose-PK-PD relationships early in drug development, effective and safe dosage regimens may be employed so as to minimize or avoid failed trials.

THE CONCENTRATION PRINCIPLE IN DRUG DEVELOPMENT

A basic tenet of biochemical pharmacology is that the intensity and duration of drug action is mediated via the time course of drug concentrations at the site of action (pharmacodynamics, PD). While this may be easiest to demonstrate in in vitro drug receptor or isolated tissue preparations, there is much evidence to suggest that drug action *in vivo* is also mediated via the time course of drug concentrations at various anatomic sites of action. Ignoring hysteresis effects, Figure 1 depicts the commonly observed sigmoidal PD relationship between drug concentration and drug effect, showing the separation between beneficial and toxic effect curves that is characteristic of clinically useful drugs. Although direct assessment of drug concentrations at actual sites of action is seldom possible, the drug concentration in blood plasma or serum often bears a proportional relation, such that blood concentrations can be used in lieu of site concentrations.

However, in clinical therapeutics and drug development, intensity and duration of drug effects must be controlled externally by the dosage regimen. Here, understanding of the relation-

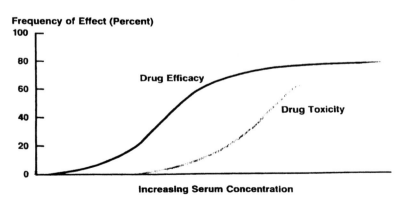

Finn et al, In "Individualizing Drug Therapy", Page 4. Gross, Townsend, Frank, Inc., N.Y., 1981.

Fig. 1. Sigmoidal relationship between drug concentration at sites of action and intensity of pharmacologic effect. Clinically useful drugs are characterized by having their drug concentration-beneficial-effect curves lie to the left of the corresponding concentration-toxicity curves.

2

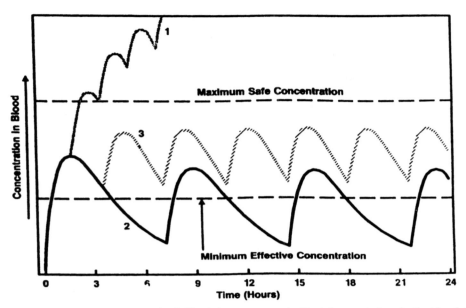

Fig. 2. Time course of drug concentration in blood plasma or serum (and by inference at sites of action) in relation to characteristics of the dosage regimen. Drug concentrations can fluctuate below, within, or above the so-called therapeutic window (defined by the minimum effective and maximum safe concentrations) depending upon the size and frequency of the dosages within a multiple dose regimen.

ship between dosage regimens and the time course of drug concentrations (pharmacokinetics, PK) is essential in order to link dosage regimens with drug effects over time (Figure 2).

If uniform dosage regimens yielded similar tissue drug concentrations among patients, then dosage control alone would yield pharmacokinetically predictable concentrations at sites of action. However, variability in PK is often high both within and between patients. As a consequence, drug concentrations in patients following exposure to a common dosage regimen often vary multiple-fold. This high variability in PK has significant implications in both drug development and clinical therapeutics. In the latter, it leads to the desirability of discovering paradigms for individualizing dosage regimens to optimize therapeutic outcome via attainment of effective and safe concentrations. In the case of drug development, high PK variability, if unappreciated, can lead to inefficient clinical trial designs when based on dosage control alone. In contrast, an appreciation of a drug's PK/PD early in drug development, despite high PK variability, can be used to advantage in designing informative clinical trials that yield dose-response information or that are based on direct control of attained drug concentrations (Sanathanan and Peck, 1991).

OPPORTUNITIES FOR INCORPORATION OF PK/PD IN DRUG DEVELOPMENT

At the present time, PK/PD techniques are used to establish required bioavailability and bioequivalence information. Beyond that, these techniques have seldom been used in such a way as to contribute to the efficiency of drug development. This is somewhat surprising since key PK/PD concepts and techniques have been evolving throughout the last 30 years. One

3

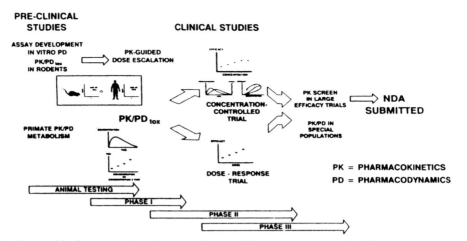

Fig. 3. Opportunities for incorporation of pharmacokinetics (PK) and pharmacodynamics (PD) in drug development. Overlaid on this time-line style chart of drug development by Phases (left to right: pre-clinical studies, Phase I, II, and III clinical studies, and NDA submission) are points in the development of a new drug where PK/PD concepts and techniques can be used to improve the efficiency of drug development. See text for detailed discussion.

technique, therapeutic drug monitoring, which entails the monitoring of blood concentrations of narrow therapeutic range drugs (e.g., aminoglycosides, anti-epileptic medications, theophylline, digoxin, etc.) has become standard medical practice.

As depicted graphically in Figure 3, key opportunities exist for incorporation of PK/PD in drug development that could contribute to improving the efficiency of drug development. Preclinical animal toxicokinetic data can be used to guide dosage selection and escalation schemes in Phase I dose-tolerance studies (Collins, Grieshaber and Chabner, 1990; Collins, page 49 of this volume), to assess adequacy of carcinogenicity testing, and to ensure drug assay development in advance of Phase I human trials. PK/PD studies in phase I dose-tolerance trials take advantage of the unique opportunity to map the PK/PD profile to determine maximum tolerated concentrations (Peck and Collins, 1990). Moreover, Phase I PK/PD data are essential for designing informative and efficient Phase II dose-response trials to establish efficacy. In Phase II, when interindividual differences in PK are large, the randomized concentration-controlled clinical trial (Sananthanan and Peck, 1991) can be an efficient alternative to the traditional dose-controlled trial as discussed subsequently on pages 239-247. In Phase III, correlation of observable patient features (e.g., sex, age, weight, organ dysfunction, etc) with PK and PD via the PK-screen (Temple, 1985) and population methods (Peck,1992; Grasela, pages 141-144) enable derivation of paradigms for individualization of dosage.

BENEFICIARIES OF IMPROVED DRUG DEVELOPMENT

If the efficiency of drug development can be improved through use of PK/PD, there are potential gains for all interested parties: patients, drug developers, and regulatory scientists.

Patients could be afforded optimal drug dosage regimens that are available within several years after initiation of development. If developers enjoy cost savings from compressed drug development times and fewer failed clinical trials, a portion of these savings could be passed on to consumers and could also be directed to R&D of additional new drugs. Moreover, drug manufacturers marketing drugs with optimal dosage regimens could expect lessened risk of liability for injury in the marketing phase. Regulatory scientists could expect to complete review of compact and persuasive NDA's within months after commencing the review.

REFERENCES

Collins, J. M., C. K. Grieshaber, and B. A. Chabner (1990). Review: Pharmacologically guided phase I clinical trials based upon preclinical drug development. J. Natl. Cancer Inst., 82, No. 16.

DiMasi, J. A., R. W. Hansen, H. G. Grabowski, and L. Lasagna (1991). Cost of innovation in the pharmaceutical industry, J. Health Econ., 10, 107-142.

Peck, C. C. (1992). Population approach in pharmacokinetics and pharmacodynamics: FDA view. In M. Rowland and L. Aarons (Eds.), New Strategies in Drug Development and Clinical Evaluation: Population Approach. Commission of European Communities, Brussels, pp. 157-168.

Peck, C. C., and J. M. Collins (1990). New drugs: The first time in man, a regulatory perspective, J. Clin. Pharmacol., 30, 210-222.

Sanathanan, L., and C. C. Peck (1991). The randomized concentration- controlled trial: An evaluation of its sample size efficiency. Controlled Clin. Trials, 12, 780-794.

Temple, R. J. (1983). Discussion Paper on Testing of Drugs in the Elderly. FDA, Rockville, Maryland.

THE CASE FOR PRECLINICAL PHARMACODYNAMICS

Gerhard Levy
Department of Pharmaceutics, School of Pharmacy
State University of New York at Buffalo, Amherst, N.Y. 14260

ABSTRACT

Pharmacodynamics concerns the relationship between drug concentration and intensity of pharmacologic effect. It includes the exploration and assessment of relevant variables such as pharmacologically active metabolites, pharmacodynamic drug interactions and effects of genetics and underlying diseases. Available (though limited) information indicates that drug concentrations required to produce a defined intensity of pharmacologic action are quite similar in man and animals. For such interspecies comparisons, consideration must be given to possible differences in drug-protein binding, active metabolites, kinetics of equilibration of drug between plasma and biophase, and definition of the pharmacologic endpoint. It is now evident that many unanticipated, pharmacodynamically relevant clinical risk factors, including some that have caused a substantial number of deaths, could have been recognized in preclinical pharmacodynamic studies. Examples based on studies in the author's laboratory include potentiation of barbiturates in renal failure, increased response to benzodiazepines in severe liver disease, increased neurotoxicity of theophylline in renal failure, increased potency of general anesthetics in hemorrhagic hypovolemia, and the steep responder syndrome in warfarin therapy. Preclinical pharmacodynamics provides a means for identifying, in advance of clinical use, potential risk factors and conditions under which drugs may be subject to profound changes in their concentration-effect relationships.

INTRODUCTION

If the process of drug development is to be productive and efficient, the various phases of this process must be designed to elicit information which is useful for the subsequent phases of development. There must be a logical continuum wherein previous information is used as a basis for the design of the next studies. This is particularly important in the planning of

Integration of Pharmacokinetics, Pharmacodynamics, and Toxicokinetics in Rational Drug Development, Edited by A. Yacobi *et al.*, Plenum Press, New York, 1993

clinical investigations and the development of clinical protocols because inadequate clinical studies can contribute substantially to the cost of a drug development and to the time required to bring a new drug on the market.

PRECLINICAL PHARMACOKINETICS AND PHARMACODYNAMICS

The place of preclinical (animal) pharmacokinetics in drug development is well established. Assessment of drug absorption and elimination kinetics is done as part of the selection of the most promising in a series of pharmacologically active compounds. Studies in animals are performed also to determine if the candidate compounds are enzyme inducers or inhibitors, or if they are subject to other time-dependent effects such as product inhibition or cosubstrate depletion. If such is the case, then future clinical studies must be designed to assess the magnitude and time course of these alterations in the therapeutically relevant drug concentration range. Determination of the pharmacokinetics of the drug candidate in several animal species is the logical precursor of well-designed animal toxicology studies and provides the opportunity to explore interspecies correlations with the ultimate aim of predicting, by appropriate extrapolation, the pharmacokinetic characteristics of the compound in man.

Unlike pharmacokinetics, the role of pharmacodynamics in the preclinical phase of drug development is barely in its beginning. This is unfortunate because pharmacodynamics, i.e. the relationship between drug concentration in plasma or certain tissue fluids and the intensity of drug action, is essential to the optimum interpretation and utilization of pharmacokinetic information. At present, only one relatively minor aspect of preclinical pharmacodynamics appears to be an established part of the drug development process. That aspect is the assessment of the pharmacologic activity of the metabolites of a drug or drug candidate. The relevance of this assessment to the drug discovery process is obvious. There are, however, other aspects of preclinical pharmacodynamics that are important and yet frequently neglected. These include in the first instance the characterization of the relationship between drug concentration and intensity of drug action(s), preferably in sufficient detail to permit modelling and to recognize time-dependent phenomena such as the development of functional tolerance. Several other aspects of preclinical pharmacodynamics can contribute substantially to the drug development process. One of these is the use of animal data to predict therapeutic and toxic drug concentrations in humans.

EFFECTIVE DRUG CONCENTRATIONS IN ANIMALS AND HUMANS

The plasma concentration of a drug required to elicit a certain (intensity of) action is often similar in experimental animals and humans. In a report on the Workshop on the Qualitative and Quantitative Comparability of Human and Animal Developmental Neurotoxicity, Francis, Kimmel, and Rees (1990) stated that "Comparisons of administered doses (resulting in similar effect levels) revealed a wide range of differences across species (up to a 10,000-fold difference). On the other hand, comparisons across species using internal measurements of dose (e.g., blood or brain levels) showed a remarkable correlation (generally, a 1 to 2-fold difference)." In the case of the antiepileptic drug phenytoin, Ramzan (1990) reported that the onset of ataxia occurred in rats at serum unbound drug concentrations of 6.3 ± 1.7 (mean ± S.D.) mg/l. The serum total phenytoin concentrations associated with ataxia in humans are between 30 and 40 mg/l (Kutt and co-workers, 1964); the corresponding concentrations of unbound drug are between 3 and 6 mg/l based on the typical phenytoin protein binding of 10 to 15 percent in human serum. In another study, neurotoxic manifestations of phenytoin in pregnant rhesus macaques occurred at plasma concentrations (total drug) in excess of 30 µg/ml, "consistent with data reported in mouse, rat, rabbit, dog, rhesus macaque and human" (Hendrie and co-workers, 1990). The plasma concentration of the antihypertensive agent nilvadipine associated with a 20 percent reduction of diastolic blood pressure was about 20 mg/ml in dogs (Wu and co-workers, 1988) and the same in humans (Cheung and co-workers, 1988). The concentration of ethanol in brain, serum and cerebrospinal fluid of rats at onset of loss of righting reflex (i.e. sleep) is between 3 and 4 mg/ml or mg/g (Danhof, Hisaoka and Levy, 1985); the hypnotic concentrations of ethanol in man are similar.

It is unfortunate that comparative information on the effective concentrations of new drugs in various species of animals and (eventually) humans is either not obtained or not fully utilized in drug development. Knowledge of effective drug concentrations in animals can greatly facilitate dose ranging in Phase I studies. There is increasing evidence that, as Gianni and co-workers (1990) have stated, "preclinical pharmacology offers reliable guidelines to safely accelerate the process of Phase I trials".

One must, however, be aware of several important considerations when making interspecies comparisons of effective drug concentrations. First, the pharmacologic endpoint used for determinations of effective concentration must be comparable in the different species. Next, attention must be paid to the appropriate fluid or tissue for concentration determination in the context of the possibility of a disequilibrium between drug in plasma and drug at the site of action (Danhof and Levy, 1984). Differences in plasma protein binding of a drug between species must be taken into consideration; concentrations of unbound drug should be compared in cases where drug-protein binding is extensive. Also, the possible contribution of active metabolites to the pharmacologic effect of a drug must be kept in mind.

ASSESSMENT OF COMPLEX PHARMACODYNAMIC RELATIONSHIPS

Studies in experimental animals can reveal and elucidate complex pharmacodynamic relationships which also occur in humans. An excellent example are the pharmacodynamics of the coumarin anticoagulants. These agents, of which warfarin and dicumarol are best known in the United States, act indirectly and their maximum clinically apparent effect (increase of prothrombin time) occurs in man about 2 days after maximum plasma concentrations produced by a single, large dose (Nagashima, O'Reilly and Levy, 1969). We have developed a pharmacodynamic model which permits resolution of the observed change in prothrombin complex activity (which is derived from the prothrombin time) into its components: the synthesis and elimination of prothrombin complex activity. The direct effect of the coumarin

9

anticoagulants is the inhibition of the synthesis of prothrombin complex activity (which reflects the inhibition of the synthesis of vitamin K dependent clotting factors) and this inhibitory effect is related linearly to the logarithm of the drug concentration in plasma without any delay (Nagashima, O'Reilly and Levy, 1969). The pharmacodynamic model includes the assumption that prothrombin complex activity declines exponentially with time after administration of a synthesis-blocking dose of the coumarin anticoagulant. Despite the complexity of the pharmacodynamic model, it was found to apply equally to humans and rats (Yacobi, Wingard and Levy, 1974). This exemplifies the possibility of exploring pharmacodynamic modelling approaches in preclinical studies for the purpose of optimizing subsequent clinical protocols.

Another of our studies of warfarin pharmacodynamics in rats provided additional, valuable information relevant to the therapeutic use of the drug in humans. Warfarin pharmacodynamics, like the pharmacodynamics of other drugs (Levy, 1985), exhibit pronounced inter-individual but relatively little intraindividual variability in humans. We observed such inter-individual variability also in rats and found a strong correlation between the slope of the anticoagulant effect-log concentration relationship of warfarin and the free fraction value of the drug in the serum (Yacobi and Levy, 1977). Based on that observation, Routledge and co-workers (1979) recognized a similar relationship in man. Since the serum or plasma free fraction value of warfarin can be determined by the in vitro addition of the drug to a drug-free serum or plasma sample, one is able to characterize "steep" and "shallow" warfarin responders before initiation of therapy.

EFFECT OF DISEASE STATES ON THE KINETICS OF DRUG ACTION

There are many reasons for the large interindividual variability in the pharmacodynamics of drugs (Levy, 1985). One such reason is the presence of underlying disease. Our group has intensively explored this aspect of pharmacodynamics in recent years. One of our first efforts in this area was stimulated by a report in 1954 by Dundee and Richards of significantly lower loading and maintenance dose requirements for thiopental-mediated general anesthesia in uremic patients as compared to patients with normal renal function. These investigators also reported that such increased sensitivity to the drug could be produced in patients with normal renal function by administration of urea before thiopental. We were able to demonstrate the same dose-sparing effect of urea on thiopental in normal rats and we established that its mechanism was pharmacokinetic rather than pharmacodynamic (Danhof and Levy, 1985). In further explorations on rats with either surgically or chemically-induced renal failure, we found that the concentrations of barbiturates required to produce sleep (loss of righting reflex) in rats were substantially decreased by renal failure (Danhof, Hisaoka and Levy, 1984). This pharmacodynamic alteration is mediated by an endogenous, dialyzable material which accumulates in renal failure (Hisaoka and Levy, 1985). Clearly, the ability to discover such effects of disease on drug action in preclinical studies is of enormous value.

Another example of the potential utility of preclinical pharmacodynamic investigations derives from a tragic occurrence following the Japanese attack on Pearl Harbor during World

War II. Surgery had to be performed on many casualties whose blood volume was severely depleted by hemorrhage. The general anesthetic agent used in these procedures was usually thiopental. As reported by Halford in 1943, "death ensued in enough cases to cause us to abandon it (thiopental) as too dangerous". We found in studies on rats that hemorrhagic hypovolemia caused a pronounced increase in central nervous system sensitivity to the depressant effect of a barbiturate, an observation which, had it been made before the use of thiopental at Pearl Harbor, might have saved hundreds of lives (Klockowski and Levy, 1988).

Theophylline is a widely used bronchodilator. Its usual therapeutic plasma concentration range is quite narrow and is frequently exceeded due to pronounced inter- and intraindividual variations in the total clearance of this drug. High concentrations of theophylline can cause neurotoxicity of which the most serious manifestation is generalized seizures that are often fatal or the cause of permanent brain damage. Noting that some patients had seizures at relatively low (but super therapeutic) plasma theophylline concentrations whereas others did not experience seizures even at ten-fold higher concentrations, we explored various potential risk factors for theophylline neurotoxicity in rats. We found one such risk factor to be renal failure; rats with bilaterally ligated ureters had convulsions at drug concentrations in cerebrospinal fluid that were about one-half those in normal controls (Ramzan and Levy, 1987). Significantly, Aitken and Martin (1985) concluded from a retrospective review of hospital records of patients with theophylline toxicity that "patients with renal dysfunction may be at higher risk for life-threatening complications of theophylline intoxication". This important observation could have been predicted (and lives could have been saved!) by appropriate preclinical studies.

As a final example of the value of preclinical pharmacodynamics for predicting effects of underlying diseases in humans, I cite our experience with the benzodiazepines. Recent clinical reports have described pronounced increases in the central nervous system depressant effect of a benzodiazepine in hepatic cirrhosis compared to the effect on individuals without liver disease at comparable plasma concentrations of unbound drug (Fisch and co-workers, 1986; Bakti and co-workers, 1987). We studied the pharmacokinetics and pharmacodynamics of desmethyldiazepam in rats with carbon tetrachloride induced liver dysfunction (Klockowski and Levy, to be published). Using rotarod performance as an index of CNS functionality, we observed that a serum concentration of about 0.04 mg/l of unbound desmethyldiazepam produced an impairment of about 20 percent in normal rats and of 100 percent in rats with liver disease. Again, the preclinical observations could have predicted the clinical effects and prevented many cases of unanticipated adverse effects due to benzodiazepines in patients with liver disease.

In conclusion, knowledge derived from preclinical pharmacodynamic studies on suitable animal models can be extraordinarily useful for the design and efficient performance of subsequent clinical studies, for the development of pharmacodynamic models and for anticipating and exploring the effects of variables such as underlying diseases on drug concentration vs. pharmacologic activity relationships. Drug development will be facilitated and human pharmacotherapy will become safer and more effective if properly conducted preclinical pharmacodynamic studies become an integral part of the drug development process.

REFERENCES

Aitken, M. L., and T. R. Martin (1985). Life-threatening complications of theophylline toxicity are not predicted by serum theophylline levels. Amer. Rev. Resp. Dis., 131, A68.

Bakti, G., H. U. Fisch, G. Karlaganis, C. Minder, and J. Bircher (1987). Mechanism of the excessive sedative response of cirrhotics to benzodiazepines: model experiments with triazolam. Hepatology, 7, 629-638.

Cheung, W. K., L. L. Sia, D. L. Woodward, J. F. Graveline, R. E. Desjardins, A. Yacobi, and B. M. Silber (1988). Importance of oral dosing rate on the hemodynamic and pharmacokinetic profile on nilvadipine. J. Clin. Pharmacol., 28, 1000-1007.

Danhof, H., M. Hisaoka, and G. Levy (1984). Kinetics of drug action in disease states. II. Effect of experimental renal dysfunction on phenobarbital concentrations in rats at onset of loss of righting reflex. J. Pharmacol. Exp. Ther., 230, 627-631.

Danhof, M., and G. Levy (1984). Kinetics of drug action in disease states. I. Effect of infusion rate on phenobarbital concentrations in serum, brain and CSF of normal rats at onset of loss of righting reflex. J. Pharmacol. Exp. Ther., 229, 44-50.

Danhof, M., and G. Levy (1985). Kinetics of drug action in disease states. V. Acute effect of urea infusion of phenobarbital concentrations in rats at onset of loss of righting reflex. J. Pharmacol. Exp. Ther., 232, 430-444.

Danhof, M., M. Hisaoka, and G. Levy (1985). Kinetics of drug action in disease states XII: Effect of experimental liver diseases on the pharmacodynamics of phenobarbital and ethanol in rats. J. Pharm. Sci., 74, 321-324.

Dundee, J. W., and R. K. Richards (1954). Effect of azotemia upon the action of intravenous barbiturate anesthesia. Anesthesiology, 15, 333-346.

Fisch, H. U., G. Baktir, G. Karlaganis, and J. Bircher (1986). Excessive effects of benzodiazepines in patients with cirrhosis of the liver: a pharmacodynamic or a pharmacokinetic problem? Pharmacopsychiatry, 19, 14.

Francis, E. Z., C. A. Kimmel and D. C. Rees (1990). Workshop on the qualitative and quantitative comparability of human and animal developmental neurotoxicity: Summary and implications. Neurotoxicol. Teratol., 12, 285- 292.

Gianni, L., L. Vigano, A. Surbone, D. Ballinari, P. Casali, C. Tarella, and J. M. Collins (1990). Pharmacology and clinical toxicity of 4'-iodo-4'- deoxydoxorubicin: An example of successful application of pharmacokinetics to dose escalation in phase I trials. J. Natl. Cancer Inst., 82, 469-477.

Halford, F. J. (1943). A critique of intravenous anesthesia in war surgery. Anesthesiology, 4, 67-69.

Hendrie, T. A., J. R. Rowland, P. E. Binkerd, and A. G. Hendrickx (1990). Developmental toxicity and pharmacokinetics of phenytoin in the rhesus macaque: An interspecies comparison. Reproductive Toxicol., 4, 257-266.

Hisaoka, M., and G. Levy (1985). Kinetics of drug action in disease states. XIII. Effect of dialyzable component(s) of uremic blood on phenobarbital concentrations in rats at onset of loss of righting reflex. J. Pharmacol. Exp. Ther., 234, 180-183.

Klockowski, P., and G. Levy (1988). Kinetics of drug action in disease states. XXIII. Effect of acute hypovolemia on the pharmacodynamics of phenobarbital in rats. J. Pharm. Sci., 77, 365-366.

Kutt, H., W. Winters, R. Kolenge, and F. McDowell (1964). Diphenylhydantoin metabolism, blood levels and toxicity. Arch. Neurol., 11, 642-648.

Levy, G. (1985). Variability in animal and human pharmacodynamic studies. In M. Rowland, L. B. Sheiner, and J.-L. Steimer (Eds.), Variability in Drug Therapy: Description, Estimation, and Control, Raven Press, New York, pp. 125-138.

Nagashima, R., R. O'Reilly, and G. Levy (1969). Kinetics of pharmacologic effects in man: The anticoagulant action of warfarin. Clin. Pharmacol. Ther., 10, 22-35.

Ramzan, I. (1990). Pharmacodynamics of phenytoin-induced ataxia in rats. Epilepsy Res., 5, 80-83.

Ramzan, I. M., and G. Levy (1987). Kinetics of drug action. XVIII. Effect of experimental renal failure on the pharmacodynamics of theophylline-induced seizures in rats. J. Pharmacol. Exp. Ther., 240, 584-588.

Routledge, P. A., P. H. Chapman, D. M. Davies, and M. D. Rawlins (1979). Pharmacokinetics and pharmacodynamics of warfarin at steady state. Br. J. Clin. Pharmacol., 8, 243-247.

Wu, W-H., B. M. Henderson, R. Lanc, D. Garnes, A. Yacobi and B. M. Silber (1988). Relationship between the pharmacokinetic and pharmacodynamic profile of nilvadipine in the dog. Drug Metab. Dispos., 16, 222-227.

Yacobi, A., and G. Levy (1977). Comparative pharmacokinetics of coumarin anticoagulants XXVIII: predictive identification of rats with relatively steep serum warfarin concentration-anticoagulant response characteristics. J. Pharm. Sci., 66, 145.

Yacobi, A., L. B. Wingard, Jr., and G. Levy (1974). Comparative pharmacokinetics of coumarin anticoagulants X: relationship between distribution, elimination, and anticoagulant action of warfarin. J. Pharm. Sci., 63, 868-872.

UTILITY OF KINETIC, DYNAMIC, AND METABOLIC DATA IN NONCLINICAL PHARMACOLOGY/TOXICOLOGY STUDIES

Judi Weissinger
Center for Drug Evaluation and Research
Food and Drug Administration
Rockville, MD 20857

ABSTRACT

Kinetic, dynamic, and metabolic data can be used to predict the appropriate studies, doses, duration, route of administration, species, and dosage interval in toxicology studies coordinated with drug development These data are used to predict starting and maximal doses in human studies, and when evaluated in conjunction with the data obtained in human pharmacokinetic studies, serve as an index for animal to human comparisons and extrapolations The optimal use of kinetic and dynamic information in standard pharmacologic and toxicologic studies will be presented. Reference will be made to problems encountered in the absence of these data and protocol development advantages where these data are incorporated. Development of pharmaceuticals, without incorporating kinetic and dynamic information, is currently associated with more costly, more time consuming, less utilizable knowledge and subsequent studies are often needed to explain anomalous results.

INTRODUCTION

The pharmaceutical development community, whether government, industry, or academia, focuses on obtaining optimal data to demonstrate the safety and effectiveness of therapeutics. With the use of appropriate scientific rationale, pivotal and critical data can be obtained when new drugs are evaluated nonclinically based upon the intended use in humans. These data can be developed most expeditiously when the nonclinical pharmacologic and toxicologic activity, disposition, and metabolism are fully characterized and can be related to expected effects in humans.

Existence of a well thought out plan, based on knowledge of the kinetics, the dynamics, and the metabolism of a drug, can increase the overall efficiency of the risk assessment process

Integration of Pharmacokinetics, Pharmacodynamics, and Toxicokinetics in Rational Drug Development, Edited by A. Yacobi *et al.*, Plenum Press, New York, 1993

by allowing more effective planning of the animal toxicity studies and providing information for extrapolation of those results across species and to humans. This knowledge is also useful in predicting and characterizing drug interactions, evaluating stereoisomeric relationships, dose adjustment in reproductive studies, evaluating the data needed for targeted drug delivery systems, and explaining anomalous results.

Here, I will discuss what is needed to establish the well thought out plan for animal studies, and the utility of nonclinical kinetic, dynamic, and metabolic data in drug development.

PREREQUISITES FOR A WELL THOUGHT OUT PLAN

Any discussion of the development of a well thought out plan based on knowledge of the kinetics, the dynamics, and the metabolism of a drug should address the terminology used, utility of concentration-response phenomena, appropriate endpoints, critical comparisons of experimental data to established physiologic and pharmacologic models, and the importance of timing the studies for optimal use of the data.

Terminology

Kinetic parameters describe the activity of the body on the course of disposition of the drug. Dynamic information addresses the activity of the drug on bodily processes. Metabolism describes the biotransformation of the drug in the body. The terms "pharmaco" and "toxico" are used to describe the effect elicited at a given exposure; "pharmaco" is the range producing desired effects and "toxico" is the range producing undesired effects. There may be a large difference in disposition, activity and metabolism depending upon the dose administered and the existence of saturable systems. It should also be understood that both types of effects may be seen in a given dose range. Thus for a given set of responses, the "pharmaco" parameters and the "toxico" parameters may be the same.

Concentration-Response vs. Dose-Response

The focus should be on concentration-response characteristics, and not solely on dose-response characteristics. Because of effects based on saturable processes in active absorption, protein binding, active secretion and reabsorption at renal tubules, induction or saturation of biotransformation enzymes and shifts in formation of biotransformation products that are concentration related, it is more accurate to consider blood or tissue levels to describe exposure than to consider dose. Similarly, relying on dose may not take into account the effects of concentration on receptor affinity, duration of receptor occupation, or reversibility.

Endpoints

Several endpoints have been described for use in kinetic evaluations.

C_{max} : Maximum systemic concentration
T_{max} : Time of maximum concentration

AUC : Area under the systemic concentration time curve
Cp-ss : Steady-state systemic concentration
F_{abs} : Absolute bioavailability
CL : Clearance
V_d : Volume of distribution

When assessing the utility of any particular endpoint, it is important to identify the active moiety and the relationship of the parent drug to metabolites. Assays chosen and ability to obtain useful data will depend upon this knowledge.

Utility of Models

It is important to evaluate how well the data correlate to known pharmacokinetic and pharmacodynamic models. Irregularities in disposition may be identified when experimental data are identified as deviating from standard pharmacokinetic models. Identification of additional compartments where accumulation might occur, saturation of a system, and alteration in metabolic profile or some other physiologic phenomena that preclude dose proportionality, can be identified by comparison of experimental data to established models. Irregularities in biologic activity may be identified when experimental data deviate from standard pharmacodynamic models. Congruence to models can be used to assess validity of determination, or suggest alternative explanations such as irreversible occupation of receptors, saturation of the enzyme responsible for receptor "clearing", or other receptor phenomena that preclude concentration-response proportionality.

Timing of Studies

We have been recommending disposition and metabolism studies be conducted early in drug development. Single dose pharmacokinetics and toxicokinetics may be used for predicting optimal exposures in humans, and for guidance in toxicity study protocol design. With additional completion of phase 1 and characterization of steady state in humans and animals, the data may be used to suggest modifications to development strategy based on the comparison to humans.

When seeking pre-IND guidance from FDA, more specific recommendations can be obtained when the preliminary information includes:

1. production method, purity, stability
2. known actions
3. proposed dose
4. proposed route of administration
5. chemical identity
6. bioactivity
7. disposition
8. metabolic profile
9. the intended clinical study, including proposed population

Many sponsors feel, and understandably so, that resources committed early to address the bioactivity, disposition, and metabolic profile information may be lost if the drug is not going to succeed when studied in phases 1 and 2 in humans. Resources include animals and time, as exemplified by the development of analytical methods, synthesis of additional drug, delay in submitting proposed protocol, and the technical time expended. However, important information may be gained to improve the outcome of drug development. For instance, a drug may not be pursued because it was not shown to be effective in phase 2. If inability to achieve or maintain appropriate concentration at the site of action was the real reason for the apparent lack of effectiveness, changes to the dosage form or dosage regimen may be appropriate. These may be proposed on the basis of animal data, that allow for display of effectiveness based on increases in absorption and distribution, or decreased metabolism and excretion. If a drug shows lack of effectiveness in phase 2, considerations such as irreversible occupation of receptors, too rapid reversibility of occupation of receptors, and/or too little selectivity for receptors, animal pharmacodynamic studies may alert the sponsor to these issues so that development will not be hindered by apparent ineffectiveness in humans.

UTILITY OF NONCLINICAL KINETIC, DYNAMIC, AND METABOLIC DATA

Here, I will discuss the utility of nonclinical kinetic, dynamic, and metabolic data in drug development. These data may increase the overall efficiency of the risk assessment process through:

1. more effective planning of animal toxicity studies
2. increased understanding of the mechanisms of toxicity
3. predicting and characterizing drug interactions
4. considering changes with age (pediatric and elderly)
5. identifying changes with pathophysiology
6. explaining stereoisomeric relationships
7. dose adjustment in reproductive studies
8. determining the data needed for targeted drug delivery systems
9. evaluating changes in formulation
10. providing information for extrapolation of animal data across species to   humans

Effective Planning of Animal Studies

Kinetic, dynamic, and metabolic data are essential to the proper design and planning of the nonclinical pharmacology/toxicology studies. These studies should be conducted in the species to be used for toxicity testing, by the same route(s) of administration plus intravenous if that is not the intended route to evaluate the fraction absorbed. It is important that the dosage regimen proposed for clinical use be evaluated. It is important that the range of doses proposed for study, including those producing toxicity, be characterized for the duration representative of the proposed clinical use. A biotransformation profile, which may be qualitative at this stage, is important. These data, collected in animals, are used to predict appropriate studies, short and long term, plus evaluation of specialized systems. The design of those studies with respect to doses that assure optimal exposure, duration, route of administration, choice of species, and dosage interval, may be based on these data. Changes to expected protocols may be justified with knowledge of the kinetics, dynamics, and metabolism.

Understanding Mechanisms of Toxicity

Kinetic, dynamic, and metabolic studies are useful in evaluating the mechanism of untoward effects. The predictability that effects observed at pharmacologic and toxicologic ranges help to define mechanisms of toxicity. Knowledge of mechanisms often allows for scientific prediction that a toxicity will or will not be expected to occur in humans. Shifts to alternate metabolic pathways may suggest an association between a new metabolite and a toxicity observed. Likewise, saturation of an excretion pathway may allow for increased levels of drug related to a toxic response.

Drug Interactions

Kinetic, dynamic, and metabolic studies are useful in predicting and characterizing drug interactions. Where two drugs are know to be absorbed, protein bound, biotransformed, excreted, or accumulated in tissues by similar mechanisms, changes in rate may identify an interaction and its mechanism. Similarly where two drugs have similar structures or are known to have activity at a common receptor, additive, synergistic, and inhibitory effects may be identified as possible mechanisms for interaction. Two drugs competing for the same metabolic pathway or one drug inducing or inhibiting the enzyme system required for metabolism of another, are also mechanisms of interaction that may be identified using metabolic profiles.

Age-Related Phenomena

Kinetic, dynamic, and metabolic effects on drugs may vary with age. The elderly and pediatric populations may have differing capabilities for absorption, protein binding, metabolism, and excretion of drugs. Receptor number, function, density, and regenerative ability may be related to age. And the reversibility of changes that occur in receptor populations may be dependent upon age.

Effect of Changes in Health Status

Kinetics, dynamics, and metabolism in pediatric and aging populations may be considered with respect to data gathered in young and aged animals and compared to the average population. Changes in disposition, activity, and metabolism of drugs are known to occur with pathophysiologic conditions such as renal impairment, hepatic compromise, obesity, and hypertension. Animal models exist that can be used to predict the alterations associated with these conditions. The accumulation of drugs in certain compartments, such as fetal tissue, milk, brain, and tumors, may vary with age and health status and can also be characterized with these studies.

Stereoisomer Development

Knowledge of the kinetics, dynamics, and metabolic fate are invaluable in the development of stereoisomers and stereoisomeric mixtures. Evaluation of the qualitative and quantitative relationships may offer insight into the ultimate response observed. The role of disposition is equally important in determining the overall activity where absorption, distribution, biotransformation, or excretion differs between enantiomers. One enantiomer may actually be more potent, or just better absorbed, less protein bound, less efficiently converted to an inactive metabolite, or be subject to competition for excretion by a less potent or inactive enantiomer. Kinetic and dynamic studies may also serve to identify the potential for interconversion from one stereoisomer to its enantiomer.

Dose Adjustment in Reproductive Studies

Because of changes in physiology during pregnancy and nursing, total exposure is rarely optimized beyond choosing a dose in normal and pregnant animals. Kinetics can be used to evaluate the exposure related to a given dose in premating animals, in pregnant animals, in nursing animals, and in offspring.

Targeted Drug Delivery Systems

Development of targeted drug delivery systems is an important improvement in delivering the drug more optimally to its site of action. New delivery systems and new drugs are subjected to intense scrutiny with respect to safety and effectiveness. Where the delivery system has been previously approved and the drug has also been previously approved, depending upon the results of pharmacokinetic studies and the relationship of those results to predictions regarding drug levels (and adequacy of previous toxicologic evaluations), phase 1 studies may be able to proceed.

Bridging (Confirmatory) Studies

Comparison of kinetic profiles is often sufficient for comparison of an old formulation or method of manufacture with a new one. These bridging studies may be used to confirm that differences in lots, differences brought about during scale up, changes in excipient, or impurities identified will not affect disposition of a drug. Dynamic studies may identify any additional biologic effect.

Preclinically, predictions to humans are made after defining the parameters related to pharmacological effect in animals, defining the parameters related to toxicity in animals, and considering the maximum exposure proposed for humans with the likelihood that similar effects will be observed. Several models have been used for these predictions based on body weight, body surface area, physiologically based pharmacokinetic modeling and allometry.

After products are evaluated in phase 1 studies, the validity of the predictions can be tested by comparing blood levels and tissue distribution (parent drug and its metabolites) in each species and then relating the effects to blood levels and effects observed in humans. Thus, drug exposure can be compared in animals and humans (either as plasma levels or AUC), clearance can be compared in animals and humans, and desired and adverse effects can be compared to dose and exposure in animals and humans.

After phase 2, revisions in extrapolations may be made to reflect changes associated with disease state for which the drug is intended.

LABELING

This presentation would not be complete if I did not address the implications of these important data to the accuracy and understanding of physician labeling. The precautions sections include nonclinical information under carcinogenicity, genotoxicity, impairment of fertility, pregnancy, overdosage, and animal toxicology (where relevant).

Current Labeling

The standard labeling might look like the following: X toxicity study of TRADENAME was conducted in Y species after Z route of administration at doses up to P mg/kg daily (Q times the maximum recommended human dose). There were no differences in E (endpoint); or A toxicity was observed at P but not at dose M or N.

Proposed Interim Labeling

A change in labeling, to reflect the actual exposure levels, might produce unscientific comparisons to drugs labeled under the standard system, which relates the studies by dose in mg/kg. Interim proposed labeling would allow for both the exposure and dose comparisons between animal studies and maximum recommended human dose or exposure related to that dose. An example of the interim labeling might look like the following:

TRADENAME was tested in X toxicity studies in Y species at doses of up to P mg/kg daily by Z route of administration. There were no differences in E (endpoint), or A toxicity was observed at Q mg/kg. At P mg/kg, exposures were N times the levels obtained after clinical administration of the maximum recommended human dose, A mg/kg. (The multiple may alternatively be calculated based on AUC or dose in mg/meter^2).

Optimal Labeling

Eventually, the goal for accurate labeling might result in the following throughout the Rx pharmaceutical industry: X Toxicity study of TRADENAME was conducted in Y species after Z route of administration at A, B, and C, (Q, R, and S) times the exposure in humans based on [blood level, AUC, tissue concentration, fluid concentration, etc.]. There were no differences in E (endpoint).

It is important to note that where an active metabolite is related to any of the observed effects, it should be so noted in the labeling, again in relationship to the appropriate parameters for comparison to humans.

Additionally, if knowledge exists regarding the disposition of the active moiety that suggests the assumption of relating blood level to concentration at the site of action is not appropriate, this should be considered in labeling.

CONCLUSIONS

The contribution of knowledge of the animal kinetics, dynamics, and metabolism of a drug to optimal and expeditious development has been highlighted. Examples of the utility of nonclinical kinetic, dynamic, and metabolic data in specific areas of drug development were offered. Since the ultimate goal is safe use and scientifically rational drug development, the following conclusions are offered:

Pharmacokinetic analysis of a drug should complement, support, and provide insight into the toxicity of the drug within the context of its clinical investigation.

Accurate, quantitative, interspecies extrapolation and comparison of pharmacologic and toxicologic effects cannot be considered in the absence of pharmacokinetic data.

These data should provide a rational basis for understanding the pharmacology and toxicology of investigational drugs, a mechanism for extrapolation to other animals and humans, and assistance in the design of toxicity studies and selection of appropriate species.

Subsequent chapters by FDA scientists, Drs. Fitzgerald and Green, will offer examples based on our experience with these data and guidance on how to conduct the studies most optimally.

PHARMACOKINETICS AND DRUG METABOLISM IN ANIMAL STUDIES (ADME, PROTEIN BINDING, MASS BALANCE, ANIMAL MODELS)

Glenna G. Fitzgerald
Division of Neuropharmacological Drug Products
Center for Drug Evaluation and Research
Food and Drug Administration
Rockville, MD 20857

ABSTRACT

A careful evaluation of the pharmacokinetics and metabolism of a new drug should play an integral and continuing role in the nonclinical workup for that drug, and should be initiated very early in the drug development program. These studies are of primary importance for the planning and design of animal toxicity studies, and for the selection of the appropriate animal model for purposes of estimating a safe clinical dose. Examples of the usefulness of nonclinical pharmacokinetic data for explaining toxicity which occurred, while allowing clinical trials to continue, are presented.

Studies of pharmacokinetics and drug metabolism in animals form an integral part of the preclinical and ongoing nonclinical evaluation of a new drug. The primary uses of such studies are for the planning and design of animal toxicity studies and for the interpretation of the results of animal toxicity studies, particularly regarding interspecies differences in toxicity and extrapolation of animal toxicity data to humans. There are no specific regulations which define the scope of pharmacodynamic, pharmacokinetic, or toxicokinetic studies which would be useful or necessary for characterizing a new drug for purposes of supporting clinical investigations or for marketing. All that is stated in the Code of Federal Regulations, 21 part 312.23, IND content and format, is the following statement under Pharmacology and Drug Disposition: "A section describing the pharmacological effects and mechanism(s) of action of the drug in animals and information on the absorption, distribution, metabolism, and excretion of the drug, if known". In the Center for Drugs and Biologics Guideline for the Format and Content of the Nonclinical/Pharmacology/Toxicology Section of a New Drug Application, published in February of 1987, only a brief listing of desirable and useful types

Integration of Pharmacokinetics, Pharmacodynamics, and Toxicokinetics in Rational Drug Development, Edited by A. Yacobi *et al.*, Plenum Press, New York, 1993

Table 1. Guidelines for the Format and Content of the Nonclinical
Pharmacology/Toxicology Section of an Application

ABSORPTION, DISTRIBUTION, METABOLISM, EXCRETION
(ADME) STUDIES

(A)   ORGANIZE AVAILABLE DATA FOR EACH SPE-
CIES/STRAIN IN THE FOLLOWING SEQUENCE IN SUM-
MARY TABLES AND
DETAILED REPORTS:

ABSORPTION, PHARMACOKINETICS, SERUM HALF-LIFE
PROTEIN BINDING
TISSUE DISTRIBUTION/ACCUMULATION
ENZYME INDUCTION OR INHIBITION
EXCRETION PATTERN

(B)   STUDY DESCRIPTIONS SHOULD CLEARLY STATE THE
DOSE(S) USED IN EACH STUDY

---

of drug disposition studies was included (Table 1). One might therefore have the impression that nonclinical pharmacokinetic and drug metabolism studies constitute a minor part of the overall characterization of a new drug, and that they more or less stand on their own and are not integrated into the overall development of the drug. In fact, nothing could be farther from the truth. Increasingly, both the pharmaceutical industry and FDA are relying upon the early pharmacokinetic and toxicokinetic characterization of drugs across species. The information obtained from these studies is providing invaluable guidance for designing subchronic and chronic animal studies which will assist us in interpreting the biological actions, both desirable and undesirable, of the drug, These studies in turn provide information about the best animal models to use as guides for designing phase 2 and phase 3 clinical trials if toxicity of the drug happens to be a problem.

The one point that cannot be overemphasized in this brief overview is that the pharmacokinetic profiling of a new drug should form an integral portion of the earliest nonclinical characterization of a drug, and these studies should be incorporated into the continuing toxicological evaluation of the drug. The data obtained should also be integrated with the clinical pharmacokinetic information as it becomes available, so that a ready comparison may be made for purposes of explaining unexpected adverse findings. The types of nonclinical pharmacokinetic studies that regulatory pharmacologists like to have submitted will first be outlined. Then a few examples of the usefulness of the pharmacokinetic data the FDA receives, both in terms of interpreting unexpected results and in terms of planning additional nonclinical studies needed to clarify these results, will be presented.

Traditionally, pharmacokinetic studies of the type being described often use relatively low doses of drug in acute or short term subacute studies. Usually the drug is radiolabeled so that its transit through the body may be readily followed. A term which is being more frequently encountered recently is toxicokinetics. It refers more specifically to the study of the same processes by which the drug is handled in the biological milieu of the body, but when studied at doses chosen for toxicity studies and usually administered for extended durations. In essence, toxicokinetics focuses on studies in which doses are higher than those used to elicit pharmacological responses, and also higher doses than those which will be used in humans. Its usefulness lies primarily in the interpretation of toxicities observed in subchronic and chronic animal studies, in establishing species differences in metabolic profile and kinetics, and in establishing a safety margin between doses used in toxicity studies and those used in clinical trials. There is no sharp delineation between pharmacokinetics and toxicokinetics from a practical point of view, since the data obtained are essentially a continuum, one data set representing nontoxic and the other representing toxic doses.

Table 2 briefly summarizes major aspects of ADME. Both the rate and extent of absorption become major factors to consider when characterizing drugs other than those intended for intravenous administration. For a drug which will be administered by the oral route, the following information is needed initially: does it disintegrate at acid pH, does it get into the gut, does it pass the gut wall? If it is not known whether or not drug is absorbed by a particular species, how can an appropriate dosing regimen be determined for toxicity studies? And if drug is poorly absorbed, that species is clearly an inappropriate one to use for future studies. In addition to the importance of knowledge about rate and extent of absorption across the gut is knowledge about bioavailability. Bioavailability is defined as that fraction of oral dose of parent drug reaching the systemic circulation relative to blood drug level after intravenous administration. If levels of parent drug are very low, it must then be determined whether or not absorption is poor or if there is extensive first pass metabolism by the liver. If there is first pass metabolism by the liver, whether or not this is a consistent effect across species and gender must be explored. Since there are diverse amounts and/or activities

Table 2. Pharmacokinetics in Animal Studies

ABSORPTION
    Rate and Extent
    Bioavailability
DISTRIBUTION
    Blood/Plasma Concentrations/Protein Binding
    Tissue Concentrations
    Volume of Distribution
METABOLISM
    First Pass Effect
    Enzyme Induction
    Pharmacologically or Toxicologically Active Metabolites
ELIMINATION
    Clearance
    Route

---

of drug metabolizing enzymes in different species, there often are differences in metabolic profile. These differences may be useful for explaining differences in toxicity across species. It is also very important, particularly if there are major metabolites as well as interspecies differences in toxicity, to determine if the metabolites are active pharmacologically or toxicologically. If there is a major active metabolite it may be prudent to conduct toxicity studies with that metabolite. The possibility that there is evidence for saturable metabolism should also be explored in early studies, and if there is, at what doses and plasma levels it occurs. If that is the case, plasma levels of parent drug may be increasing disproportionately as dose increases. Alternatively, there may be enzyme induction with associated increases in levels of metabolites. Particularly for any drug that is extensively metabolized, it should be determined as soon as possible whether or not the pattern in humans is similar. Within the realm of possibility, the species with a metabolic profile for the drug which follows a pattern that is most like that seen in humans should be the one used for subchronic and chronic toxicity studies.

Several parameters are examined for the purpose of obtaining a picture of the distribution of the drug in the body. Early in development the usually measured plasma parameters consist of C_{max}, or maximum observed plasma concentration; T_{max}, or the time for the plasma level to reach C_{max}; AUC, or total area under the plasma concentration time curve from time zero to infinity; and $T_{1/2}$ or time for drug plasma level to decline by 50%. After repeated dosing, estimation of C_{ss}, or concentration at steady state, may be made. All of these measures are useful for choosing dosing regimens and appropriate dose ranges for toxicity studies. For example, if half life is very short, once a day dosing would not appropriately define the toxic potential of the drug in animals. Clearly a drug with a short half life will be given to people more frequently than once a day. Which of the concentration measures provides better correlation with therapeutic or toxic effects? AUC may more accurately reflect the body burden or exposure than C_{max} or C_{ss}. One important reason for obtaining peak plasma levels is for determination of the most appropriate timing of physiological measurements which are to be incorporated into the study, such as blood pressure, ECG, heart rate. The volume of distribution relates the amount of drug in the body to blood or plasma concentrations . It is a hypothetical volume of body fluid which would be required to dissolve the total amout of drug at the same concentration as that found in blood, and it reflects the distribution of drug beyond the circulating blood. It is a useful measure because a very large volume of distribution is indicative of extensive extravascular distribution. It may reflect tissue pools or binding which could conceivably result in slow clearance and/or toxicity in the organ(s) where drug accumulates. Drug distribution studies, in which animals are given labeled drug, with serial examination of levels of radioactivity in tissues at a variety of time points, provide us with the information which may explain why there is a large volume of distribution, because drug may be remaining in some tissue compartments for a long period of time. These studies are usually conducted by giving acute doses of drug and then following the radioactivity in tissues until it has declined to minimal levels. They also include examinations at several early time points when drug levels are expected to be high. They may be useful for explaining differences in toxicity between species because of drug accumulation, for explaining target organ toxicity, and also simply for the purpose of demonstrating that the drug is actually reaching the pharmacologically desirable target site in an appropriate time frame. This type of study is also useful for measuring placental transfer of drug in reproduction studies. The plasma protein binding of drugs, like a careful examination of bioavailability, is one of those extremely important measurements that sometimes isn't given full attention. Protein binding studies are usually done in an in vitro setting, and measure the nonspecific binding of drug, primarily to serum albumin for acidic drugs and to α_1-acid glycoprotein for basic drugs. This is a particularly important concept because it is only free drug which is available to diffuse across membranes and reach the appropriate receptors. If a drug is highly protein bound, very little will be available to exert the desired pharmacodynamic action. If it is given with another drug which is also protein bound, one drug may displace the other from its binding site and there can be unexpected and relatively large increases in available plasma levels of one or the other drug, which may in turn lead to unexpected toxicity that requires dose adjustment. Usually when drug plasma levels are measured in preclinical toxicity studies and also in clinical studies, it is total drug that is measured, with no distinction between free and bound. This is an important point to remember when relating drug plasma levels to observed toxicities if significant protein binding of that drug was shown in in vitro studies.

The parameters that describe absorption, distribution and metabolism of a drug are useful for designing toxicity studies which characterize the biological and toxicological actions of a drug in the body. The kinetics relating to elimination of the drug from the body are equally important and complex. Clearance is the rate of elimination by all routes. Kidney and liver play a major role in excretion of many drugs either as unchanged drug or water soluble metabolites. Biliary excretion into the feces is also a major route. Mass balance studies are used, not only to examine route and rate of clearance but also to shed light on how complete absorption may have been. The data obtained may indicate that drug is being stored in tissue or that a low bioavailability may have been due to metabolism. These studies are similar to tissue distribution studies, in which radiolabeled drug is given, preferably by both oral and intravenous routes, and urinary and fecal samples are collected over a series of time points. The mean cumulative recovery of drug and metabolites provides additional information about the extent of the bioavailability of the drug in addition to identifying organs that are involved in its clearance. A drug that is cleared by the renal route may tend to accumulate in chronic toxicity studies in which older animals may have compromised renal function. The results could be an apparent shift in the dose response curve for toxicity which would not be relevant to normal animals or people.

All of these studies, if carefully planned, and conducted at appropriate doses and times, can be most useful for the planning of an efficient toxicology program which may speed clinical development of the drug. At the very minimum, they should provide answers to many perplexing toxicology questions that arise. For example, if there are changes in such parameters as clearance, volume of distribution, and half-life as a function of dose or concentration of drug, it is helpful to know that these effects may have been due to saturation of protein binding, if drug binds extensively, or to hepatic metabolism, if drug is extensively metabolized, or to saturation of active renal transport of the drug. In short, the more the pharmacokinetic profile has been characterized, the easier it is to explain changes in kinetic parameters or toxicity that may occur.

Table 3. Differences in Margin of Safety Based on Dose versus Plasma Concentrations

SPECIES	DOSE mg/kg	C_{max} µg/ml
RAT	250	24
	1000	52
	2000	85
HUMAN	15	8

A few representative examples of pharmacokinetic data from nonclinical studies which were submitted to the FDA, and which provided some insight into toxicological problems, will serve to illustrate the usefulness of ADME studies. These examples are based on actual drugs but some of the facts have been somewhat altered in the interest of confidentiality. The data in Table 3 represent a chronic study in which a carcinogenic response, consisting of a rare tumor type in rats, occurred in a dose related manner in one sex of rat. The question becomes how to evaluate these results. This drug is not metabolized by either human or rat, and is essentially not protein bound. If one looks only at dose on a mg/kg basis, there appears to a margin of safety of between 70 and 140 fold. With the type of toxicity involved, that margin may or may not provide a measure of comfort. However, when one examines plasma drug concentration, the margin of safety shrinks to 6 to 10 fold. Currently, additional information is being generated, including an examination of drug disposition and accumulation, with special attention to the organ in question, in both sexes of rat as well as in other species. These data, together with additional plasma level data in all species involved, will hopefully provide useful information for purposes of regulatory decision making.

It is important to emphasize in relation to this example that the extrapolation of data between animals and humans, for purposes of establishing a safety margin, based on mg/kg doses, can result in very misleading results. Invariably, there appears to be a much greater safety margin than when plasma level data, which represent actual drug exposure, are used. Either mg/m^2 or the allometric equation for body surface area, $W^{0.67}$, provide a better estimate of relative exposure than mg/kg because they reflect, at least to some extent, differences between species in metabolism and clearance.

In a second example, the importance of measuring drug and metabolite levels at several time points is apparent. Sudden death following convulsions occurred within approximately one month in a subchronic study in monkeys. There was no similar toxicity after acute dosing, or in a rat study using higher doses. These deaths occurred at doses of 45 and 100 mg/kg but not at lower doses of 20 mg/kg or less. The major metabolite of this drug had already been identified, and it occurred in both species. It had also been determined that the metabolite was inactive. The subchronic study protocols had fortunately been designed to include plasma level measurements of both parent and metabolite on day 1 and after 1,2 and 3 months of dosing. Figures 1 and 2 illustrate the levels of metabolite and of parent in the monkey after one dose and after one month of dosing.

It is clear that after one month of dosing, the level of metabolite (Figure 1) was decreasing relative to day 1. However, the level of parent drug (Figure 2) was increasing after

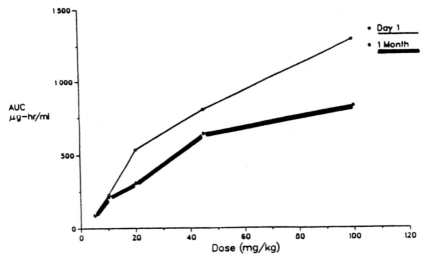

Fig. 1. Mean AUC Values of Metabolite in Rhesus Monkeys Given Drug Orally

repeated dosing, especially at high dose. There was apparently saturation of the metabolic pathway in the monkey, but not in the rat. The fact that the metabolite had already been identified, and that both parent and metabolite had been measured in the subchronic studies, meant that the sponsor did not need to go back and re- examine these parameters in nonclinical studies. There was already adequate information to allow the sponsor to proceed with limited clinical trials in order to obtain information about the metabolic profile in humans.

Tables 4 and 5 contain data from another example in which the use of tissue distribution studies proved useful for explaining toxicity in one species which did not occur in another. Dogs receiving the high dose of that drug all developed cardiac and skeletal muscle necrosis, and some receiving the middle dose were also affected, but those receiving low dose were

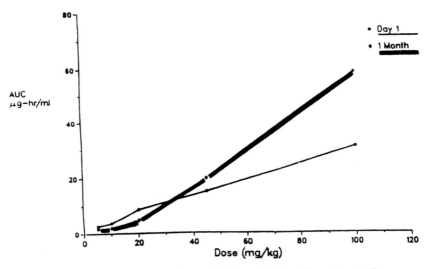

Fig. 2. Mean AUC Values of Parent in Rhesus Monkeys Given Drug Orally

Table 4. Pharmacokinetic Parameters in Two Species

| | DOSE (mg/kg) | | |
	20	40	60
DOGS			
AUC (μg-hr/ml)	20	75	115
C_{max} (μg/ml)	8	24	35
C_{ss} (μg/ml)	3	12	19
CL(ml/min/kg)	4	2.6	2.3
Vd (l/kg)	47	55	43
MONKEYS			
AUC (μg-hr/ml)	6	13	20
C_{max} (μg/ml)	3	6	9
C_{ss} (μg/ml)	1	2	3
CL(ml/min/kg)	14	13	14
Vd (l/kg)	24	20	30

not. These lesions did not occur in monkeys. When pharmacokinetic parameters were examined (Table 4) it could be seen that there was a non-linear accumulation of drug in plasma in dogs receiving the middle and high doses, with disproportionate increases in AUC, C_{max} and C_{ss}. Monkeys were not similarly affected. Clearance appears to be somewhat decreased in dogs, and there is no information about metabolism. However, when tissue distribution studies were done (Table 5), it was clear that drug was accumulating in heart and skeletal muscle of the dog where the lesions had occurred, and in the liver which was also a target

Table 5. Tissue Concentrations in 4 Week Study at 60 mg/kg/day

TISSUE	MONKEY	DOG
HEART*	1.8	38.7
MUSCLE*	1.0	94.9
LIVER*	2.2	83.1
PLASMA C_{SS}**	3.35	19.2

*(microgram/gram tissue)
**(microgram/ml plasma)

Table 6. Comparison of Plasma Levels in Two Species Receiving the Same Doses

SPECIES	DOSE (mg/kg)	PLASMA LEVELS OF PARENT DRUG AUC (ng-hr/ml) DAY		
		1	7	14
RAT	1	9	2	3
	3.3	42	35	43
	10	190	1215	2847
BABOON	1	7	-	5
	3.3	12	-	17
	10	34	-	78

organ. There was no accumulation in tissues in the monkey. Although we cannot monitor tissue levels in humans, monitoring for dose accumulation in plasma in clinical trials could provide a useful marker for potential toxicity until additional metabolism information is obtained so that it may be determined whether the dog or the monkey represents the better animal model.

In a final example (Table 6), plasma levels were disproportionately high in rats receiving high dose, and increased in a non linear fashion between days 1 and 7 and days 7 and 14. The rapid accumulation of parent drug was associated with serious toxicity and was thought to occur because the drug inhibits its own metabolism in that species. Toxicity in baboons was minimal, and drug did not accumulate. As in the previous example, it should be determined in early clinical trials which species provides the better model for humans. If there is an indication that plasma levels may become non-linear with increasing dose or repeated dosing, particular care should be exercised to avoid the rapid and precipitous elevations of plasma levels observed in the rat.

Regulators rely increasingly on data obtained from pharmacokinetic and toxicokinetic investigations to aid them in determining which animal models are most appropriate, and to provide explanations and suggest solutions for difficult toxicological problems which might otherwise interrupt clinical development.

NONCLINICAL CONSIDERATIONS: DISPOSITION OF DRUGS

Martin D. Green
Division of Antiviral Drug Products
Center for Drug Evaluation and Research
FDA, Rockville, MD 20857

ABSTRACT

In the design and conduct of pharmacokinetic and toxicokinetic studies, several features should be considered to maximize the utility of the resultant data. Recommendations will be offered regarding the conduct of studies relating the advantages of using the same species, route of administration, and frequency of administration, where possible, as that proposed for pharmacologic and toxicologic testing. The period of dosing should be representative of the proposed clinical duration. Possible "endpoints" to be considered include area under the curve, maximum plasma concentration, volume of distribution, time to maximum plasma concentration, clearance, and half-life of elimination. As suitable, the absolute fraction absorbed should be determined following the administration of the drug at various doses. If a drug will be used under steady state or special physiological conditions, additional pharmacokinetic and toxicokinetic studies if conducted under similar conditions offer useful information. It is also important to evaluate the potential to form metabolites and their contribution to the overall activity profile. Pharmacokinetic and toxicokinetic data has "utility" because it provides a rational and scientific basis crucial to understanding the biological effects of a drug, in identifying and designing appropriate nonclinical studies, and in validating extrapolations between animal studies and humans. Pharmacokinetic and toxicokinetic studies play an integral role in assessing safety and effectiveness.

INTRODUCTION

In the two previous chapters, Drs. Weissinger and Fitzgerald described the value of performing dispositional studies that include pharmacokinetics and toxicokinetics in nonclini-

Integration of Pharmacokinetics, Pharmacodynamics, and Toxicokinetics in Rational Drug Development, Edited by A. Yacobi *et al.*, Plenum Press, New York, 1993

cal studies. In addition, they have presented examples that illustrate the advantages of collecting these data. Here, I will continue with important considerations regarding the conduct of these studies, useful endpoints, and the application of animal pharmacokinetic and toxicokinetic studies to drug development.

To provide a more rational and scientifically valid approach to the analysis of nonclinical efficacy and safety studies, pharmacokinetic and toxicokinetic studies should be considered based on the intended use of the drug. These kinetic studies make use of concentration and time relationships in determining endpoints useful for understanding the connection between a dose and its biological effects.

CONDUCT OF STUDIES

The pharmacokinetics and toxicokinetics of single and repeat dose administrations of a drug are useful tools in the investigation of its biological properties. With the repeated administration of a drug at a given dose, changes may occur in the systemic level of exposure. In some cases, untoward accumulation of a drug may lead to unanticipated toxicities or alterations in various physiological systems. Conversely in some cases, with repeated dosing the systemic levels of a drug may be lowered through increased rates of metabolism or decreased absorption.

Pharmacokinetic and toxicokinetic studies may be conducted either as an integral part of toxicity or efficacy studies or as separate, independent studies. Kinetic studies are often conducted using satellite groups of animals rather than in animals being evaluated for a drug's efficacy or toxicity to avoid confounding variables.

Nonclinical pharmacokinetic and toxicokinetic studies of a new drug are best conducted using the same species, dose range, and route of administration as that used in pharmacological and toxicological studies. A sufficient number of animals should be included at each dose to ensure that inherent variation does not obscure meaningful results in the scientific determination of various kinetic endpoints.

Dosing regimens are important in determining the relationships between a drug, its dose and biological effects. To the greatest extent practical and based on a knowledge of drug disposition, the dosing regimens used in pharmacological and toxicological studies should be representative of those proposed for clinical use.

In larger, non-rodent species, the possibility of once, twice or three times, daily administration may provide sufficient flexibility to mimic levels of drug intended for use in the clinic. Particularly in longer term rodent studies, a practical maximum of twice daily administration of a drug may be the maximum feasible limit on the frequency of dosing. In some cases, an increase in the amount of drug administered per dose may offset the effect of less frequent dosing regimens. Depending upon the absorption and metabolic profile, administration of a drug through the diet may be shown to provide adequate levels of exposure.

The design of kinetic studies should take into account a drug's potential to undergo biotransformation. Where the biological activity of a drug resides in its metabolites, the pharmacokinetics and toxicokinetics of the metabolites may be of more value than that of the parent drug. Early in the development of a drug, a qualitative metabolic profile should be established. This qualitative profile should provide a basis for making comparisons across various species that are used in nonclinical studies. In vitro studies using either tissue homogenates or tissue cultures may also provide useful information in assessing the likelihood that metabolites may be formed.

During the conduct of pharmacokinetic and toxicokinetic studies, various types of samples can be collected including blood, plasma, serum, or urine; however, several problems exist in using urinary samples that limit their value. For example, since the cumulative amount of drug excreted through the urine is calculated through a summation of all previous determinations, cumulative errors may result. Also as the drug is held in the bladder for varying times, the cumulative amount of drug excreted relative to a specific time is uncertain. Lastly, practical difficulties exist in accurately collecting uncontaminated urine.

Pharmacokinetic and toxicokinetic samples should be taken at appropriate intervals to characterize periods of significant changes in the in vivo levels of a drug. Pilot studies may be necessary to determine optimal sampling time points. Due to the practical limitations imposed during the conduct of nonclinical studies, these studies may be conducted as a pragmatic compromise between the limited number of samples that can be collected and the information necessary to characterize the kinetics of a drug. In particular for drugs that are very quickly or very slowly absorbed or eliminated, adjustments to a sampling plan can be made as information becomes available regarding its kinetics. These drugs may be identified a priori by their chemical nature or similarity to known compounds with established kinetics.

In designing kinetic studies, a group size should be selected that produces scientifically useful data and uses a minimum number of animals. In selecting a group size for kinetic studies, two major factors should be considered: 1) variability among animals due to sex, age, or physiological status and 2) the analytical assay.

In general, serial sampling from individual animals provides the most accurate data; however, in cases where this method may introduce significant physiological effects, sampling from pooled groups of animals is an acceptable alternative. Pooling of samples from different animals will yield less precise estimates. Obviously when drug and tissue distribution studies are performed, inter-animal variability is unavoidable.

Before initiating pharmacokinetic and toxicokinetic studies, analytical methods for quantifying systemic levels of a drug must be developed and validated. Assays for active metabolites should be developed as soon as possible. Analytical assays should be validated with regard to their reproducibility, sensitivity, and specificity. In the design and conduct of kinetic studies, the impact of assay requirements, for example sample volume, on the sampling strategy must be considered. For rodent studies, volume, number, and frequency of samples taken may be problematic to the conduct of kinetic studies. In rodent studies, small groups of animals, may be used to achieve reasonable precision. In some rodent studies, the total number of animals involved in a study may be reduced, by staggering the sampling from animals during the course of a study. In kinetic studies using larger animals such as dogs or monkeys, serial samples may be obtained; therefore a smaller total number of animals may be utilized in these studies.

ENDPOINTS

The following endpoints are considered useful products of kinetic studies: maximum observed concentration of drug (C_{max}), time to C_{max} (T_{max}), area under the concentration curve (AUC), clearance, half-life, and bioavailability. C_{max} is defined as the observed peak concentration of the drug substance over time. T_{max} is defined as that time at which the observed peak concentration occurs. Although highly dependent on sampling times, C_{max} and T_{max} are suggestive of the rate of drug absorption. Both C_{max} and T_{max} are subject to substantial timing error and unless an accurate knowledge of the time course of change is established, these endpoints may be of little value. If these endpoints are critical variables, studies should be conducted to accurately assess C_{max} and T_{max}.

AUC is defined as the area under the concentration-time curve and may be stated as a value over a fixed period of time such as 24 hours or extrapolated to infinity. AUC provides an excellent means of assessing the combined influences of time and concentration.

Total clearance may be defined as the proportionality factor and relates the rate of elimination to a drug's concentration. Clearance is a highly useful indicator of the rate of a drug's systemic removal.

The half-life of a drug may be determined from empirical data. Half-life has the advantage that it is both a familiar term and provides a ready means of relating drug levels to dosing regimens. If the terminal elimination phase of the drug's kinetic profile is measured, it should be followed until the concentration falls below detectable limits or for at least four half-lives.

Bioavailability quantifies the proportion of a drug that is absorbed and available to exert its systemic effects. Bioavailability is defined in terms of both the extent and rate of a drug's absorption. During the course of pharmacological and toxicological studies, absolute and relative bioavailability may be determined. Absolute bioavailability refers to the systemic measurement of a drug following its intravenous administration whereas relative bioavailability refers to a comparison between two or more formulations. The intravenous administration of a drug and measurement of absolute bioavailability may pose special problems. Following the intravenous administration of a drug, high tissue concentrations may be produced that result in various toxic effects. Hence in some cases, measurement of a drug's absolute bioavailability may be precluded by toxicity.

In addition to those endpoints that are cited above, other endpoints should be determined as appropriate. The extent of plasma protein binding should be measured if a large fraction of drug may be bound. Similarly the rate and extent of a drug's uptake into red blood cells may be important in understanding the biological effects of some drugs. The volume of distribution should be reported in cases where it provides interpretable information. The minimum concentration of drug (C_{min}), defined as the concentration observed immediately prior to administering a given dose, should be measured, if feasible, in repeated dose studies. C_{min} may be used as an indicator of a drug's propensity for accumulation.

To calculate the pharmacokinetic and toxicokinetic endpoints as cited above, standard references should be consulted regarding various methods and procedures.

APPLICATION

The information gained from pharmacokinetic and toxicokinetic studies can be used to optimize and improve the design of nonclinical studies and extrapolate the results of these studies to clinical situations.

Early in the development of a drug, kinetic studies can be used to design rational and scientifically valid nonclinical studies. From an understanding of the relationship between the applied and the internal dose of a drug, more efficient and effective studies can be devised. For example if an applied dose is expected to yield only marginal changes in systemic exposure, it may be deleted from study. In addition, simply increasing the systemic level of a drug beyond that producing meaningful biological changes would also be unlikely to provide useful information in evaluating the relationship between a dose and its pharmacological or toxicological activity.

As drug development approaches the initiation of clinical studies, pharmacokinetic and toxicokinetic studies provide a means of extrapolating the results of toxicity or efficacy testing across species. Measurement of pharmacokinetics and toxicokinetics can provide a means of identifying and quantifying differences between species. An understanding of pharmacology and toxicity in terms of kinetic factors may provide a scientific basis upon which to predict the frequency and degree of response from one species to another. Conclusions drawn from the assumption that an applied dose is proportionate to an internal dose may lead to a false appreciation of a drug's margin of safety. Except in those cases where pharmacodynamic or toxicodynamic differences may confound an appropriate scientific interpretation, drug equivalency of effects across species is best stated on the basis of pharmacokinetic or toxicokinetic endpoints.

CONCLUSION

In conclusion, the rational and scientific application of pharmacokinetic and toxicokinetic principles to drug development will provide an enhanced basis for assessing and evaluating the results of nonclinical studies. Kinetic studies are best carried out through an integrative approach and are most useful when conducted within the range of doses used to establish the safety and effectiveness of investigational drugs. In the design and conduct of kinetic studies, careful consideration should be given to the route of administration, animal species, and dosing schedule. Early in the development of a drug, pharmacokinetic and toxicokinetic studies can be employed to guide the selection of doses used to establish initial safety and effectiveness. As a drug is developed, kinetic studies are of great value in devising a means of establishing the equivalence of a drug across species. If used appropriately, pharmacokinetic and toxicokinetic studies will increase the scientific merit and integrity of nonclinical investigations.

USE OF ACUTE TOXICITY DATA IN THE DESIGN AND INTERPRETATION OF SUBCHRONIC AND CHRONIC TOXICITY STUDIES

Karl K. Rozman
Department of Pharmacology, Toxicology & Therapeutics
University of Kansas Medical Center
Kansas City, Kansas 66160 U.S.A.
and
Section of Environmental Toxicology
GSF-Institut für Toxikologie
8042 Neuherberg, F.R.G.

ABSTRACT

This contribution shows that the relative toxic potency of 4 chlorinated dibenzo-p-dioxins (CDDs) is similar in 2 species with different sensitivities (guinea pig, rat). More importantly, it also demonstrates that the relative toxic potencies of these homologues and their mixture is essentially identical for acute, subchronic and chronic dosing in the same species (rat). The importance and usefulness of careful considerations of toxicokinetic and toxicodynamic data obtained in acute experiments for the design of subchronic and chronic toxicity studies is discussed.

INTRODUCTION

Most subchronic and chronic toxicity studies are driven by the need to satisfy regulatory requirements. As a result scientific considerations (e.g. dose responses) become secondary to concepts of limited value such as the maximum tolerated dose (MTD). Most often for carcinogenicity bioassays the second dose is selected as one-half of the MTD which represents a disregard of the considerable variability in shape and slope of dose response curves resulting from the administration of various compounds. Using four chlorinated dibenzo-p-dioxins (CDDs) as examples, the importance and usefulness of scientific considerations in preclinical

Integration of Pharmacokinetics, Pharmacodynamics, and Toxicokinetics in Rational Drug Development, Edited by A. Yacobi *et al.*, Plenum Press, New York, 1993

toxicity studies will be demonstrated as well as the pitfalls when regulatory considerations prevail over science.

Results and Discussion

A comparison of the relative potencies of 7 homologues of 2,3,7,8-tetrachlorodibenzo-p-dioxin (tetra-CDD) shows several interesting features (Table 1). First, the relative acute potency of tetra-CDD homologues is quite similar in 2 species with considerably different sensitivities to this class of compounds (for tetra-CDD guinea pig LD_{50}: 2 µg/kg; rat LD_{50}: 43 µg/kg). This suggests that the underlying mechanism of acute toxicity is most likely the

Table 1. Acute Subchronic and Chronic (carcinogenic) Potency of Various Homologues of Tetra-CDD in Guinea Pigs and Rats

RELATIVE POTENCY OF DIOXIN ISOMERS

Isomer	LD_{50}[a] Guinea Pig	LD_{50}[b] Rat	Subchronic Rat	Carcinogenicity Rat
2,3,7,8-Tetra-CDD	1.0	1.0	1.0	1.0
1,2,3,7,8-Penta-CDD	0.7	0.2	0.4[c]	ND
1,2,3,4,7,8-Hexa-CDD	0.03	0.05	0.05[d]	0.04[d]
1,2,3,6,7,8-Hexa-CDD	0.03-0.02	ND		
1,2,3,7,8,9-Hexa-CDD	0.03-0.02	ND	ND	ND
1,2,3,4,6,7,8-Hepta-CDD	0.003	0.007	ND	ND
1,2,3,4,6,7,8,9-Octa-CDD	--	(0.001)[e]	0.001-0.01[f]	ND

ND is not determined.
[a]*From McConnel et al. (1978).*
[b]*From Stahl et al. (1991).*
[c]*From Pluess et al. (1988).*
[d]*From EPA/600/8-84/014F (1985).*
[e]Estimated.
[f]*From Wermelinger et al. (1990)* and *Couture et al. (1988).*

same or very similar in these 2 species. Second, and more importantly, the relative potencies of the various congeners (as far as data are available) are essentially identical for acute, subchronic and chronic toxicities (carcinogenicity) in the Sprague-Dawley rat. It would be highly improbable for a correlation to be coincidental for this many variables. It is more likely that the relative potencies remain the same because the mechanism of acute, subchronic and chronic toxicities of CDDs is identical. Third, the 3 hexa-CDDs are equipotent in the guinea pig and probably also in the rat as a mixture of 2 hexa-CDDs resulted in the same subchronic and chronic relative potency as did a single hexa-CDD acutely. This suggests a highly symmetrical interaction site (receptor) being the critical mediator of toxicity.

The question then arises why and how CDDs might exert a diverse profile of toxic effects (e.g. lethality, porphyria, carcinogenicity) by the same mechanism? The first relevant consideration is that of dose.

Table 2. Cumulative Doses and Associated Mortality for Acute, Subchronic and Chronic Toxicities of Tetra-CDD in the Sprague-Dawley Rat

	Dose (μg/kg)		Mortality (% of controls)	
	Male	Female	Male	Female
Acute[a] (single iv dose)	72.7	ND	100	ND
Subchronic[b] (1 μg/kg/5 days a week for 13 weeks orally)	65.0	65.0	17	50
Chronic[c] (Carcinogenicity) (0.1 μg/kg/day for 104 weeks orally)	72.8	72.8	0	72

ND is not determined.
[a]Rozman et al. (1989).
[b]Kociba et al. (1976).
[c]Kociba et al. (1978).

Table 2 illustrates that subchronic and chronic dosing with tetra-CDD cause mortality at similar cumulative doses as does an acute dose, although some minor differences (at the most 2 to 3-fold) are present due to differences in route of administration and sex. The dose is, however, only a crude measure of exposure because of considerable differences in the toxicokinetics of tetra-CDD after acute, subchronic and chronic administration. A better measure for the target specific exposure is a comparison of the AUCs (area under the curve) in the target organ (liver). AUCs for acute (Fig. 1), subchronic (see appendix) and chronic (see appendix) exposure were calculated and found to be remarkably similar for all three circumstances (Table 3).

Unfortunately, these studies were not designed to prove conclusively the similarity of the AUCs with mortality as an end point of toxicity. However, the fact that the quotient between an LD_{80} and LD_{20} of tetra-CDD and the sex difference is only about a factor of 2

Table 3. AUC's for Acute, Subchronic and Chronic (carcinogenicity) Studies of Tetra-CDD in the Sprague-Dawley Rat

	Dose (μg/kg)		AUC (ppb x days)	
	Male	Female	Male	Female
Acute[a] (single iv dose)	72.7	ND	17,570	ND
Subacute (1 μg/kg/5 days a week for 13 weeks)	65.0	65.0	21,419	18,770
Chronic[c] (Carcinogenicity) (0.1 μg/kg/day for 104 weeks)	72.8	72.8	ND	17,515

ND is not determined.
[a]Rozman et al. (1989).
[b]Kociba et al. (1976).
[c]Kociba et al. (1978).

for each suggests that the AUCs for acute, subchronic and chronic toxicities of tetra-CDD would be fairly close if not identical also under optimum conditions of comparison.

Similar AUCs after different dosing regimens can lead to similar toxicities only if the mechanism of action is the same and if the lesion is essentially irreversible. We have demonstrated earlier that the inhibition of hepatic phosphoenolpyruvate carboxykinase (PEPCK) activity satisfies the criteria for a mechanistic cause-effect relationship in the toxicity of CDDs and that it is indeed irreversibly inhibited for up to 32 days after dosing (Weber et al., 1991). The link between inhibition of PEPCK activity and body weight change has been firmly established by Stahl et al. (1991) and Lebofsky et al. (1991). Hence the finding of Peterson et al. (1984) that the body weight gain of rats is impaired at a roughly constant increment for up to 90 days after a single nonlethal dose of tetra-CDD may be viewed as further evidence of an essentially irreversible inhibition of PEPCK by tetra-CDD.

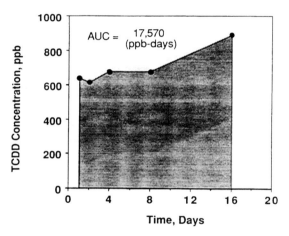

Fig. 1.The AUC (area under the curve) of the liver concentration of tetra-CDD after a single iv dose (72.7 µg/kg) in the Sprague-Dawley rat.

Similar arguments can be advanced for the possibility that other end points of tetra-CDD toxicity are related to an irreversible and hence cumulative inhibition of PEPCK activity. Elevated porphyrin levels have been reported after both subchronic and chronic exposure to tetra-CDD (Kociba et al. 1976, 1978). Interestingly, elevated tryptophan levels have been associated with porphyrias and related serotonergic mechanisms (Essman, 1979). Inhibition of PEPCK-activity by CDDs and elevated plasma levels of tryptophan show a high correlation (Rozman et al., 1990) suggesting that inhibition of PEPCK activity or a related event may be the underlying fundamental lesion leading to chemically induced porphyria by an indirect mechanism.

A similar association and the possibility of a cause-effect relationship between inhibition of PEPCK activity and liver cancer has been discussed previously (Rozman et al., 1990).

These considerations allow some fundamental conclusions about the mechanism of toxicity of this class of compounds and of all other chemicals acting by the same mechanism:

1. Average tissue concentration × time = cumulative toxicity

This point has been demonstrated by Tables 2 and 3. However, this principle appears to be expandable (and probably generalizable) to other end points of toxicity (e.g. porphyria, cancer) because comparable AUCs for tetra-CDD-induced porphyria caused similar elevations in the urinary excretion of coproporphyrin in female rats after subchronic and chronic administration (compare Tables 2 and 3 with Kociba et al., 1976 and 1978). It is now also understandable why Goldstein et al. (1982) were unable to induce porphyria with acute doses of tetra-CDD. The dose of tetra-CDD required to cause porphyria, acutely kills most animals before porphyria becomes manifest. However, unlike Goldstein et al. (1982), we have occasionally observed porphyric rats after acute doses of tetra-CDD particularly in animals with prolonged time to death. These considerations further imply that the dose responses regarding lethality and porphyria in acute, subchronic and chronic studies are identical when plotted versus the cumulative dose. The 3-dimensional presentation (Fig. 2) illustrates this concept, where the word toxicity may be substituted by lethality or urinary porphyrins or for that matter by tumor incidence.

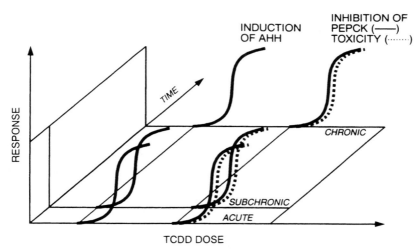

Fig. 2. Schematic presentation of the concept: average tissue concentration × time = cumulative toxicity and illustration of identical and parallel dose responses between inhibition of PEPCK activity and toxicity and between PEPCK activity/toxicity and AHH induction, respectively.

This latter point is of crucial importance for the design of carcinogenicity bioassays. The Kociba et al. (1978) study is a case in point. Acute dose-responses of tetra-CDD are shown for male and female Sprague-Dawley rats in Fig.3. These dose-responses indicate that male rats are acutely 1.67 times less sensitive to tetra-CDD than female rats. Yet, Kociba et al. (1978) administered the same per kg dose to both sexes and found that tetra- CDD caused liver and lung tumors only in female rats. It is important to note that tumors occurred only in female rats and only at a dose which was associated with excess mortality, thus exceeding the

MTD. Males, which did not show excess mortality did not display excess tumor incidence. However, according to acute studies the male equivalent dose of the female dose is 72.8 x 50/30 = 121.6 µg/kg. When VanMiller et al. (1977) gave 125.6 µg/kg tetra- CDD to male rats in a chronic study, they found comparable liver and lung tumor incidences in male rats as did Kociba et al. (1978) in female rats. Again, tumors in male rats occurred only together with excess mortality. This example illustrates the pitfalls of disregarding acute potencies in the

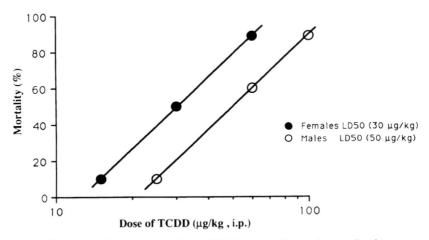

Fig. 3. Acute dose responses of tetra-CDD in male and female Sprague-Dawley rats.

dose selection for carcinogenicity bioassays. The end result was that many toxicologists misinterpreted tetra-CDD as a female-specific rat carcinogen. The need to do the bioassay at MTD also obscured the fact that the dose responses to tumor formation and mortality are identical.

Another frequently encountered fundamental misunderstanding in the interpretation of dose responses is also illustrated in Fig. 2. The mechanism of toxicity of CDDs was thought to be mediated by binding to the Ah-receptor, which appears necessary for the induction of certain enzymes such as arylhydrocarbon hydroxylase (AHH) because this biological effect displays a parallel dose response to dose-responses of toxicity. This is a fundamental misunderstanding of the mathematical meaning of a dose-response statement. For one compound and for a specific effect there is only one dose response, no matter by how many steps the target specific dose is separated from the effect (e.g. interaction with DNA, altered transcription of mRNA and translation of enzyme protein, decreased enzyme activity, blockage of a biochemical pathway, derailment of intermediary metabolism, lethality). Any and all of these steps that are cause-effect-related to the dose have to have identical dose responses. Parallel dose responses can have only two meanings, either it is a different substance (agonist, antagonist) or it is a different effect. Thus Ah-receptor-mediated biological effects are not fundamental to the mechanism of toxicity of CDDs but represent a different biological effect.

2. A threshold dose is implicit in the concept of relative potency

Evidence presented by Stahl et al. (1991) and Lebofsky et al. (1991) and by others indicate that the mechanism of action for all 4 CDDs and their mixture is identical. This means that the dose-response curves are parallel at any and all doses. In the absence of complete understanding of tumor formation the alternative and currently accepted extrapolation forces all dose response curves through zero (at least for carcinogenicity) ignoring the shape of the dose response curves which rise very sharply near a threshold dose (Fig. 4). This amounts to abolishing the validity of the relative potency and requires the assumption that the mechanism of action of toxicity (e.g. formation of preneoplastic foci) is different at very low doses (at which all carcinogens would become equipotent) than at somewhat higher doses.

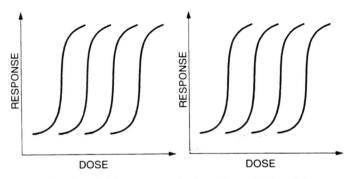

Fig. 4.Schematic presentation of parallel dose responses for four different CDDs and the consequence of assuming threshold vs. no threshold for viewing relative potency.

The data and interpretations presented here suggest that dose response curves for chronic effects (carcinogenicity) of CDDs have the same shape and equivalent cumulative dose response characteristics as subchronic and acute dosing regimens. Therefore, the chronic (carcinogenicity) dose response curves will still rise sharply from threshold doses as they do after subchronic or acute dosages. This point is well illustrated by an earlier discussion of the carcinogenicity of tetra-CDD in male and female rats in this text. Tumor and mortality dose-responses begin to rise in female rats at a dose which is a subthreshold dose in male rats. At just slightly higher doses (1.67 times) both mortality and tumor dose responses begin to rise sharply for male rats as well.

In conclusion, these considerations demonstrate that the relative potency concept is a powerful tool on which to base regulatory action and that at the same time it is internally inconsistent with the no-threshold concept for CDDs and most likely for all compounds and for all end points of toxicity including cancer.

APPENDIX

Areas Under Curve (Liver Dose) for Subchronic and Chronic Studies of TCDD

$t_{1/2}$ for liver estimated as 19 days

$k = \ln(2)/t_{1/2} = \ln(2)/19 \text{ days} = 0.0365/\text{day}$

For a continuous input (compound in feed)

$X(t) = X_{ss}(1-e^{-kt})$ $\qquad$ X_{ss} = steady-state concentration

Subchronic Study (90 Days)

Dose = 1.0 µg/kg/5 days a week for 13 weeks

$X(t)$ is very near, but not quite at steady state:

$X(90) = 324$ ppb for males and 284 for females in the liver

$$X(90) = X_{ss}(1-e^{-0.0365(90)}) = X_{ss}(0.9625)$$

$$X_{ss} = X(90)/0.9625 = \frac{284ppb}{0.9625} = 295\ ppb$$

$$\int_0^{90} X(t)dt = X_{ss}\int_0^{90} (1-e^{-kt})dt = X_{ss}[t + \frac{e^{-kt}}{k} \Big|_0^t]$$

$$= X_{ss}[t + \frac{1}{k}(e^{kt}-1)] \quad \begin{aligned} &= 18{,}770\ ppb\ x\ days\ for\ females \\ &= 21{,}419\ ppb\ x\ days\ for\ males \end{aligned}$$

Average Concentration

$$\frac{\int_0^{90} X(t)dt}{90\,days} = 208\ ppb$$

Chronic Study (104 wks = 728 days)

Dose = 0.1 µg/kg/day

$X(728) = 25$ ppb for females in the liver

$$\int_0^{728} X(t)dt = X_{ss}[t + \frac{1}{k}(e^{-kt}-1)] = 17{,}515\ ppb\ x\ days$$

Average Concentration

$$\frac{\int_0^{728} X(t)dt}{728\,days} = 24.06\ ppb$$

REFERENCES

Couture, L. A., M. R. Elwell, and L. S. Birnbaum (1988). Dioxin-like effects observed in male rats following exposure to octachlorodibenzo-p-dioxin (OCDD) during a 13- week study. Toxicol. Appl. Pharmacol., 93, 31-46.

EPA (1985) Health assessment document for polychlorinated dibenzo-p-dioxins, EPA/600/8-84/014F.

Essman, W. B. (1979). Serotonin in skin and skin disorders. In W. B. Essman (Ed.), Serotonin in Health and Disease Volume V: Clinical Applications SP Medical & Scientific Books, New York/London, pp. 321-287.

Goldstein, J.A., P. Linko and H. Bergman (1982). Induction of porphyria in the rat by chronic versus acute exposure to 2,3,7,8-tetrachlorodibenzo-p- dioxin. Biochem. Pharmacol., 31, 1607-1613.

Kociba. R. J., P. A. Keeler, C. N. Park, and P. J. Gehring (1976). 2,3,7,8- Tetrachlorodibenzo-p-dioxin (TCDD): results of a 13-week toxicity study in rats. Toxicol. Appl. Pharmacol., 35, 553-574.

Kociba, R. J., D. G. Keyes, J. E. Beyer, R. M. Carreon, C. E. Wade, D. A. Dittenber, R. P. Kalnins, L. E. Frauson, C. N. Park, S. D. Barnard, R. A. Hummel, and C. G. Humiston (1978). Results of a two-year chronic toxicity and oncogenicity study of 2,3,7,8-tetrachlorodibenzo-p-dioxin in rats. Toxicol. Appl. Pharmacol., 46, 279-303.

Lebofsky, M., L. W. D. Weber, and K. Rozman (1991). Polychlorinated dibenzo-p-dioxin inhibit key enzymes of gluconeogenesis: dose responses and in vivo structure activity relationships in rats. Toxicologist, 11, 263.

McConnell, E.E., J. A. Moore, J. K. Haseman, and M. W. Harris (1978). The comparative toxicity of chlorinated dibenzo-p-dioxins in mice and guinea pigs. Toxicol. Appl. Pharmacol., 44, 335-356.

Peterson, R. E., M. D. Seefeld, B. J. Christian, C. L. Potter, Ch. K. Kelling, and R. E. Keesey (1984). The wasting syndrome in 2,3,7,8- tetrachlorodibenzo-p-dioxin toxicity: basic features and their interpretation. In A. Poland and R. O. Kimbrough (Eds.), Banbury Report 18: Biological Mechanisms of Dioxin Action. Cold Harbor Laboratory, pp. 291-308.

Pluess, N., H. Poiger, C. Hohbach, and Ch. Schlatter (1988). Subchronic toxicity of some chlorinated dibenzofurans (PCDFs) and a mixture of PCDFs and chlorinated dibenzo dioxins (PCDDs) in rats. Chemosphere, 17, 973-984.

Rozman, K., S. W. Ernst, and L. W. D. Weber (1989). Disposition of TCDD in rats after intravenous injection. Toxicologist, 9, 118.

Rozman, K., L. W. D. Weber, B. Pfeiffer, M. Lebofsky, B. U. Stahl, L. Kerecsen, R. H. Alper, and H. Greim (1990). Evidence for an indirect mechanism of acute toxicity of 2,3,7,8-tetrachlorodibenzo-p-dioxin in rats. In O. Hutzinger and H. Fiedler (Eds.), Dioxin '90, Vol. I, Eco-Informa Press, Bayreuth, F.R.G., pp. 133-136.

Stahl, B. U., M. Lebofsky, A. Kettrup, and K. Rozman (1991). Comparative acute toxicity of four polychlorinated dibenzo-p-dioxins (PCDDs) and their mixture in the male Sprague-Dawley rat. Toxicologist, 11, 263.

Van Miller, J. P., J. J. Lelich, and J. R. Allen (1977). Increased incident of neoplasms in rats exposed to low levels of 2,3,7,8-tetrachlorodibenzo-p-dioxin (TCDD). Chemosphere, 6, 537-578.

Weber, L. W. D., M. Lebofsky, B. U. Stahl, J. R. Gorski, G. Muzi, and K. Rozman (1991). Reduced activities of key enzymes of gluconeogenesis as possible cause of acute toxicity of 2,3,7,8-tetrachlorodibenzo-p-dioxin (TCDD) in rats. Toxicology, 65, 97-107.

Wermelinger, M., H. Poiger, and Ch. Schlatter (1990). Results of a 9-month feeding study with OCDD in rats. In O. Hutzinger and H. Fiedler (Eds.), Dioxin '90. Eco-Informa Press, Bayreuth, F.R.G., pp. 221-224.

USE OF PHARMACOKINETICS AND PHARMACODYNAMICS IN PRECLINICAL STUDIES TO GUIDE DOSAGE ESCALATION SCHEMES IN PHASE I STUDIES OF ANTICANCER DRUGS

Jerry M. Collins
Division of Clinical Pharmacology
Food and Drug Administration
Rockville, MD 20857

ABSTRACT

For the concept of pharmacologically-guided clinical trials with new anticancer drugs, the principal focus has been development of links between preclinical testing and Phase I clinical trials. Recent experiences with very lengthy Phase I trials for at least 8 drugs have provided particular impetus for the project. The specific concept was that dose-limiting toxicity is predicted by drug concentrations in plasma, and that the quantitative relationship between drug exposure (as measured by plasma drug concentration times time, or CxT) and toxicity holds across species. As a consequence, dose escalations in man could safely be based on measurements of drug levels in plasma, rather than on empirical escalation schemes. Although the concept is still relatively new, practical results have already been achieved. Examples will be given of Phase I trials which were completed with a savings of 12-24 months. Overall, there is now a substantial collection of data which demonstrates that coordination with preclinical pharmacology and toxicology studies can save both time and resources in early clinical trials without a loss of safety.

INTRODUCTION

Phase I testing of new drugs has never attracted as much attention as the definitive trials of efficacy. Phase I trials are briefer, involve fewer subjects, and generally provide little information about the ultimate efficacy of drugs. The two major elements are the selection of a safe starting dose and some procedure for escalating doses until an endpoint of toxicity (or another goal) is reached.

Integration of Pharmacokinetics, Pharmacodynamics, and Toxicokinetics in Rational Drug Development, Edited by A. Yacobi *et al.*, Plenum Press, New York, 1993

In most therapeutic areas, Phase I testing is conducted with healthy volunteers. In the development of drugs for diseases such as cancer and AIDS, patients are used. Although the primary scientific goal of Phase I testing is the determination of safe doses for further testing, patients volunteer for these trials when there are no acceptable therapeutic alternatives. Realistically, the probability of successful treatment is very low, especially for tumors which have already proven to be refractory to established agents. Nonetheless, because of the life-threatening nature of the disease, and the nature of the risks incurred by the patients, investigators have an obligation to maximize the potential benefit to these subjects.

Since these drugs have severe toxicities which in themselves may be life- threatening, there is a desire to move slowly and cautiously. This creates a fundamental conflict with the goal of avoiding the use of doses which are too low to provide any possible benefit. The compromise between these conflicting goals has been to escalate doses rapidly at the outset of a trial, then to decrease the rate of escalation as the trial proceeds. The "modified Fibonacci" escalation scheme is the most frequently used approach of this type in anticancer drug development. The initial escalation step is 100%, with a gradual decrease in escalation size to 25-35% increases over the previous step.

Recently, our interest in ways to improve the current system of Phase I testing has been further stimulated by the relatively long time that a variety of drugs have spent in Phase I testing. As listed in Table 1, a series of 8 drugs have recently completed Phase I trials of exceptional length.

The ratio of the final dose (MTD) to the entry dose determines the number of steps required to complete the trial. Each step requires about 2 months to complete, so all of these drugs required at least 2 years to finish.

Low entry doses are a sign of poor correlation between toxic doses in animals and in humans. In each of these cases, human tissues are apparently less sensitive than murine tissues. As described by Collins and co-workers (1986), examples also exist of poor corelations due to more sensitivity in humans.

Table 1. Recent Examples of Very Lengthy Phase I Trials

Drug Name	Sponsor	Entry Dose mg/m^2	MTD mg/m^2	Fibonacci Steps
Acodazole	NCI[a]	20	1184	12
Didemnin B	NCI	0.03	2.0	12
Amonafide	NCI	10	625	12
Brequinar	DuPont	6	2600	19
Sulfonylurea	Lilly	30	2250	13
Crisnatol	Wellcome	7.5	516	12
Datellipticinium	Sanofi	1.3	220	16
SM-108	Japan	20	2500	15

[a] NCI, National Cancer Institute

Data from Collins, Grieshaber, and Chabner (1990)

Table 2. Comparison of Dose Ratios and CxT Ratios

Drug	MTD/LD10 Dose Ratio	CxT at MTD CxT at LD10
5-Azacytidine	6.0	1.1
Doxorubicin	5.0	0.8
Teroxirone	4.3	0.8
PALA	2.8	3.3
Pirozantrone	2.1	0.8
Dihydroazacytidine	1.2	0.3
Diaziquone	1.0	1.0
Indicine-N-Oxide	0.9	0.6
Amsacrine	0.8	1.3
Tiazofurin	0.7	0.9
Pentostatin/DCF	0.7	1.1
Thio-TEPA	0.4	1.0
F-Ara-AMP	0.1	0.1

Our first goal is to determine the basis for interspecies differences; then, we need to use this information to change the way testing is done.

We began with the pharmacodynamic hypothesis that similar biological effects (toxicity) would be elicited at similar plasma levels in mice and humans. This assumption has a long history in various therapeutic fields, but had never been specifically applied to anticancer drugs. To test this hypothesis, we compared plasma levels of various anticancer drugs which were measured in mice at the LD10 and humans at the MTD. As shown in Table 2, the ratio of MTD/LD10 has greater variation than the ratio of plasma levels. There are a few outliers (F-Ara-AMP, dihyroazacytidine, and PALA), but otherwise there is considerable support for the pharmacodynamic hypothesis.

Not all drugs have a mechanism of action which is dependent upon CxT or AUC. For other drugs, some threshold concentration determines the incidence of dose-limiting toxicity (Collins, Leyland-Jones, and Grieshaber, 1987). When such a threshold exists, the MTD depends strongly upon the rate of drug administration, that is, there is schedule-dependence. Careful attention to matching of delivery schedules between human and preclinical testing is required.

Regardless of whether thresholds or AUC values are controlling, the next step is to determine a strategy for customizing the Phase I trial based upon the information determined in murine toxicology and pharmacology studies. While the escalation steps in a modified Fibonacci scheme are pre-programmed before the Phase I trial begins, a pharmacologically-guided dose escalation scheme adjusts the size of the escalation step based upon plasma levels. Examples of alternative escalation schemes have been presented by Collins and co-workers

Table 3. Impact of Closer Preclinical-Clinical Collaboration

Name[a]	MTD Entry	Fibonacci Steps	Clinical Impact
Acodazole	60	12	None[b]
Didemnin B	70	12	None[b]
HMBA	7 (30)	4 (10)	Entry Dose Increased
Amonafide	60	12	None[b]
Flavone AA	100	10 (14)	Escalation Accelerated
Merbarone	15 (120)	7 (15)	Entry Dose Increased
Deoxysperg	28 (700)	9 (21)	Entry Dose Increased
Pirozantrone	20	6 (8)	Escalation Accelerated

[a] Eight consecutive NCI drugs entered into Phase I.

[b] Planning too far advanced for any impact.

The numbers in parentheses correspond to the requirements of the standard system, without pharmacologic/toxicologic matching.

(1986). The "extended factors of two" scheme permits doubling of doses at each escalation step, until the AUC approaches the value measured at the murine LD10.

The combination of improved escalations schemes and more careful attention to schedule-dependence has already yielded tangible results. Table 3 presents a summary of our experience with eight consecutive drugs entered into clinical testing via the NCI drug development program.

For the 3 of the first 4 drugs, development had proceeded without utilization of these concepts, and the Phase I trials were quite lengthy. For 3 of the other drugs, the entry dose was increased, with impressive savings in time and resources. For deoxyspergualin, 12 fewer escalation steps were required, which translates into a time savings of two years. For the two cases of altered escalation patterns, the savings were more modest, but generated considerable support for the overall concept.

Although far from universally applied, these concepts have been picked up by commercial firms in this country. Currently, there are underway a number of pharmacologically-guided Phase I trials of both anticancer and anti-retroviral drugs.

In addition to the interest in these concepts in the United States, there has been substantial activity in this area in Europe (EORTC group, 1987; Foster and co-workers, 1988; Graham and co-workers, 1989; Gianni and co-workers, 1990; Newell, 1990).

ACKNOWLEDGEMENT

The work described herein has been an outgrowth of collaborative efforts with the staff of the National Cancer Institute and the Food and Drug Administration.

REFERENCES

Collins, J. M., D. S. Zaharko, R. L. Dedrick, and B. A. Chabner (1986). Potential risks for preclinical pharmacology Phase I clinical trials. Cancer Treat. Rep., 70, 73-80.

Collins, J. M., B. Leyland-Jones, and C. K. Grieshaber (1987). Role of preclinical pharmacology in Phase I clinical trials: considerations of schedule-dependence. In F. M. Muggia (Ed.), Concepts in Cancer Chemotherapy. Martinus Nijhoff, Boston. pp. 129-140.

Collins, J. M., C. K. Grieshaber, and B. A. Chabner (1990). Pharmacologically guided Phase I clinical trials based upon preclinical drug development. J. Nat. Cancer Inst., 82, 1321-1326.

EORTC Pharmacokinetics and Metabolism Group (1987). Pharmacokinetically guided dose escalation in Phase I clinical trials. Commentary and proposed guidelines. Eur. J. Cancer Clin. Oncol., 23, 1083-1087.

Foster, B.J., M. A. Graham, D. R. Newell, L. A. Gumbrell, and A. H. Calvert (1988). Clinical pharmacokinetics of antrapyrazole CL-941 factors compromising the implementation of a pharmacokinetically guided dose escalation scheme. Proc. Amer. Soc. Clin. Oncol., 7, 64.

Gianni, L., L. Vigano, A. Surbone, D. Ballinari, P. Casali, C. Tarella, J. M. Collins, and G. Bonadonna (1990). Pharmacology and clinical toxicity of 4'-iodo-4' deoxydoxorubicin: an example of a successful application of pharmacokinetics to dose escalation in Phase I trials. J. Natl. Cancer Inst., 82, 469-477.

Graham, M. A., D. R. Newell, B. J. Foster, and A. H. Calvert (1989). The pharmacokinetics and toxicity of the anthrapyrazole anti-cancer drug C1-941 in the mouse: a guide for rational dose escalation in patients. Cancer Chemother. Pharmacol., 23, 8-14.

Newell, D. R. (1990). Phase I clinical studies with cytotoxic drugs: pharmacokinetic and pharmacodynamic considerations. Brit. J. Cancer, 61, 189-191.

van Hennik, M.B., W. J. F. van der Vijgh, I. Klein, F. Elferink, J. B. Vermorken, B. Winograd, and H. M. Pinedo (1987). Comparative pharmacokinetics of cisplatin and three analogues in mice and humans. Cancer Res., 47, 6297-6301.

USE OF TOXICOKINETIC PRINCIPLES IN DRUG DEVELOPMENT: BRIDGING PRECLINICAL AND CLINICAL STUDIES

Mauricio Leal, Avraham Yacobi and Vijay K. Batra
Medical Research Division, American Cyanamid Company
Pearl River, N.Y. 10965

ABSTRACT

Toxicokinetics has gained wide acceptance in validating dose related drug exposure in safety evaluation studies. Although exposure is confirmed by measuring blood levels, the concept of comparing safe/toxic blood concentrations in animals to those in man has not been fully realized. Furthermore, in many cases, the frequency of dosing in animal safety studies may not match with that proposed for use in man. Many examples exist demonstrating that the efficacy, safety and toxicity of a drug are influenced by the mode and frequency of drug administration. Although physiological differences between various animal species and man make direct extrapolations to man difficult, new techniques have been proposed which may allow for reasonably good estimates of pharmacokinetic parameters in man. A successful extrapolation would be very useful in planning and expediting early clinical trials. The relationship between safe dosages, pharmacologic-toxicologic activities, and blood levels can guide in selecting early dosages for initial administration to man and in subsequent dosing escalation strategy.

INTRODUCTION

Toxicokinetics is widely utilized in validating dose related drug exposure in animals and ensuring that exposure is greater in animals than that expected in man at therapeutic doses (Barry and Yacobi, 1984; Batra and Yacobi, 1989; de la Iglesia and Greaves, 1989). Regulatory agencies have recognized the usefulness of toxicokinetics and are in strong support of substantiating safety evaluation studies with drug disposition data (Glocklin and Chah, 1989) Today, most pharmaceutical companies have established toxicokinetic programs to document drug exposure in animals during safety evaluation studies.

Integration of Pharmacokinetics, Pharmacodynamics, and Toxicokinetics in Rational Drug Development, Edited by A. Yacobi *et al.*, Plenum Press, New York, 1993

Toxicokinetics may be defined as the application of pharmacokinetic principles to the design, conduct and interpretation of safety evaluation studies. Toxicokinetic data help understand the nature of drug accumulation or possible enzyme induction/inhibition. The scope of toxicokinetics has the potential to evolve from its current state to one that aids in the reliable interpretation of toxicology findings and extrapolation of the resulting data to man (Cambell and Ings, 1988; Hawkins and Chasseaud, 1985; Ings, 1990; Voisin and co-workers, 1990).

This chapter will focus on concepts of toxicokinetics that help in drug development and in bridging preclinical and clinical studies. Examples will be presented to show the use of animal data in the design and dose selection for early phase I clinical trials.

ROUTE OF ADMINISTRATION

The route of drug administration in toxicology studies should mimic that intended for man. If a drug is to be given to man by IV bolus then toxicology studies should also employ the IV bolus route. Toxicity may be related to peak plasma concentrations or to continuous drug exposure over an extended period. For example, a single bolus dose of valproic acid to pregnant mice produced 10 fold greater teratogenicity than when the same mg/kg/day dose was given as a continuous infusion (Nau, 1983). In this case, the effect was probably related to higher peak plasma concentrations after the bolus administration. On the other hand, the teratogenicity of cyanide was greater after continuous and prolonged drug delivery than after a bolus injection (Doherty, Fern and Smith, 1982). In another study, dogs given gentamicin showed a reduction in glomerular filtration rate by 86% after a continuous infusion and by 29% when given by bolus injections every 4 hours (Powell and co-workers, 1983).

FREQUENCY OF DOSING

The frequency of dosing in safety evaluation studies need to mimic that intended for man (US FDA, 1989). Because of physical or practical constraints, however, the frequency of dosing in animal safety evaluation studies may not be identical to that proposed for use in man. Many studies have demonstrated that the efficacy, safety and toxicity of a drug are determined by the route and frequency of drug administration (Nau, 1983; Doherty, Fern and Smith, 1982; Powell and co-workers, 1983; Levy, 1989; Nau, 1991; Boyd and Crinsky, 1970).

One of the earlier examples in this area is from the work of Boyd and Crinsky (1970) who administered 6 g/kg/day of captan to rats by gavage either once daily or twice daily. After two days of treatment, percent mortality was 25% for the twice daily dosing and 10% for the once daily administration.

Hottendorf and coworkers (1976) reported a computer simulation of an aminoglycoside given in one single dose, or as two and three divided doses over 8 hours (Fig. 1). As expected the single dose exhibited the highest peak plasma concentration. The duration of body exposure at a mean plasma level, however, was highest when the drug was given in three divided doses. Thus, depending upon whether toxicity is related to the peak plasma concen-

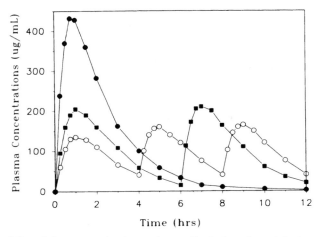

Fig. 1. Computer-simulation of plasma concentration vs. time profiles in dogs after a daily dose of an aminoglycoside given in 3 different regimens. The closed circle (●) represents a single dose of 200 mg/kg, the closed square (■) represents 100 mg/kg given b.i.d., and the open circle (O) represents 67 mg/kg given t.i.d. From Hottendorf and co-workers (1976) Published with permission.

trations or duration of exposure, different dosing regimens may produce different degrees of toxicity.

An experimental case was recently noted with compound A which was given to dogs once daily (Q24H) or as a divided dose given three times a day (every eight hours, Q8H) for one month. The pharmacokinetic data were linear and there was dose proportionality after these regimens. However, the Q8H regimen resulted in greater toxicity than the Q24H regimen. The concentration vs. time profile for compound A suggested that toxicity was not related to the peak plasma concentration but probably to the duration of exposure to plasma concentrations over a given threshold level. To demonstrate this, theoretical threshold plasma concentrations of 0.5 and 1 µg/ml were selected. Dogs given compound A as a Q8H dosing regimen had an exposure time of 50-100% longer than those receiving the Q24H regimen (Table 1). Although the same daily dose was given, comparison of the dosing regimens and their relationship to toxicity maximized the use of the toxicokinetic information for the design of future safety evaluation studies with compound A.

TABLE 1. Exposure Time of Compound A After a Once Daily (Q24H) or Three Times Daily (Q8H) Dosing

Dosing Regimen	Exposure Time (hours) Spent Over	
	0.5 mg/ml	1.0 mg/ml
Q8H	17	9
Q24H	8	6

A clinical dosing regimen is designed to maintain an effective plasma concentration range and to minimize peak to trough fluctuation. In safety evaluation studies, the often used single daily dose regimens produce fluctuations of drug plasma concentrations between very high peak and very low nadir concentrations over most of the dosing interval (Hawkins and Chasseaud, 1985; Nau, 1983; Levy, 1989). In order to avoid extensive drug plasma concentration fluctuations new delivery systems have been introduced to decrease frequency of dosing; such as transdermal devices (scopolamine, nitroglycerin and nicotine), sustained release oral drug delivery systems (theophylline, lithium and procainamide), continuous infusion therapy (bleomycin, doxorubicin and fluorouracil) and osmotic minipumps (valproic acid). Similar drug delivery systems could be used in safety evaluation studies in animals under similar conditions as intended for therapeutic use in man.

SAFETY EVALUATION STUDIES OF METABOLITES

Measuring plasma concentrations of major metabolites in safety evaluation studies may be as important as measuring unchanged drugs (de la Iglesia and Greaves, 1989). Most compounds undergo some degree of metabolism to active or inactive metabolites which may directly or indirectly affect the safety findings. An inactive metabolite may accumulate in the body particularly in patients with impaired renal or hepatic impairment and may exert indirect effects by interacting with other concomitantly administered drugs or with endogenous compounds. Therefore, in safety evaluation studies it would be necessary to document exposure to adequate plasma concentrations of the drug and its major metabolite(s).

An experimental case is the accumulation of a major inactive metabolite of compound B in patients with renal impairment. Compound B is intended for intravenous use (given Q6H) and is excreted in urine unchanged (60-70%) and as an inactive metabolite (20%). During a

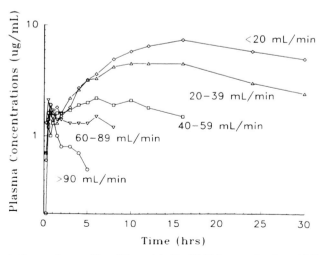

Fig. 2. Plasma concentration vs. time profiles of the metabolite (M-B) in normal and renal failure patients (grouped by creatinine clearance) after a single dose of 375 mg Compound B.

clinical study, the plasma concentration vs. time profiles of the major metabolite (M-B) showed accumulation in patients with low creatinine clearance (Fig. 2).

The clearance of the unchanged drug was proportional to creatinine clearance. A decrease in clearance resulted in a modest accumulation of the drug in plasma. Based on the profile of the unchanged drug, the dosing frequency was adjusted and patients with severe renal failure received a BID treatment. Based on pharmacokinetic analyses of the metabolite data, it was expected that the BID dosing regimen would lead to elevation of M-B concentration in plasma. In the safety evaluation studies the estimated concentrations of the metabolite were very low in both rats and dogs for all doses tested (Table 2). Thus, it was deemed necessary to evaluate the safety of the metabolite by direct administration to animals. Enrollment of renally impaired patients in clinical trials was temporarily postponed until safety was confirmed at high plasma concentrations of the metabolite in animals.

TABLE 2. Comparison of Predicted Peak Plasma Concentrations of Compound B and its Metabolite M-B in Patients with Renal Failure with those Observed in Safety Evaluation Studies in Rats and Dogs after Dosing with Compound B

Species	Dose	C_{max} B (µg/mL)	C_{max} M-B (µg/mL)
MAN	375 mg	40	160
RATS	160 mg/kg	66	7
DOGS	500 mg/kg	2423	27

Using superposition principles, peak plasma concentrations of compound B and M-B were estimated to be 40 and 160 µg/mL, respectively, following a BID regimen in patients. Based on these concentrations and a safety margin of 10-15 fold, the desired peak plasma concentration of M-B in the dog was predicted to be about 2400 µg/ml. Then by conducting a metabolite pharmacokinetic study (where a dose of 66 mg/kg resulted in a peak plasma concentration of 426 µg/mL), the metabolite dose needed was estimated to be 400 mg/kg. This information and the results of the earlier range finding studies with the metabolite, helped in dosing selection for the safety evaluation study in the dog. The metabolite was proven to be safe and the clinical trials in patients with renal impairment resumed successfully.

The experience with compound B demonstrates that testing of the safety of the metabolites needs to be considered. It requires early metabolism work and availability of appropriate bioanalytical methodologies to measure metabolite concentrations in biological fluids. Although not always feasible, early metabolism information in animals in many cases would help reduce the cost and time of the development of a new drug.

EXTRAPOLATION TO MAN

Interspecies scaling is a method of interpolation and extrapolation based on the underlying anatomical, physiological and biochemical similarities in mammals(Mordenti and Chappell, 1989). Interspecies scaling concepts can be incorporated into experimental design and preclinical data analyses, allowing some extrapolation from animal to man (Mordenti and Chappell, 1989). If successful, these extrapolations can help in designing early phase I studies.

Two approaches may be used in extrapolating animal data to man based on interspecies similarities in: a) the physiology; and b) the size (allometry) of the animals. The physiological approach is mechanistic in nature and requires establishing models that are based on anatomical, biochemical and physiological parameters such as blood flow rates, tissues and fluid volumes, protein binding, tissue to blood partition coefficients and enzyme kinetics (Ings, 1990; Mordenti and Chappell, 1989; Chappell and Mordenti, 1991; Gabrielsson, 1991) These models can predict the influence of disease, concomitant medications, age or pregnancy on drug disposition and have been applied and used predictively in environmental toxicology (Gabrielsson, 1991; Paustenback and co-workers, 1988), developmental toxicology (Chappell and Mordenti, 1991; Reitz and co-workers, 1988; Gabrielsson and Larsson, 1987) and in chemotherapy (Ings, 1990; Mordenti and Chappell, 1989). The physiological models, however, have found limited use in drug development due to their complexity, inadequate reliability of data and cost (Ings, 1990).

In contrast to the mechanistic approach, the allometric approach is empirical and does not attempt to give physiological meaning to the pharmacokinetic parameters. However, it is simple and utilizes data which are commonly available during preclinical drug development. Allometric scaling is based upon the principle that physiological variables among species can be related to their body weight. Mathematically the relationship is expressed as follows:

TABLE 3. The Allometric Relationship Between Physiological Variables (Y) and Body Weight (W) in Mammals

Physiological Variables	Relationship
Blood weight (g)	$Y = 0.055\ W^{1.0}$
Liver weight (g)	$Y = 0.082\ W^{0.87}$
Kidney weight (g)	$Y = 0.021\ W^{0.85}$
Cardiac circulation (min)	$Y = 0.44\ W^{0.21}$
Creatinine clearance (ml/hr)	$Y = 8.72\ W^{0.69}$
Inulin clearance (ml/hr)	$Y = 5.36\ W^{0.77}$
Hepatic blood flow (L/min)	$Y = 0.0554\ W^{0.89}$
Heart beat (beat/sec)	$Y = 0.296\ W^{-0.28}$
Respiratory cycle	$Y = 0.169\ W^{-0.28}$

Adapted from Campbell and Ings (1988). Published with permission.

$$Y = A * W^b \qquad\qquad (Eq.\ 1)$$

where Y is the physiological (or pharmacokinetic) variable, A is the allometric coefficient (intercept on the y axis), W is the body weight and b is the allometric exponent (slope) (Campbell and Ings, 1988; Mordenti and Chappell, 1989; Fisher and co-workers, 1989; Mordenti, 1985; Boxenbaum, 1982). Basically, the equation indicates that the value of a physiological variable increases with the size of species when the allometric exponent is positive or decreases with body weight when the allometric exponent is negative. Using the allometric power equation, many anatomical and physiological variables in animals and man can be predicted (Table 3).

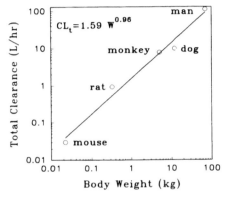

Fig. 3. Allometric relationship between body weight and total clearance of AZT. From Patel and co-workers (1990). Published with permission .

An excellent review of allometry has been provided by Mordenti and Chappel (1989, 1991). In many instances, allometric scaling of pharmacokinetic parameters have proven successful. Most of these examples involve drugs which are highly dependent on: a) renal clearance, such as methotrexate (Ings, 1990; Gabrielsson, 1991; Boxenbaum, 1982), b) hepatic blood flow, such as cyclophosphamide with high hepatic clearance (Boxenbaum, 1982); or c) metabolic clearance by reactions other than the MFO system, such as theophylline (Gaspari and Bonati, 1990). Other recent examples of successful scaling include AZT (Patel and co-workers, 1990) (Fig. 3) and the combination product YP-14 (Komuro and co-workers, 1990).

For compounds which are metabolized by the MFO system and which are low clearance compounds (where elimination is independent of hepatic blood flow), allometric scaling is reliable for most species. The predicted value for man, however, is usually overestimated. For example, for phenytoin and antipyrine the value of the physiological variables depend not only on the body weight but also on brain weight. This modification is based on the principles of evolutionary adaptation associated with neoteny (Boxenbaum, 1982). Relationships were developed to correct for maximum lifespan potential (MLP) by Sacher (1959):

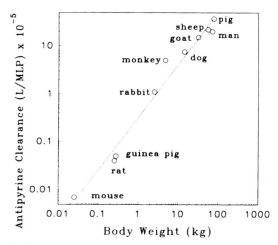

Fig. 4. Allometric relationship between body weight and clearance of antipyrine when corrected for maximum lifespan potential (MLP). From Campbell and Ings (1988). Published with permission.

$$MLP = 10.839 \, (BW)^{0.636} \cdot (B)^{-0.225} \qquad\qquad (Eq.\ 2)$$

and adapted to the allometric equation by Ings (1990) to correct for brain weight:

$$CL = A(BW)^{b} \cdot (B)^{a} \qquad\qquad (Eq.\ 3)$$

where b and a are the allometric exponents (slopes) derived from the scaling relationship between clearance (CL) and brain weight (BW) or clearance and body weight (B), respectively. Values for MLP and brain and body weights for common laboratory animals can be

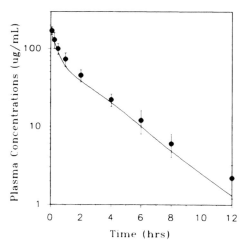

Fig. 5. Comparison of predicted (—, --) and observed (•) concentrations of cefodizime in human plasma. The solid (—) and dashed (- -) lines represent the predicted values with and without correction for protein binding, respectively. From Matsushita and co-workers (1990). Published with permission.

found in a review by Boxenbaum (1982). Normalizing data for MLP brings the clearance of low extraction drugs eliminated by oxidative metabolism in man (such as antipyrine) in line with those from other species (Fig. 4).

Bachmann (1989) attempted to determine half-lives in man using kinetic data acquired from three animal species. Allometric scaling was done on the basis of species weight and maximum lifespan potential. The predicted clearance and volume of distribution were used to determine half-lives. Bachmann (1989) concluded that half-lives could be allometrically estimated with sufficient accuracy and could be adequate predictors in man.

Another factor that can influence the allometric relationship is protein binding. For compounds which exhibit interspecies variability of unbound fraction in plasma, such as ß-lactam antibiotics, plasma protein binding should be considered in scaling (Matsushita and co-workers, 1990; Mordenti, 1986).

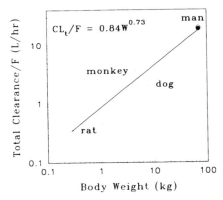

Fig. 6. Allometric scaling of compound A using oral clearance (CL/F) from one month safety evaluation studies in rats, dogs and monkeys. The open circles ○ represent observed values and the closed circle ● represents the predicted value in man.

Matsushita and coworkers (1986) reported the excellent allometric relationship for cefodizime and cefotetan between both renal and hepatic clearance of unbound drug and body weight. As seen in Fig. 5, the predicted concentration vs. time profile of cefodizime in man was closer to the observed profile after correction for protein binding.

An advantage of toxicokinetics is the ability to collect data from safety evaluation studies in which several species are given a wide range of doses over an extended period of time. The predictions made from allometric scaling of toxicokinetic data will be subjected to variability, yielding more realistic estimates. For example, as part of one-month safety evaluation studies for compound A, toxicokinetic parameters were obtained from rats, dogs and monkeys over a wide range of oral doses. The data from the monkey study were subjected to variability, much like what would be expected in early phase I clinical trials. Toxicokinetic parameters were adjusted for dose (in mg) and regressed against body weight on a log-log scale. Oral clearance values from toxicokinetic studies showed good correlation across species and provided a good estimate of the oral clearance in man (Fig. 6).

BRIDGING PRECLINICAL AND CLINICAL

In order to extrapolate animal data to man, it would be preferable to use the concept of safe/toxic plasma concentration range rather than to rely on safe/toxic dose range. Using the relationships proposed by Mordenti and Chappell (1989), equivalent doses between animals and man can be calculated based on allometric scaling of clearance values. For these relationships to be valid, it is important to know whether it is the plasma concentration at steady state or the peak plasma concentration or the area under the plasma concentration vs. time curve that correlate to the therapeutic or toxic effect. If such information is available, allometric extrapolation and derived mathematical relationships can be used to predict doses across species. For example, to determine a dose that would give a particular AUC which is associated with an effect in animals and a clinically relevant effect in man, the following equations can be formulated:

$$AUC_{animal} = \frac{(F_{animal} \cdot D_{animal})}{CL_{animal}} \qquad\qquad (Eq.4)$$

$$AUC_{man} = \frac{(F_{man} \cdot D_{man})}{CL_{man}} \qquad\qquad (Eq.\ 5)$$

where F is bioavailability (fraction of drug reaching systemic circulation unchanged), D is dose (mg/kg), and CL is clearance. To attain equal AUCs in animal and man, Equations 4 and 5 can be simplified to give the following equation:

$$D_{man} = D_{animal} \cdot \frac{(F_{animal})}{(F_{man})} \cdot \frac{(CL_{man})}{(CL_{animal})} \qquad\qquad (Eq.\ 6)$$

The case of Compound A may be used as an example. Safety evaluation studies suggested that a dose of 5 mg/kg/day was associated with a clinically relevant toxicity in monkeys. Allometric scaling of oral clearance values from rats, dogs and monkeys, predicted an oral clearance of 0.3 L/hr/kg for a 70 kg man as compared to the observed value of 0.9 L/hr/kg in monkeys. Based on the completeness of absorption, uniformity and linearity of the toxicokinetic data across species, F in monkeys and man was assumed to be equal. Thus, the dose in man which results in an equal AUC to that after a dose of 5 mg/kg/day in monkeys was calculated by equation 6:

$$D_{man} = 5 mg/kg/day \cdot (1) \cdot \frac{(0.3 L/hr/kg)}{(0.9 L/hr/kg)}$$

The predicted dose in man was, therefore, 1.7 mg/kg/day which was chosen for the multiple dose safety and tolerance clinical trials.

CONCLUSION

Toxicokinetics is gaining continuous acceptance by drug development scientists within the industry and regulatory agencies. By fully extending the basic pharmacokinetic principles to safety evaluation studies, toxicokinetics can aid in the interpretation and extrapolation of animal data to man. The importance of pharmacokinetics in interspecies scaling is one of the primary reasons for conducting early preclinical studies as part of safety evaluation testing (Ings, 1990; Voisin and co-workers, 1990). Extrapolation from animals to man based on dose may not be effective. Better estimates may be obtained from plasma drug concentrations and allometric scaling (Ings, 1990).

It is important that safety evaluation studies reflect the clinical situation. Since toxicity findings may differ between regimens depending on the frequency of dosing, the dosing regimen tested within animals should be consistent with that intended for use in man. Measurement of metabolites should also be considered in animal safety evaluation studies. This can circumvent unexpected delays in drug development time. Furthermore, allometric extrapolation along with the understanding of the relationship between pharmacokinetics and drug effect (pharmacodynamics) can help to bridge preclinical and clinical studies.

ACKNOWLEDGMENT

The authors thank E. Halperin-Walega, D. Ganes, A. Dutta, G. Nicolau, E. Burden, D. Johnson and many other scientists in the Pharmacodynamics and Toxicology Research Sections who contributed to this manuscript and to the presentation.

REFERENCES

Bachmann, K. (1989). Predicting toxicokinetic parameters in humans from toxicokinetic data acquired from three small mammalian species. J. Appl. Toxicol., 9, 331-338.

Barry, H., and A. Yacobi (1984). Preclinical toxicokinetics. In A. Yacobi and H. Barry, III, (Eds.), Experimental and Clinical Toxicokinetics, American Pharmaceutical Association, APS, Washington, DC, pp. 1-7.

Batra, V. K., and A. Yacobi (1989). An overview of toxicokinetics. In A. Yacobi, J. P. Skelly, and V. K. Batra (Eds.), Toxicokinetics and New Drug Development, Pergamon Press, New York, NY, pp. 1-20.

Boxenbaum H. (1982). Interspecies scaling, allometry, physiological time, and the ground plan for pharmacokinetics. J. Pharmacokinet. Biopharm., 10, 201-227.

Boxenbaum, H. (1984). Interspecies pharmacokinetic scaling and the evolutionary-comparative paradigm. Drug Metab. Rev., 15, 1071-1121.

Boyd, E. M., and E. Crinsky (1970). The 100-day LD_{50} index of Captan. Acta Pharmacol. Toxicol., 29, 226-240.

Campbell, D. B., and R. M. J. Ings. (1988) New approaches to the use of pharmacokinetics in toxicology and drug development. Human Toxicol., 7, 469- 479.

Chappell, W. R., and J. Mordenti (1991). Extrapolation of toxicological and pharmacological data from animals to humans. In B. Testa (Ed.), <u>Advances in Drug Research</u>, Academic Press, London. pp. 1-116.

de la Iglesia, F. A., and P. Greaves (1989). Role of toxicokinetics in drug safety evaluations. In A. Yacobi, J. P. Skelly, and V. K. Batra (Eds.), <u>Toxicokinetics and New Drug Development</u>, Pergamon Press, New York. pp. 21- 32.

Doherty, P. A., V. H. Fern, and R. P. Smith (1982). Congenital malformations induced by infusion of cyanide in the golden hamster. <u>Toxicol. Appl. Pharmacol.</u>, <u>64</u>, 456-464.

Fisher, J. W., T. A. Whittaker, D. H. Taylor, H. J. Clewell III, and M. E. Andersen (1989). Physiologically based pharmacokinetic modeling of the pregnant rat: a multiroute exposure model for trichloroethylene and its metabolite, trichloroacetic acid. <u>Toxicol. Appl. Pharmacol.</u>, <u>99</u>, 395-414.

Gabrielsson, J. L. (1991). Utilization of physiologically based models in extrapolating pharmacokinetic data among species. <u>Fund. Appl. Toxicol.</u>, <u>16</u>, 230-232.

Gabrielsson, J. L., and K. S. Larsson (1987). The use of physiological pharmacokinetic models in studies on the disposition of salicylic acid in pregnancy. In H. Nau and W. J. Scott (Eds.), <u>Pharmacokinetics in Teratogenesis</u>, CRC Press, Boca Raton, Florida. pp. 13-26.

Gaspari, F. and M. Bonati (1990). Interspecies metabolism and pharmacokinetic scaling of theophylline disposition. <u>Drug Metab. Rev.</u>, <u>22</u>, 179-207.

Glocklin, V. C., and C. C. Chah (1989). Toxicokinetics in preclinical evaluation of drug safety. In A. Yacobi, J. P. Skelly and V. K. Batra, (Eds.), <u>Toxicokinetics and New Drug Development</u>. Pergamon Press, New York, NY, pp. 33-41.

Hawkins, D. R., and L. F. Chasseaud (1985). Reasons for monitoring kinetics in safety evaluation studies. <u>Arch. Toxicol. Suppl.</u>, <u>8</u>, 165-172.

Hottendorf, G. H., D. R. VanHarken, H. Madissoo, and B. E. Cabana (1976). Pharmacokinetic considerations in toxicology. <u>Proc. Eur. Soc. Toxicol.</u>, <u>17</u>, 255-262.

Ings, R. M. J. (1990). Interspecies scaling and comparisons in drug development and toxicokinetics. <u>Xenobiotica</u>, <u>20</u>, 1201-1231.

Komuro, M., H. Matsushita, T. Maeda, T. Shindo, and Y. Kawaguchi (1990). <u>Pharmacokinetic considerations of YP-14</u>. ISSX, San Diego.

Levy, G. (1989). Some pharmacodynamic aspects of toxicokinetics. In A. Yacobi, J. P. Skelly, and V. K. Batra (Eds.), <u>Toxicokinetics and New Drug Development</u>, Pergamon Press, New York. pp. 97-107.

Matsushita, H., H. Suzuki, Y. Sugiyama, Y. Sawada, T. Iga, M. Hanano, and Y. Kawaguchi (1990). Prediction of the pharmacokinetics of Cefodizime and Cefotetan in humans from pharmacokinetic parameters in animals. <u>J. Pharmacobio. Dyn.</u>, <u>13</u>, 602-611.

Mordenti, J. (1985). Pharmacokinetic scale-up: accurate prediction of human pharmacokinetic profile from animal data. <u>J. Pharm. Sci.</u>, <u>74</u>, 1097-1099.

Mordenti, J. (1986). Man versus beast: pharmacokinetic scaling in mammals. <u>J. Pharm. Sci.</u>, <u>75</u>, 1028-1040.

Mordenti, J., and W. Chappell (1989). The use of interspecies scaling in toxicokinetics. In A. Yacobi, J. P. Skelly and V. K. Batra, (Eds.), <u>Toxicokinetics and New Drug Development</u>, Pergamon Press, New York. pp. 42- 96.

Nau, H. (1983). The role of delivery systems in toxicology and drug development. <u>Pharm. Internat.</u>, <u>4</u>, 228-231.

Nau, H. (1991). Pharmacokinetic considerations in the design and interpretation of developmental toxicity studies. Fund. Appl. Toxicol., 16, 219-221.

Patel, B.A., F. D. Boudinot, R. F. Schinazi, J. M. Gallo, and C. K. Chu (1990). Comparative pharmacokinetics and interspecies scaling of 3'-azido- 3'deoxythymidine (AZT) in several mammalian species. J. Pharmacobio. Dyn., 13, 206-211.

Paustenback, D. J., H. J. Clewell, III, M. L. Gargas, and M. E. Andersen (1988). Physiologically based pharmacokinetic model for inhaled carbon tetrachloride. Toxicol. Appl. Pharmacol., 96, 191-211.

Powell, S. H., W. L. Thompson, M. A. Luthe, R. C. Stern, D. A. Grossniklaus, D. D. Bloxham, D. L. Groden, M. R. Jacobs, A. O. DiScenna, H. A. Cash, and J. D. Klinger (1983). Once daily vs. continuous aminoglycoside dosing: efficacy and toxicity in animal and clinical studies of gentamicin, nethilmicin and tobramycin. J. Infect. Dis., 147, 918-932.

Reitz, R. H., J. N. McDougal, M. W. Himmelstein, R. J. Nolan, and A. M. Shumann (1988). Physiologically based pharmacokinetic modeling with methylchloroform: implications for interspecies, high dose/low dose and dose route extrapolations. Toxicol. Appl. Pharmacol., 95, 185-199.

Sacher, G. A. (1959). Relation of lifespan to brain weight and body weight in mammals. In G. E. W. Wolstenholme, and M. O'Connor (Eds.), Ciba Foundation Colloquia on Aging. Vol. 5., Churchill, London, pp. 115-133.

US FDA, Division of Antiviral Drug Products (1989). Reference guide for the nonclinical toxicity studies of antiviral drugs indicated for the treatment of non-life threatening diseases: evaluation of drug toxicity prior to Phase I clinical studies.

Voisin, E. M., M. Ruthsatz, J. M. Collins, and P. C. Hoyle (1990). Extrapolation of animal toxicity to humans: interspecies comparisons in drug development. Regul. Toxicol. Pharmacol., 12, 107-116.

PRECLINICAL PHARMACODYNAMICS OF CENTRAL NERVOUS SYSTEM ACTIVE AGENTS

M. Danhof, J.W. Mandema and A. Hoogerkamp
Center for Bio-Pharmaceutical Sciences
Division of Pharmacology
University of Leiden, Sylvius Laboratory
P.O. Box 9503, 2300 RA Leiden, The Netherlands

ABSTRACT

In preclinical drug development power spectral analysis of drug induced changes in the electroencephalogram (EEG) is often used to characterize the pharmacological properties of new psychotropic drugs. In this chapter a new approach is proposed for this type of investigations, which allows additional quantitative pharmacodynamic information (i.e. potency, intrinsic efficacy, rate of biophase equilibration) to be derived.

The feasibility of determining concentration-pharmacological effect relationships in individual rats was determined using midazolam as a model drug. The increase in amplitudes in the 12- 30 Hz frequency band of the EEG was used as a pharmacodynamic measure. The results show that the pharmacodynamics of midazolam can be characterized on the basis of the sigmoidal Emax model thus allowing estimation of the pharmacodynamic parameters Emax and EC50.

Subsequent model studies were conducted to determine the relevance of the obtained pharmacodynamic parameter estimates. For a number of full benzodiazepine receptor agonists (flunitrazepam, midazolam, oxazepam and clobazam) significant differences in potency (expressed as EC50) were observed. These differences were found to be closely correlated to differences in their affinity for the benzodiazepine receptor in vitro. In addition a close correlation was observed with values of the pharmacodynamic parameter estimates obtained in the PTZ model of anticonvulsant effect. For benzodiazepine receptor ligands which differ in intrinsic efficacy (midazolam, bretazenil, flumazenil and Ro 19-4603) significant differences in Emax were observed, which were in agreement with the known differences between these compounds in other test systems.

Integration of Pharmacokinetics, Pharmacodynamics, and Toxicokinetics in Rational Drug Development, Edited by A. Yacobi *et al.*, Plenum Press, New York, 1993

The pharmacodynamics of baclofen were determined using the decrease in amplitudes in the 12-30 Hz frequency band as a pharmacodynamic measure. For the enantiomers, marked differences in pharmacodynamic parameter estimates were observed. However the rate of biophase equilibration was quite similar with a half-life of approximately 30 minutes.

In conclusion, by the proposed alternative procedure for pre-clinical pharmaco-EEG studies, relevant quantitative pharmacodynamic information on new psychotropic drugs can be obtained. It is suggested that the availability of this type of information may be of value in the early phases of drug development and may facilitate the subsequent clinical development process.

INTRODUCTION

The purpose of preclinical pharmacodynamic investigations is to obtain information on the pharmacological properties of new chemical entities, usually on the basis of data obtained in a variety of different pharmacological test systems both in vivo and in vitro. Generally the emphasis in this type of investigations is on determining the nature of the pharmacological actions of these compounds and much less on obtaining quantitative pharmacodynamic information such as the potency and the intrinsic efficacy or the rate of biophase equilibration. Availability of the latter type of information may be of great value however in the early development process and in the selection of compounds for further clinical development. In addition if pharmacodynamic parameter estimates obtained in an animal model would have predictive value with regard to the human situation, this information may be expected to facilitate greatly the design of phase 1-3 clinical trial protocols and thus the clinical develop-ment process. It appears important therefore to explore the feasibility of obtaining relevant quantitative pharmacodynamic parameter estimates in preclinical pharmacodynamic studies and to determine their predictive value with regard to the situation in man.

For CNS active drugs, quantitative EEG monitoring is often used to characterize and classify the pharmacodynamic properties of new compounds with psychotropic action (Itil, 1974a, 1974b, 1981; Itil et al., 1982; Herrmann, 1982). In this type of investigations generally no drug concentrations are determined and consequently no quantitative pharmacodynamic information is obtained. Recently however a chronically instrumented rat model was devel-oped which allows simultaneous monitoring of the EEG effect (through permanently im-planted cortical electrodes) in conjunction with arterial blood concentrations (through a permanently implanted cannula in the femoral artery) in conscious rats. (Mandema and Danhof, 1990; Ebling et al., 1991). Utilizing this technique it is possible to obtain, following the administration of a single intravenous dose, data sets that can be subjected to simultaneous pharmacokinetic-pharmacodynamic modelling and thus be used to obtain information on for example the potency and intrinsic efficacy and the rate of biophase equilibration. In this chapter the technical aspects of this approach will be discussed on the basis of model studies with benzodiazepines and baclofen. In addition potential applications with regard to pharma-codynamic drug-drug and drug-ethanol interactions and the characterization of the rate and extent of functional tolerance development will be discussed.

PHARMACOKINETIC-PHARMACODYNAMIC MODELLING OF THE EEG EFFECT OF MIDAZOLAM

In order to determine the feasibility to derive quantitative pharmacodynamic parameter estimates of benzodiazepines in the chronically instrumented rat model, the pharmacokinetics and pharmacodynamics of midazolam were studied (Mandema et al., 1991a). The plasma concentration and the EEG effect versus time profile were determined following intravenous administration of 10 mg/kg in 5 minutes. The characteristic changes in the EEG in this experiment are shown in Figure 1. In this figure the upper trace shows the baseline EEG pattern. As the concentration of midazolam increases during the intravenous infusion, initially an increase in the high frequency (beta) activity of the EEG is observed (trace 2), which is followed by an increase in the slow wave (delta) activity (trace 3) at higher concentrations.

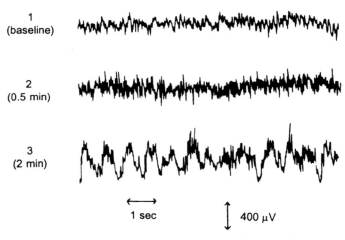

Fig. 1. Characteristic EEG changes observed during intravenous administration of 10 mg/kg of midazolam in 5 minutes. Trace 1 represents the baseline EEG pattern. As the concentration of midazolam increases first an increase in high frequency (beta) activity is observed (trace 2; 0.5 min after the start of the infusion), followed by an increase in the slow wave (delta) activity at higher concentrations of the drug (trace 3; 2 minutes after the start of the infusion). (From: Mandema et al., 1991a).

Of these characteristic changes in the EEG pattern the change in amplitudes in the high frequency range (11.5-30 Hz) was determined by aperiodic analysis [Gregory and Pettus, 1986] and used as the pharmacological effect parameter. The time course of the concentrations of midazolam in plasma and of the pharmacological effect in one individual rat is given in Figure 2.

No measurable delay (hysteresis) between the plasma concentration and the EEG effect was observed and the two were therefore directly correlated to each other. Figure 3 shows the derived concentration effect relationship of the same rat as presented in Figure 2. It shows that the pharmacodynamics can be satisfactorily characterized on the basis of the sigmoidal Emax model. The average pharmacodynamic parameter estimates of midazolam were Emax = 92 ± 5 μV/s, EC50 = 38 ± 4 ng/ml and Hill factor 0.76 ± 0.08. By examination of the influence

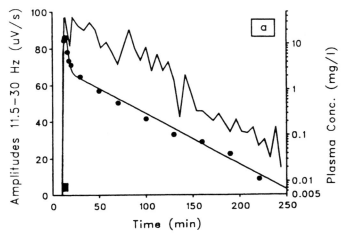

Fig. 2. Midazolam plasma concentration ● and EEG effect (change in amplitude in the 12-30 Hz frequency band) versus time profiles in an individual rat following intravenous administration of 10 mg/kg of midazolam in 5 minutes. (Mandema et al., 1991a)

of rate and route of administration it could be demonstrated that the parameter estimates are indeed unique and not confounded by the presence of interactive metabolites and/or the development of acute functional tolerance during the experiments. The results of this study demonstrate therefore the feasibility of obtaining quantitative pharmacodynamic parameter estimates in individual rats following the administration of a single dose of midazolam.

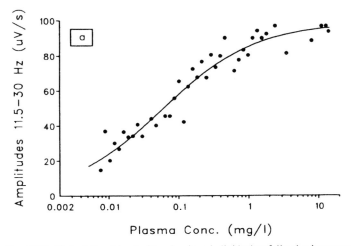

Fig. 3. Concentration-EEG effect relationship of midazolam in an individual rat following intravenous administration of 10 mg/kg in 5 minutes. The solid line represents the best fit of the actual data points according to the sigmoidal Emax pharmacodynamic model (Mandema et al., 1991a).

72

PHARMACODYNAMICS OF BENZODIAZEPINE RECEPTOR LIGANDS: FULL AGONISTS, PARTIAL AGONISTS AND INVERSE AGONISTS

From the foregoing it appears that the EEG effect of midazolam and therefore probably of benzodiazepines in general, fulfills many of the requirements of an ideal pharmacodynamic measure in that it provides a continuous, sensitive, reproducible and objective quantification of the effect on the central nervous system. However the relevance of the EEG parameter is yet unclear and needs to be validated. The mechanism of action of benzodiazepines is well described and involves the interaction with the specific GABA-benzodiazepine receptor complex (Haefely et al., 1985; Haefely, 1989). It has been demonstrated that different drugs can differ widely in their affinity to and intrinsic efficacy at this receptor complex (Haefely, 1989; Villar et al., 1989). An important question is now whether EEG effect parameters can indeed reflect such differences in affinity and intrinsic activity. Therefore the pharmacodynamics of different benzodiazepines were studied. Initially four benzodiazepines were studied which are known to be full agonists but which differ widely in their affinity for the benzodiazepine receptor: flunitrazepam, midazolam, oxazepam and clobazam. For each of these drugs the pharmacodynamics were studied following the administration of a single intravenous dose. It was found that the concentration EEG effect relationships could in each case be described satisfactorily by the sigmoidal Emax pharmacodynamic model (Figure 4). The average Emax values of these 4 different compounds were similar, although the value for flunitrazepam was slightly higher than for the other 3 drugs. The average EC50 values based on total drug concentration however showed a highly significant difference between all drugs and ranged from 26 ± 3 ng/ml for flunitrazepam to 859 ± 98 mg/ml for clobazam (Table 1). Correction of the EC50 value for protein binding in individual rats (resulting in the unbound value

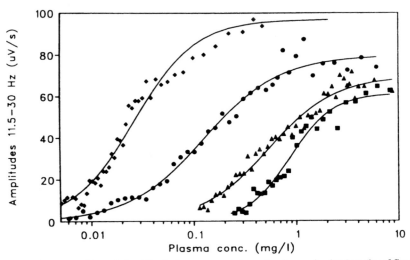

Fig. 4. Concentration EEG effect relationships in four representative rats who received 2.5 mg/kg of flunitrazepam ♦, 5 mg/kg of midazolam ●, 10 mg/kg of oxazepam ▲, or 20 mg/kg of clobazam ■, as an intravenous bolus injection. The solid lines represent the best fits to the data points according to the sigmoidal Emax model (Mandema et al., 1991b).

Table 1. Comparison of the potency estimates (EC50 values) derived from the EEG model and the Pentylenetetrazol (PTZ) threshold model, a model to measure the anticonvulsant activity of benzodiazepines (Mandema et al., 1991b)

	EEG model	PTZ model	EEG/PTZ
Flunitrazepam	26 ± 3	51 ± 18	0.51
Midazolam	105 ± 10	158 ± 35	0.66
Oxazepam	559 ± 37	708 ± 133	0.79
Clobazam	859 ± 98	1113 ± 240	0.77

EC50,u) gave values for which no significant difference between flunitrazepam and midazolam could be detected (Table 2).

In order to assess the relevance of the obtained parameter estimates a comparison was made with the receptor binding characteristics in vitro and with pharmacodynamic parameter estimates obtained in the pentylenetetrazol (PTZ) model of anticonvulsant effect. In this respect it is important that the PTZ seizure model has been widely used as a sensitive measure to compare the relative activity of anticonvulsants (Nutt et al., 1986) and to screen for benzodiazepine like activity which is mediated by the interaction at the GABA benzodiazepine receptor complex (Haefely et al., 1981). The results of the comparative studies are summarized in Table 1 and Table 2, respectively.

The values in Table 2 indicate that affinity to the benzodiazepine receptors is the highest for midazolam and flunitrazepam, while oxazepam and clobazam show a much lower affinity. Furthermore it appears that there is a close correlation between the potency of the four benzodiazepines in the EEG model and their affinity for the receptor, as is reflected by the constant ratio of EC50,u and Ki, ranging from 0.6 to 0.8. The values in Table 1 indicate that there are also wide differences in the potency of the four benzodiazepines in the pentylenetetrazol threshold model of anticonvulsant effect. Again a close correlation between the EC50 values in both models was observed. Thus it can be concluded that on the basis of the EEG model realistic estimates of the potency of different benzodiazepines can be obtained, which reflect differences in affinity to the central GABA-benzodiazepine receptor complex.

Table 2. Comparison of the potency estimates (EC50,u) determined on basis of EEG activity and benzodiazepine receptor affinity (Ki) of 4 benzodiazepines (Mandema et al., 1991b)

	EC50,u (ng/ml)	Ki (ng/ml)	EC50,u/Ki
Midazolam	3.7 ± 0.5	4.9 ± 0.5	0.76
Flunitrazepam	4.2 ± 0.7	7.0 ± 0.5	0.60
Oxazepam	49 ± 4	86 ± 15	0.57
Clobazam	277 ± 34	350 ± 61	0.79

In order to determine whether EEG effect parameters can also be used to determine differences in intrinsic efficacy at the benzodiazepine receptor, the concentration EEG effect relationships of a full benzodiazepine agonist (midazolam), a partial agonist (bretazenil), a competitive antagonist (flumazenil) and an inverse agonist (Ro 19-4603) were determined in a comparative study. The observed concentration effect relationships are shown in Figure 5. Apart from differences in EC50, especially important differences in Emax were observed. Compared to midazolam the values of the relative intrinsic efficacy of bretazenil was 0.26, whereas the intrinsic efficacy of flumazenil in a relevant concentration range was found not to be significantly different from zero and for Ro 19-4603 a negative value was observed. This agrees well with the known pharmacological properties of these compounds (Mandema et al., 1992a).

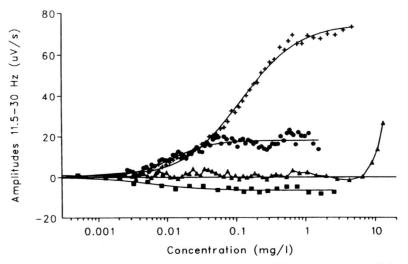

Fig. 5. Averaged concentration EEG effect relationships in rats obtained following intravenous administration of 5 mg/kg of midazolam (+), 2.5 mg/kg of bretazenil ●, 10 mg/kg of flumazenil ▲ and 2.5 mg/kg of Ro 19-4603 ■ (Mandema et al., 1992a).

Thus, in summary, it can be concluded that on the basis of the new approach of quantitative pharmaco EEG studies, relevant quantitative pharmacodynamic parameter estimates on benzodiazepines can be obtained which reflect differences in affinity and intrinsic efficacy at the central GABA-benzodiazepine receptor complex.

PHARMACOKINETICS-PHARMACODYNAMICS OF BACLOFEN ENANTIOMERS

Baclofen is a gamma-amino-butyric acid (GABA) derivative which has been shown to selectivity interact with a specific class of GABA receptors (the GABA-b receptor) and which is used clinically in the treatment of spasticity (Faigle, 1980; Bowery, 1982). Because of the fact that its site of action is located in the brain, baclofen has to cross the blood-brain barrier before exerting its pharmacological action. The transport of baclofen into the central nervous system has been shown to be relatively slow, presumably as result of the fact that the drug has the physicochemical properties of a zwitter-ion at physiological conditions and possesses only a moderate lipophilicity. In addition baclofen is a chiral compound and its enantiomers have been demonstrated to possess different pharmacological properties with the R-enantiomer exhibiting a much more profound muscle relaxant effect than the S-enantiomer. With baclofen quantitative pharmaco-EEG studies were performed to determine the feasibility of characterizing the pharmacodynamic properties of the individual enantiomers. In addition special attention was given to the characterization of the kinetics of equilibration with the site of action (Mandema et al., 1992c).

The pharmacodynamics of baclofen were determined following intravenous administration of the separate enantiomers as well as the racemate and the decrease of the amplitudes in the 12- 30 Hz frequency band of the EEG was used as measure of the pharmacological response. The time course of the plasma concentration and the pharmacological response following administration of the R-enantiomer is given in Figure 6.

A profound delay between the plasma concentrations and the EEG effect was observed and therefore simultaneous pharmacokinetic-pharmacodynamic modelling on the basis of postulation of an effect compartment was necessary to derive time independent pharmacodynamic parameter estimates. The pharmacodynamics of the R-enantiomer could be described on the basis of the sigmoidal Emax pharmacodynamic model. The values of the pharmacodynamic parameter estimates were: Emax = 20 ± 2 μV/s, EC50 = 0.61 ± 0.11 mg/L and N = 3.7 ± 0.7. For the R-enantiomer only modest EEG changes were observed which were best characterized on the basis of a linear pharmacodynamic model. Thus important differences in the potency of the enantiomers of baclofen were observed in the quantitative EEG model which appear to reflect the known differences in clinical efficacy. The equilibration delay between plasmaconcentrations and EEG effect was best modelled by a mono-exponential conductance function (Veng-Pedersen et al., 1991). No differences were observed with respect to the rate of equilibration between plasma concentration and EEG effect for racemic, R- and S-baclofen, with values of the time to reach 50% equilibrium of 23 ± 4 min, 35 ± 6 min and 32 ± 7 min, respectively.

Recently it has been suggested that on basis of the monitoring of cerebrospinal fluid concentrations of drugs in conjunction with plasma concentrations, the blood-brain barrier transport characteristics of drugs can be determined utilizing the technique of numerical deconvolution(Van Bree et al., 1989).

Therefore a comparison was made with the rate of equilibration of baclofen between plasma and cerebrospinal fluid (Van Bree et al., 1991). The results of this comparison show that the rate of equilibration of baclofen with the site of action is considerably slower than with the cerebrospinal fluid compartment and that, therefore, cerebrospinal fluid concentrations do not accurately reflect concentrations at the site of action. Thus on basis of simultaneous pharmacokinetic-pharmacodynamic modelling some unique information with regard to the rate of biophase equilibration of drugs can be obtained, that can not be derived on the basis of more traditional pharmacokinetic approaches.

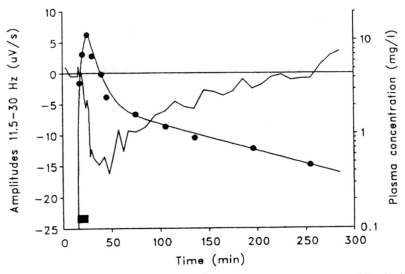

Fig. 6. Time course of the plasma concentrations ● and the EEG effect for an individual rat following intravenous administration of 0.63 mg of R-Baclofen. A bi-exponential function was fitted through the plasma concentrations. The solid bar represents the duration of the infusion (Mandema et al., 1992c)

CONCLUSIONS AND PERSPECTIVES

The purpose of the investigations described in this paper was to determine the feasibility to determine relevant pharmacodynamic parameter estimates of psychotropic drugs in pre-clinical pharmacodynamic investigations in small laboratory animals. Quantitative EEG monitoring was used as a model in this respect. The results of the investigations with midazolam demonstrate the utility of a chronically instrumented rat model in obtaining quantitative pharmacodynamic parameter estimates in individual rats. The findings with the different benzodiazepines confirm that on the basis of the EEG, indeed relevant pharmacody-namic information (potency, intrinsic efficacy) is obtained. In addition the studies with baclofen demonstrate the feasibility of obtaining estimates of the rate of biophase equilibra-tion of different drugs. An important question is now how this type of information can be used in the drug development process. In the preclinical phase a potential application is in the area of the selection of drugs for further development. Potency and intrinsic efficacy of different analogues can in principle be an important selection criterion. This also holds for the rate of biophase equilibration, which is especially relevant for drugs acting on the central nervous system due to the presence of the blood-brain barrier. In many instances preference is given to drugs which cross the blood-brain barrier relatively easily. The findings with baclofen show that the rate of equilibration with the biophase may be quite different from the rate of equilibration with the cerebrospinal fluid compartment. This indicates that it may be difficult to obtain relevant information with regard to the kinetics of biophase equilibration on the basis of traditional pharmacokinetic techniques (i.e. determination of concentration profiles in brain tissue or cerebrospinal fluid) and that the application of simultaneous pharmacokinetic/phar-macodynamic modelling concepts may offer distinct advantages. An important criterion in the selection of drugs for further development is also the selectivity of the effects with regard to different organs. In this respect it should be realized that this selectivity is not only dependent on pharmacodynamic factors (i.e. selectivity in binding to certain receptor types) but that pharmacokinetic factors (i.e. drug distribution) can also play an important role. Therefore integrated pharmacokinetic-pharmacodynamic studies may be expected to yield valuable information with regard to the selectivity of drug effects on different organ systems. Currently this approach is applied for purinergic drugs where the selectivity of the effects on the cardiovascular system versus the central nervous system is under investigation (Mathôt, Ijzerman and Danhof, unpublished observations). Recently, studies have been carried out on the pharmacodynamic interactions between different benzodiazepine analogues (Mandema et al., 1992b), and these investigations are currently extended to the pharmacodynamic interactions with ethanol (Hoyo-Vadillo, Mandema and Danhof, unpublished observations). It is believed that especially early determination of the quantitative aspects of the pharmacodynamic interactions with ethanol may be an important selection criterion in the development process of CNS active drugs. Finally, pharmacodynamic models have been developed which allow assessment of both the rate and extent of functional tolerance development (Sheiner, 1989). This type of methodology can easily be transferred to studies in small laboratory animals and thus information on quantitative aspects of functional tolerance development of different drug analogues can in principle also be obtained early in the preclinical development phase. Application of these techniques is currently being examined for midazolam and other benzodiazepines (Mandema, Hoogerkamp and Danhof, unpublished observations).

From the foregoing it appears that by application of pharmacokinetic-pharmacodynamic modelling, information can be obtained on different drug analogues which can be of value in the selection of compounds for further clinical development. Another interesting question is whether the values of the parameter estimates obtained in animal models have predictive value with regard to the values in humans. Thus far very little information is available in this respect. However preliminary findings suggest that at least for the benzodiazepines and anticonvulsants pharmacodynamic parameter estimates have quite similar values in laboratory animals and in humans (Mandema et al., 1992d). If future investigations would reveal that pharmacodynamic parameter estimates of CNS active drugs obtained in small laboratory animals do indeed have similar values in man, this could facilitate greatly the clinical development process (for example dose finding) in humans. Also this would facilitate the design of other clinical studies in phases 1-3, like for example drug interaction studies.

ACKNOWLEDGMENTS

The investigations described in this paper were supported by the Netherlands Medical and Health Research Foundation (MEDIGON, grant 900-521-106). The benzodiazepines used in the investigations were donated by Hoffmann La Roche, Basle, Switzerland; Wyeth Laboratories, Hoofddorp, The Netherlands and Hoechst Pharma, Amsterdam, The Netherlands. Racemic baclofen and the R- and S- enantiomers were a gift from Ciba-Geigy, Basle, Switzerland.

REFERENCES

Bowery, N. G. (1982). Baclofen: 10 years on. Trends Pharmacol.Sci.Oct, 400- 403.

Ebling, W. F., M. Danhof, and D. R. Stanski (1991). Pharmacodynamic modeling of the electroencephalographic effects of thiopental in rats. J. Pharmacokinet. Biopharm., 19, 123-143.

Faigle, J. W., H. Keberle, and P. H. Degen (1980). Chemistry and pharmacokinetics of baclophen. In R. G. Feldman, R. R. Young, and W. P. Koella (Eds.), Spasticity: Disordered Motor Control. Year Book Medical Publishers, Chicago, pp 461-475.

Gregory, T.K. and D. C. Pettus (1986). An electroencephalographic processing algorithm specifically intended for analysis of cerebral activity. J. Clin. Monit. 2, 190-197.

Haefely, W., (1989). Pharmacology of the benzodiazepine receptor. Eur. Arch. Psychiatr. Neurol. Sci.238, 294-301.

Haefely, W., E. Kyburz, M. Gerecke, and H. Mohler (1985). Recent advances in the molecular pharmacology of benzodiazepine receptors and in the structure activity relationships of their agonists and antagonists. Adv. Drug Res.14, 165-322.

Haefely, W., L. Pieri, P. Polc, and R. Schaffner (1981). General pharmacology and neuro-pharmacology of benzodiazepine derivatives. In F. Hoffmeister and G. Stille (Eds.), Handbook of Experimental Pharmacology. Vol. 55/II Springer, Berlin, pp 13-262.

Herrmann, W. M. (1982). Development and critical evaluation of an objective procedure for the electroencephalographic classification of psychotropic drugs. In W. M. Herrmann (Ed.), Electroencephalography in Drug Research Gustav Fisher Verlag, Stuttgart, pp. 249-351.

Itil, T. M. (1974a). Digital computer analyzed EEG in psychiatry and psychopharmacology. In G. Dolce and H. Kunkel (Eds.), CEAN Computerized EEG Analysis Gustav Fischer Verlag, Stuttgart, pp. 289-308.

Itil, T. M. (1974b). Quantitative pharmaco-electroencephalography. Use of computerized cerebral biopotentials in psychotropic drugs. In T. M. Itil, (Ed.), Modern Problems in Pharmacopsychiatry. Vol. 8: Psychotropic Drugs and the Human EEG Karger, Basel, pp. 43-75.

Itil, T. M. (1981). The discovery of psychotropic drugs by computer- analyzed cerebral bioelecric potentials (CEEG). Drug Development Research, 1, 373-407.

Itil, T. M., G. N. Menoh and K. Z. Itil (1982). Computer EEG drug data base in psychophar-macology and in drug development. Psychopharmacol. Bull., 18, 165-172.

Mandema, J. W., and M. Danhof (1990). Pharmacokinetic-pharmacodynamic modelling of the CNS effects of heptabarbital using aperiodic EEG analysis. J. Pharmacokinet. Biopharm., 18, 459-481.

Mandema, J. W., Tukker, E., and M. Danhof (1991a). Pharmacokinetic- pharmacodynamic modeling of the EEG effects of midazolam in individual rats: influence of rate and route of administration. Br. J. Pharmacol., 102, 663- 668.

Mandema, J. W., L. N. Sansom, M. M. C. Dios-Vietez, M. Hollander-Jansen, and M. Danhof (1991b). Pharmacokinetic-pharmacodynamic modelling of the electroencephalographic effects of benzodiazepines. Correlation with receptor binding and anticonvulsant activity. J. Pharmacol. Exp. Ther., 257, 472-478.

Mandema, J. W., M. T. Kuck, and M. Danhof (1992a). Differences in intrinsic efficacy of benzodiazepines are reflected in their concentration-EEG effect relationships. Br. J. Pharmacol, 105, 164-170.

Mandema, J. W., E. Tukker, and M. Danhof (1992b). In vivo characterization of the pharmacodynamic interaction of a benzodiazepine agonist and antagonist: midazolam and flumazenil. J. Pharmacol.Exp. Ther., 261, 56-61

Mandema, J. W., C. D. Heijligers-Feijen, E. Tukker, A. G. de Boer, and M. Danhof (1992c). Modeling of the effect site equilibration kinetics and pharmacodynamics of racemic baclofen and its enantiomers using quantitative EEG measures. J. Pharmacol Exp. Ther., 261, 88-95.

Mandema, J. W., B. Tuk, A. L. van Steveninck, D. D. Breimer, A. F. Cohen, and M. Danhof (1992d). Pharmacokinetic-pharmacodynamic modelling of the CNS effects of midazolam and its main metabolite alpha-hydroxymidazolam in healthy volunteers. Clin. Pharmacol Ther., 51, 715-728.

Nutt, D. J., S. C. Taylor, and H. J. Little (1986). Optimizing the pentetrazol infusion test for seizure threshold measurement. J. Pharm. Pharmacol., 38, 697-698.

Sheiner, L. B. (1989). Clinical pharmacology and the choice between theory and empiricism. Clin. Pharmacol. Ther., 46, 605-615.

Van Bree, J. B. M. M., A. V. Baljet, A. Van Geyt, A. G. de Boer, M. Danhof, and D. D. Breimer (1989). The unit impulse response theory for the pharmacokinetic evaluation of drug entry into the central nervous system. J. Pharmacokinet. Biopharm., 17, 441-462.

Van Bree, J. B. M. M., C. Heijligers-Feijen, A. G. de Boer, M. Danhof, and D. D. Breimer (1991). Stereoselective transport of baclofen across the blood-brain barrier in rats as determined by the unit impulse response methodology. Pharm. Res., 8, 259-262.

Veng-Pedersen, P., J. W. Mandema, and M. Danhof (1991). A system approach to pharmacodynamics III: an algorithm and computer program "COLAPS" for pharmacodynamic modelling. J. Pharm. Sci., 80, 488-495.

Villar, H. O., E. T. Uyeno, L. Toll, W. Polgar, M. F. Davies, and G. H. Loew (1989). Molecular determinants of benzodiazepine receptor affinities and anticonvulsant activities. Mol. Pharmacol., 36, 589-600.

PRECLINICAL PHARMACODYNAMICS OF ANTIHYPERTENSIVES

Robert A. Branch and Edwin K. Jackson
Center for Clinical Pharmacology
University of Pittsburgh Medical Center
Pittsburgh, PA 15261

OBJECTIVES OF RESEARCH IN THE ANTIHYPERTENSIVE AREA (A SPECULATIVE LOOK OVER THE HORIZON)

The objective of research in the antihypertensive area, and therefore the objective of preclinical studies with potential antihypertensive drugs, is to identify therapeutic entities with: increased efficacy, decreased toxicity, increased ease and convenience of administration, an improved profile on metabolic, hemodynamic and cellular parameters, and defined and unique mechanisms of action.

Increased efficacy may be defined as a higher percentage of patients responding with a specified fall in arterial blood pressure ("broad-spectrum" antihypertensives), as a greater decline in arterial blood pressure in an easily identifiable subgroup (targeted therapy), or as an improved clinical outcome (reduction in overall morbidity and mortality). Importantly, the latter definition of efficacy blurs the distinction between increased efficacy and decreased toxicity in as much as improved clinical outcome depends as much on the absence of adverse drug effects as it does on the blood pressure lowering ability of a given antihypertensive drug.

Regarding decreased toxicity, in a pragmatic sense the toxicity of antihypertensive drugs defines hypertension. For the practicing physician, the useful definition of hypertension is what level of arterial blood pressure warrants therapeutic intervention, not what level of arterial blood pressure is optimal for the patient. Pressure-induced damage to the cardiovascular system occurs at levels of arterial blood pressure far below 140/90 mmHg. In fact, the optimal level of systolic blood pressure may be under 110 mmHg (Stamler, 1991), and only 6 % of men over 35 years old have such readings (Stamler, 1991). Unfortunately, because of the unwanted effects of antihypertensive drugs (a risk factor that can be improved through development of new antihypertensive drugs) the fixed benefit of lowering arterial blood pressure may be more than offset by the adverse effects caused by drug therapy. However, as

Integration of Pharmacokinetics, Pharmacodynamics, and Toxicokinetics in Rational Drug Development, Edited by A. Yacobi *et al.*, Plenum Press, New York, 1993

81

the toxicity of therapy decreases, benefits of "antihypertensive" therapy may extend to patients with "high-normal" or even "normal" arterial blood pressure. Therefore, it is not inconceivable that the discovery of safer antihypertensive drugs will actually redefine hypertension such that a majority of individuals over the age of 35 will be considered hypertensive.

The inconvenience of taking medication daily for a lifetime and the likelihood that doses will be skipped due to financial pressures and/or simple forgetfulness leads to patient noncompliance. Therefore, another extremely important parameter that has a major impact on the success or failure of antihypertensive therapy is the convenience and ease of drug administration.

In this regard, once-a-day oral therapy is the current gold standard; however, it is possible that oral therapy eventually will be supplanted by constant delivery systems such as transdermal patches or subcutaneous implants. The ultimate, of course, would be a one-shot cure. Although the notion that hypertension could be "cured" may seem far-fetched, this goal theoretically could be achieved via vaccination or gene therapy. Immunization against renin has been suggested as a possible vaccination against high blood pressure (Bouhnik and co-workers, 1987), and gene therapy with a mutated angiotensinogen gene has been proposed as a conceivable strategy for gene therapy of hypertension (Jackson, 1992). Creativity in the area of strategies for a permanent cure for hypertension and advances in constant-rate, long-term delivery systems for antihypertensive drugs may revolutionize therapy for high blood pressure.

Although reduction of arterial blood pressure is the short-term goal of therapy, the long-term objective is to decrease morbidity and mortality. The optimization of this objective will be achieved only with drugs that do not adversely alter metabolic parameters (serum cholesterol, triglycerides, glucose, uric acid and potassium) (Maxwell, 1988), that cause regression of cardiac (Weinberger, 1990) and vascular smooth muscle hypertrophy (Adams, Bobik and Korner, 1990) and that reduce glomerular capillary hydrostatic pressure (Anderson, Rennke and Brenner, 1986). Again, progress in this area will cause an ever increasing percentage of the population to be redefined as hypertensive. Ultimately, antihypertensives may be developed that are not only neutral with respect to metabolic parameters, but also improve other risk factors for cardiovascular disease (antiplatelet drugs, antiatherosclerotic drugs, anti-sudden death drugs). The long-term evolution of cardiovascular drug therapy may be away from therapy for arbitrarily defined cut-offs of various risk factors. Instead, molecular entities that optimize a battery of cardiovascular risk factors may be the focus for future generations of pharmacologists.

One objective of antihypertensive therapy is to match pathophysiological mechanism with therapeutic approach. Almost all hypertensionologists accept the thesis that there exist many subgroups of essential hypertensives with different mechanisms causing blood pressure to be elevated. Therefore, such individualization of drug therapy can only be achieved when the various subtypes of hypertension have been elucidated. In this regard, discovery of new antihypertensive agents that have well-defined and unique mechanisms of action participates in a positive feedback loop of ever increasing knowledge. This positive feedback loop begins with studies on the mechanism of action of new therapeutic entities. Definition of the mechanism of action then provides a new pharmacological tool that aids in the elucidation of the pathophysiology of hypertension. This new information regarding the pathophysiology of hypertension in turn provides impetus to develop new classes of antihypertensives. Investigations on the mechanism of action of these new agents completes the postive feedback loop and the cycle continues.

An illustrative example of this positive feedback loop is the sequence of events that followed the serendipitous discovery of the antihypertensive activity of beta-adrenoceptor blockers. Research on the antihypertensive mechanisms of beta-blockers provided support for the hypothesis that excess renin release participates in some forms of essential hypertension (Buhler and co-workers, 1972). This information contributed greatly to the enthusiasm to identify new ways to block the renin- angiotensin system, and these efforts resulted in the discovery of peptidic angiotensin receptor blockers and converting enzyme inhibitors, both of which contributed greatly to our understanding of the role of the renin-angiotensin system in various types of hypertension. Research with converting enzyme inhibitors revealed a possible role for angiotensin II not only in high-renin hypertension, but also in normal-renin hypertension (Antonaccio, Rubin and Horovitz, 1979; Laragh, 1978). The hypothesis that angiotensin II has broad significance in the pathophysiology of hypertension fueled additional research to find ways to block the renin-angiotensin system. This research recently culminated in the discovery of nonpeptide angiotensin receptor antagonists (Timmermans and co-workers, 1990) and continues to motivate research directed towards developing orally active renin inhibitors with desirable pharmacokinetic profiles (Haber and Hui, 1990). Due to the development of nonpeptide angiotensin receptor blockers and renin inhibitors, we are now postured as never before to define precisely the role of the renin-angiotensin system in various types of experimental and clinical hypertension.

METHODS FOR PRECLINICAL STUDIES: SELECTING THE SPECIES

Although any new antihypertensive drug should be investigated in several species before attempting studies in man, the rat remains the cornerstone of antihypertensive drug development for several reasons. First, the rat provides a range of pathophysiological models that are not readily available in other species. An extensive literature is published on numerous rat models of hypertension including various strains of genetically hypertensive rats, as well as several types of surgically-induced hypertension. Therefore, using the rat, a given drug can be studied in a wide array of pathophysiological settings in well-described and reproducible models.

In addition to the advantage of having a range of pathophysiological models, the monetary costs associated with experimentation in the rat is low compared to most other alternatives. The rat is inexpensive to purchase, house, and maintain. In addition, the facilities to conduct both acute and chronic studies in the rat are generally less expensive compared to what is needed for experimentation on other species. Thus, a broader range of studies can be conducted on a limited research budget. This is particularly important in the early phases of drug development and while screening hypotheses concerning the mechanism of action of novel compounds.

Ultimately, new antihypertensive drugs must be evaluated in vivo, and unfortunately such experimentation is associated with ethical costs. Although professional philosophers may disagree, many think that the humane use of the rat as a laboratory model carries less ethical concerns than the employment of higher species.

Other advantages of the rat as a model for experimental hypertension include: 1) Robustness—The rat is a robust animal that tolerates well both acute and chronic studies; 2) Potential for genetic manipulation—Production of transgenic rats will permit the testing of hypotheses regarding the pathophysiology of hypertension with a precision unimaginable by past generations of researchers; 3) Conservation of pharmacological probes—Often only small quantities of new pharmacological agents are initially available for study so that experiments in larger species are impractical.

Despite these advantages, the rat is not a perfect model for evaluation of antihypertensive agents. Although a given model of experimental hypertension in rats may be well characterized, the correspondence between that experimental model of hypertension and a particular type of clinical hypertension in humans may be unclear. For instance, whether or not genetic hypertension in the rat is relevant to essential hypertension in man is controversial (Trippodo and Frohlich, 1981; McGiff and Quilley, 1981). Further, differences in the absorption, distribution, metabolism, and elimination of antihypertensive drugs in rats versus humans complicates extrapolation of studies in rats to the human situation. Finally, there may be important differences in neural and hormonal systems controlling blood pressure in humans compared with rats leading to substantially different responses to antihypertensive drugs. However, these several disadvantages are not unique to the rat, and similar objections could be raised against the use of any non-human species.

METHODS FOR PRECLINICAL STUDIES: SELECTING THE TECHNOLOGY

Measurement of blood pressure. Although blood pressure can be measured by a variety of techniques in animal models, it is difficult to obtain highly accurate measurements in completely unstressed animals, particularly in smaller species such as the rat. Recent advancements in commercially available and user-friendly technology now permit on-line, time-integrated and computerized measurement of blood pressure in unrestrained, conscious animals over several weeks by telemetry even by physiologists without training in electrical engineering and computer science. This technique should allow a precise definition of the efficacy of new drugs free of artifacts secondary to more manipulative methodology (e.g., tail cuff method, catheters protected by jackets, etc.)

Measurement of organ blood flows and the distribution of cardiac output. As mentioned earlier, an increasing emphasis will be placed on designing new antihypertensives that favorably influence various physiological and biochemical parameters. An important aspect of research on antihypertensive drugs is the determination of the effects of drugs on both regional absolute blood flow and the relative tissue distribution of cardiac output. As with blood pressure, various methods exist to quantitate these variables. However, the introduction of micro-thermistors and transit-time flow probes now permits a stable, on-line and accurate measurement of absolute cardiac output and absolute organ blood flows even in conscious rats.

Measurement of renal hemodynamics. Of increasing concern is the effects of antihypertensive drugs on afferent and efferent arteriolar resistance and glomerular capillary pressure (Tolins and Raij, 1990). A given drug may lower arterial blood pressure yet increase the percentage of the arterial blood pressure that is transmitted to the glomerulus so that glomerular hypertension is worsened by drug therapy. In the future, more information about the impact of antihypertensive drugs on the kidney should and will be required. Consequently, the modern investigation of antihypertensive drugs should include a detailed analysis of the effects of drugs on the microcirculation of the kidney using renal micropuncture techniques.

Measurement of biochemical parameters. In addition to the obvious variables such as serum cholesterol, triglycerides, glucose, uric acid and electrolytes, the impact of antihypertensive drugs on cell function at the DNA level may become an important part of antihypertensive drug research. Hypertension causes changes in the morphology and structure of blood vessels due to hyperplasia and hypertrophy of vascular smooth muscle and due to deposition of extracellular matrix material. The reversal of these processes may not be a common feature of all antihypertensive drugs (Schwartz, Majesky and Dilley, 1990). Therefore, determining the consequences of drug therapy on expression of both oncogenes and tumor-suppressing genes by vascular smooth muscle cells may help optimize drug therapy for hypertension. Technologies such as in situ hybridization and PCR should find an increasing role in this regard.

METHODS FOR PRECLINICAL STUDIES: SELECTING THE EXPERIMENTS

Confronted with a potential new antihypertensive drug, what experiments should the cardiovascular pharmacologist perform in animal models to assess whether or not expensive, time consuming and potentially risky studies should be performed in man?

Assessing Antihypertensive Potential

Chronic versus acute studies. Hypertensionologists have been extraordinarily cautious in adopting Guytonian concepts of the long-term control of arterial blood pressure. However, slowly but surely, cardiovascular physiologists are accepting the fact that the long-term regulation of arterial blood pressure is ultimately controlled by the kidney, i.e., the shape and position of the renal pressure-natriuresis curve (Guyton, 1990). This concept is extremely important to remember when designing experiments to assess the antihypertensive potential of new chemicals. For instance, assume that a drug reduces acutely cardiac output and/or total peripheral resistance without altering, either directly or indirectly, the renal pressure-natriuresis curve. The anticipated result would be an immediate antihypertensive response that would completely disappear over several days as the renal pressure-natriuresis system slowly restores long-term average blood pressure levels to the renal set-point. Conversely, assume that a drug increases the slope of the renal pressure–natriuresis curve and/or shifts this relationship to the left, but does not alter acutely either cardiac output or total peripheral resistance. In this situation, the anticipated result would be no immediate antihypertensive response, but over several days the renal pressure-natriuresis system would slowly lower long-term average blood pressure levels to the new renal set-point.

Usually, drugs that interfere with vascular, sympathetic and hormonal regulation alter blood pressure both acutely and chronically. Nonetheless, acute studies may markedly overestimate or underestimate the chronic antihypertensive activity of a potential therapeutic agent. A case in point is the class of drugs that inhibit angiotensin converting enzyme. In conscious, sodium replete spontaneously hypertensive rats (SHR), acute administration of converting enzyme inhibitors has only a modest effect on arterial blood pressure (Sweet and co-workers, 1981), whereas chronic administration will completely normalize blood pressure in this genetic model of hypertension (Koike and co-workers, 1980). Similarly, acute administration of beta-adrenoceptor blockers does not lower blood pressure in SHR, whereas chronic administration does (Antonaccio and co-workers, 1986). The antihypertensive activity of a new drug should always be assessed after administration of the drug for at least 1 week, preferably longer.

Animal models. As indicated earlier, our bias is that the rat is the most appropriate species for preclinical investigations of the antihypertensive potential of new drugs. In this species a wide array of hypertensive models are available so the question becomes which model(s) to use. A lesson to be learned from research performed with beta-adrenoceptor blockers and converting enzyme inhibitors is that logic is not always the best guide for selecting an appropriate model. For instance, the 2-kidney/1-clip Goldblatt hypertensive rat is a high-renin model of experimental hypertension that does not respond to beta-adrenoceptor antagonists (drugs that as a class inhibit renin release) (Gulati and Liard, 1979). On the other hand, the spontaneously hypertensive rat (SHR) has a normal plasma renin activity, yet chronic administration of converting enzyme inhibitors completely prevents and reverses hypertension in this model (Koike and co-workers, 1980) and chronic administration of beta-adrenoceptor antagonists lowers blood pressure in the SHR (Antonaccio and co-workers, 1986).

The primary lesson to be learned from past experience is that potential antihypertensive agents should be examined chronically in a variety of models of experimental hypertension including renovascular hypertensive rats, genetically hypertensive rats, rats with salt-induced hypertension (DOCA/salt hypertension) and rats with compromised renal function (renoprival hypertension). Unless new agents are examined in several different experimental models of hypertension, the researcher runs the risk of missing important therapeutic advances. Also, the use of several types of experimental hypertension will provide an early indication of whether the new therapeutic entity is a broad-spectrum versus a targeted antihypertensive.

Other Studies

Once a drug with potential antihypertensive activity is identified in preclinical studies, what next? As mentioned earlier, preclinical studies should assess the chronic effects of antihypertensive drugs not only on blood pressure but also on organ blood flow, cardiac output, renal function and microcirculation, metabolic parameters, and vascular smooth muscle and cardiac muscle hypertrophy. Also, investigations on the mechanism of action should be launched after the efficacy of the drug has been demonstrated.

Discovering the mechanism of action of a new class of antihypertensive drugs is important for several reasons. First, this information can be used to design yet additional therapeutic entities. Second, knowledge about how a given antihypertensive agent lowers blood pressure may suggest the strengths and limitations of the drug (e.g., drug-drug interactions, side- effects, contraindications), as well as how best to target the drug for the most appropriate subclass of patients. Third, antihypertensive drugs with well-defined mechanisms of action are useful for further investigating the pathophysiology of experimental and clinical hypertension. A fixed formula for delineating the mechanism of action of a given antihypertensive drug cannot be stated. In this regard, the creativity, ingenuity and skill of many investigators are required.

DO ANIMAL STUDIES ACCURATELY PREDICT THE EFFICACY OF ANTIHYPERTENSIVE DRUGS IN MAN?

To date there does not exist a class of antihypertensive drugs that are not effective in at least some animal models. This is true for the diuretics, beta- blockers, vasodilators, central sympatholytics, peripheral sympatholytics, converting enzyme inhibitors, calcium channel blockers and potassium channel openers. It seems unlikely, therefore, that drugs that are properly evaluated in animal models will escape detection (i.e., few false negatives would occur). Conversely, drugs which are effective in animal models are usually effective in man (i.e., few false positives are detected).

CONCLUSION

The stated objective of preclinical studies with antihypertensive drugs is to identify chemicals with increased antihypertensive efficacy, decreased toxicity, increased ease of administration, improved effects on metabolic, cardiac and renal parameters, and unique mechanisms of action. By employing the proper technology and experimental design to a range of animal models of hypertension most of these objectives can be adequately addressed with preclinical studies. However, an important caveat must be kept in mind. Because of the complex relationship between dose of an antihypertensive drug and time to full antihypertensive effect, and because of interspecies differences in drug disposition, preclinical studies with antihypertensive drugs will seldom provide useful information regarding clinical dosages of new antihypertensive agents.

REFERENCES

Adams, M. A., A. Bobik, and P. I. Korner (1990). Enalapril can prevent vascular amplifier development in spontaneously hypertensive rats. Hypertension, 16, 252-260.

Anderson, S., H. G. Rennke, and B. M. Brenner (1986). Therapeutic advantage of converting enzyme inhibitors in arresting progressive renal disease associated with systemic hypertension. J. Clin. Invest., 77, 1993-2000.

Antonaccio, M. J., B. Rubin, Z. P. Horovitz, R. J. Laffoa, M. E. Goldberg, J. P. High, D. N. Harris, and I. Zaidi (1979). Effects of chronic treatment with captopril (SQ 14,225), an orally active inhibitor of angiotensin I- converting enzyme, in spontaneously hypertensive rats. Japan J. Pharmacol., 29, 285-294.

Antonaccio, M. J., J. High, J. M. Deforrest, and E. Sybertz (1986). Antihypertensive effects of 12 beta adrenoceptor antagonists in conscious spontaneously hypertensive rats: Relationship to changes in plasma renin activity, heart rate and sympathetic nerve function. J. Pharmacol. Exp. Ther., 238, 378-387.

Bouhnik, J., F. X. Galen, J. Menard, P. Corvol, R. Seyer, J. A. Fehrentz, D. Le N'Guyen, P. Falorand, and B. Castro (1987). Production and characterization of human renin antibodies with region-oriented synthetic peptides. J. Biol. Chem., 262: 2913-2918.

Buhler, F. R., J. H. Laragh, L. Baer, E. D. Vaughan, and H. R. Brunner (1972). Propranolol inhibition of renin secretion: a specific approach to diagnosis and treatment of renin-dependent hypertensive diseases. N. Engl. J. Med., 287, 1209-1214.

Gulati, O. P., and J. F. Liard (1979). Effects of propranolol in chronic two-kidney goldblatt hypertension in rats. Arch. Int. Pharmacodyn., 240, 285-293.

Guyton, A. C. (1990) Personal and historical perspectives: The surprising kidney- fluid mechanism for pressure control - its infinite gain! Hypertension, 16, 725-730.

Haber, E., and K. Y. Hui (1990). Specific renin inhibitors: The concept and the prospects. In J. H. Laragh, and B. M. Brenner (Eds.), Hypertension: Pathophysiology, Diagnosis, and Management, Raven Press, New York. pp. 2343- 2350.

Jackson, E. K. (1992). In vivo evaluation of the antagonist activity of angiotensin I analogs. J. Pharmacol. Exp. Ther., 260, 223-231.

Koike, H., K. Ito, M. Miyamoto, and H. Nishino (1980). Effects of long-term blockade of angiotensin converting enzyme with captopril (SQ14,225) on hemodynamics and circulating blood volume in SHR. Hypertension, 2, 299-303.

Laragh, J. H. (1978). The renin system in high blood pressure, from disbelief to reality: converting-enzyme blockade for analysis and treatment. Progress in Cardiovascular Diseases, 21, 159-166.

Maxwell, M. H. (1988). Beyond blood pressure control: effect of antihypertensive therapy on cardiovascular risk factors. Am. J. Hyper., 1, 366S-371S.

McGiff, J. C., and C. P. Quilley (1981). Controversies in cardiovascular research: the rat with spontaneous genetic hypertension is not a suitable model of human essential hypertension. Circ. Res., 48, 455-463.

Schwartz, S. M., M. W. Majesky, and R. J. Dilley (1990). Vascular remodeling in hypertension and atherosclerosis. In J. H. Laragh, B. M. Brenner (Eds.), Hypertension: Pathophysiology, Diagnosis, and Management, Raven Press, New York. pp. 521-539.

Stamler, J. (Comments by), and T. Kotchen (Session Chairman) (1991). Panel Discussion: Session VII. Research and Public Health Directions: Public Health and Clinical Perspectives: Is salt restriction for everyone? Hypertension, 17 (Suppl I), I-216 - I-221.

Sweet, C. S., P. T. Arbegast, L. S. Gaul, E. H. Blaine, and D. M. Gross (1981). Relationship between angiotensin I blockade and antihypertensive properties of single doses of MK-421 and captopril in spontaneous and renal hypertensive rats. Eur. J. Pharmacol., 76: 167-176.

Timmermans, P. B. M. W. M., D. J. Carini, A. T. Chiu, J. V. Duncia, W. A. Price, G. J. Wells, P. C. Wong, R. R. Wexler, and A. L. Johnson (1990). The discovery and physiological effects of a new class of highly specific angiotensin II-receptor antagonists. In J. H. Laragh and B. M. Brenner (Eds.), Hypertension: Pathophysiology, Diagnosis, and Management, Raven Press, New York. pp. 2351-2360.

Tolins, J. P., and L. Raij (1990). Comparison of converting enzyme inhibitor and calcium channel blocker in hypertensive glomerular injury. Hypertension, 16, 452-461.

Trippodo, N. C., and E. D. Frohlich (1981). Controversies in cardiovascular research: Similarities of genetic (spontaneous) hypertension: Man and rat. Circ. Res., 48, 309-319.

Weinberger, M. H. (1990). Clinical Conference: Optimizing cardiovascular risk reduction during antihypertensive therapy. Hypertension, 16, 201-211.

PRECLINICAL PHARMACODYNAMICS OF ANXIOLYTICS: EFFECTS OF CHRONIC BENZODIAZEPINE ADMINISTRATION

Lawrence G. Miller
Division of Clinical Pharmacology, Depts. of Pharmacology and Psychiatry
Tufts University School of Medicine and New England Medical Center
Boston, MA 02111

ABSTRACT

Benzodiazepine anxiolytics act at specific receptors located on the $GABA_A$ receptor complex on post-synaptic neurons. We developed a mouse model to assess pharmacodynamics and neuro-chemical effects during chronic benzodiazepine administration. During chronic lorazepam administration, animals developed behavioral tolerance and benzodiazepine receptor downregulation in several brain regions after 1 week of treatment. Similar results were observed for clonazepam. However, for alprazolam, these alterations occurred more rapidly, after 2-4 days, and neurochemical changes occurred primarily in cortex. In contrast to results with benzodiazepine agonists, chronic antagonist and "inverse agonist" treatment had opposite effects on behavior and were associated with receptor upregulation. After benzodiazepine agonist discontinuation, behavioral and neurochemical effects were also opposite to those observed during chronic administration, suggesting the presence of a "withdrawal" syndrome. Administration of carbamazepine after lorazepam discontinuation attenuated the behavioral and neurochemical withdrawal effects. Studies to determine the cellular mechanisms of these receptor alterations indicated that receptor increases after drug discontinuation were likely to be due to enhanced receptor production. During chronic administration, receptor mRNAs were decreased, but this change occurred after the development of tolerance and receptor downregulation.

Benzodiazepine anxiolytics act at a specific binding site in the central nervous system to exert their pharmacodynamic effects. This site is located on the $GABA_A$ receptor complex on post-synaptic neurons (Olsen and Tobin, 1990). Binding of benzodiazepine agonists enhances GABA binding, which in turn opens a ligand-gated chloride channel producing neuronal hyperpolarization. Since the introduction of benzodiazepines into clinical practice almost thirty years ago, pharmacodynamic alterations have been reported during chronic administration. In particular, tolerance occurs to most benzodiazepine actions during chronic treatment (Greenblatt and Shader, 1978). Tolerance has been especially problematic in the use of benzodiazepines as anticonvulsants and sedatives. In addition, discontinuation of benzodiazepines after chronic use is associated with the development of "withdrawal" or discontinuation syndromes (Greenblatt et al., 1990). Withdrawal has limited the use of benzodiazepines as anxiolytics and hypnotics.

Behavioral tolerance and a behavioral discontinuation syndrome have been reported in animals exposed to chronic benzodiazepines (Miller, 1991). However, relatively little information has been available concerning the neurochemical substrate of these chronic benzodiazepine effects. To elucidate the basis for pharmacodynamic alterations during chronic benzodiazepine administration, we developed a mouse model of benzodiazepine tolerance and withdrawal. Results of studies in this model are described briefly below.

Initial studies of chronic benzodiazepine administration used lorazepam (Miller et al., 1988a). This compound is intermediate in half-life, potency, and receptor binding and has no active metabolites in the mouse or human. Lorazepam was delivered by subcutaneously implanted osmotic pumps. This method provides continuous serum concentrations analogous to those obtained in humans receiving multiple daily doses of a benzodiazepine, as is common clinically. Using a simple measure of ataxia, mice developed tolerance to lorazepam over a broad dose range (1-10 mg/kg/d) after 7 days of administration. Tolerance persisted to 14 days of administration. Plasma and brain concentrations of lorazepam remained constant during this period. Benzodiazepine receptor binding determined by in vivo uptake of [^{3}H]flumazenil also decreased in several brain regions at day 7 of administration. Binding determined in vitro in cortex exhibited a similar pattern. Finally, GABA$_A$ receptor function was determined by stimulation of chloride uptake into cortical preparations by the GABA analog muscimol. Uptake was decreased after 7 days of lorazepam administration.

These data indicate that downregulation of the benzodiazepine receptor, and decreased function of the GABA$_A$ receptor complex, are temporally associated with the development of tolerance. Similar findings with regard to receptor downregulation have been reported by Tietz and co-workers (1986) using chronic flurazepam, and by Marley and Gallager (1989) using chronic diazepam. Although these results do not establish that neurochemical changes cause behavioral effects, the temporal association suggests a causal role or a common response to another factor.

Subsequently, we have evaluated effects of chronic administration of several other benzodiazepine agonists, alprazolam and clonazepam. Alprazolam is a triazolobenzodiazepine with efficacy in panic disorder as well as anxiety. Some clinical reports suggest that discontinuation syndromes are more common and more severe with alprazolam (Roy-Byrne and Hommer, 1988). Chronic alprazolam administration in mice is associated with behavioral tolerance at 4 days of administration (Miller et al., 1989b). Benzodiazepine receptor binding in vivo and in vitro in cortex is also decreased after 4 days, as is GABA-dependent chloride uptake. Thus, alprazolam appears to be similar to lorazepam except that behavioral and neurochemical alterations occur more rapidly. In addition, effects of alprazolam are largely confined to cortex, whereas lorazepam-induced alterations occur in hippocampus as well (Galpern et al., 1990). Clonazepam is similar to lorazepam in producing tolerance and neurochemical changes after 1 week of administration (Galpern et al., 1992).

To shed additional light on GABA$_A$ receptor modulation, we also examined effects of chronic administration of a benzodiazepine antagonist, flumazenil, and an inverse agonist, FG 7142. The latter compound has effects opposite to benzodiazepine agonists, e.g. pro-convulsant, anxiogenic, and arousal effects. Chronic flumazenil administration produced effects opposite to those of agonists such as lorazepam: behavioral indices suggested increased activity compared to controls at 1 week, accompanied by upregulation of benzodiazepine binding and GABA-dependent chloride uptake (Miller et al., 1989a). Similar results were observed during chronic FG 7142 administration (Pritchard et al., 1991). These studies indicate that both behavioral and neurochemical parameters associated with benzodiazepine administration can be modulated in either direction, and confirm the plasticity of this system.

Finally, effects of a benzodiazepine "partial agonist" were evaluated in this model (Miller et al., 1990). Partial agonist compounds are characterized by incomplete efficacy regardless of dose, and by selectivity of effects (Haefely, 1988). That is, such compounds may have primarily anticonvulsant or anxiolytic effects with little sedation, ataxia, etc. The putative partial agonist bretazenil, over 14 days of administration across a broad dose range, produced no apparent behavioral tolerance using a simple motor paradigm. Similarly, no changes were observed in benzodiazepine or GABA$_A$ receptor function using this compound. It should be pointed out that despite high receptor affinity, bretazenil had very low potency. Nonetheless, these data suggest that partial agonist compounds might in part avoid tolerance associated with "full" benzodiazepine agonists. The results also support the role of neurochemical alterations in the development of tolerance.

In view of the clinical importance of benzodiazepine discontinuation syndromes, we also evaluated effects of drug discontinuation in this model (Miller et al., 1988b). After administration of lorazepam at a dose and interval which produced tolerance (2 mg/kg/d for 1 week), behavior remained unchanged at 12 hours to 2 days. Lorazepam concentrations in brain fell rapidly to undetectable levels, and binding returned to control levels in 24 hours. However, at 4 days after discontinuation activity increased above control values, and benzodiazepine receptor binding and GABA-dependent chloride uptake also increased. By 7 days after discontinuation, all parameters had returned to control levels. Similar results were observed with alprazolam and clonazepam (Galpern et al., 1992; Lopez et al., 1990).

These results indicate that a model of a benzodiazepine discontinuation syndrome could be produced in the mouse, with both behavioral and neurochemical components. Again, neurochemical alterations paralleled changes in behavior. Results using alprazolam were similar, except that behavioral and neurochemical changes occurred somewhat more rapidly with alprazolam. Clonazepam discontinuation produced changes similar to those observed with lorazepam.

The mouse model described above provides opportunities to assess interventions designed to attenuate or reverse benzodiazepine tolerance or withdrawal, and to investigate the molecular mechanisms of these phenomena. Several clinical studies suggested that carbamazepine administered after benzodiazepine discontinuation could limit the development of discontinuation symptoms (Klein et al., 1986; Schweizer et al., 1991). We evaluated this proposed treatment in the mouse model (Galpern et al., 1991). Anticonvulsant doses of carbamazepine alone did not alter benzodiazepine receptor binding or GABA$_A$ receptor function. However, when administered after alprazolam discontinuation, carbamazepine reduced the behavioral and neurochemical manifestations of "withdrawal". It should be pointed out that some behavioral and neurochemical changes persisted during carbamazepine treatment. Nonetheless, these were significantly reduced, supporting the efficacy of carbamazepine in the treatment of discontinuation.

With regard to the mechanism underlying tolerance, it is possible that the observed downregulation in binding is due to decreased receptor protein production due in turn to decreased gene expression. To evaluate this hypothesis, we measured mRNAs for the most abundant GABA$_A$ receptor subunits in cortex and cerebellum (Kang and Miller, 1991). Using Northern hybridization, mRNAs for the alpha1 and gamma2 subunits were unchanged from controls up to 10 days of administration of lorazepam, 2 mg/kg/d. However, at day 14 a substantial (50%) reduction in both mRNAs occurred in cortex, and this alteration persisted for 28 days of administration. These data indicate that chronic benzodiazepine administration can affect mRNA levels for subunits likely to be involved in benzodiazepine receptor binding. However, changes in mRNAs occur well after changes in binding (14 days compared to 10 days) and thus it is unlikely that these alterations are involved in the initial receptor downregulation. Rather, changes in mRNAs appear to represent a novel effect of a ligand on its receptor expression. Similar results have been reported in another laboratory (Heninger et al., 1990).

With regard to benzodiazepine discontinuation, the observed increase in receptor binding might be due to enhanced receptor synthesis. To address this hypothesis, we used the irreversible benzodiazepine receptor inactivating agent, EEDQ, to assess receptor recovery after drug discontinuation (Miller et al., 1991a). EEDQ was used to inactivate approximately 50% of benzodiazepine receptors 1 day after lorazepam discontinuation (Miller et al., 1991b). Receptor recovery occurred over the subsequent 48 hours in both lorazepam and vehicle-treated animals. However, the half-life for receptor recovery was significantly decreased in lorazepam-treated mice, suggesting enhanced receptor production or decreased receptor removal. This finding is consistent with the increase in receptor binding during lorazepam discontinuation.

In summary, we have addressed pharmacodynamics and neurochemistry of chronic benzodiazepine administration in a mouse model. Behavioral tolerance was associated with receptor downregulation, and a discontinuation syndrome was associated with receptor upregulation. Development of tolerance and discontinuation effects was similar for several benzodiazepine agonists, although the time course varied somewhat and the regional distribution of neurochemical changes also varied among agonists. Chronic effects of a benzodiazepine antagonist and an inverse agonist were opposite to alterations produced by agonist compounds. A partial agonist produced no behavioral or neurochemical changes during chronic administration.

This model was used to evaluate the effects of carbamazepine on alprazolam withdrawal. Carbamazepine attenuated both behavioral and neurochemical alterations after discontinuation, suggesting a possible treatment for withdrawal symptoms. With regard to mechanisms for tolerance and discontinuation syndromes, molecular biological studies indicated that mRNAs for several GABA$_A$ receptor subunits were decreased during chronic lorazepam administration, but that this effect followed rather than preceded receptor down-regulation. For benzodiazepine discontinuation, use of an irreversible receptor inactivator indicated that receptor recovery was accelerated after lorazepam discontinuation. This finding is consistent with receptor upregulation after lorazepam discontinuation.

The study of chronic benzodiazepine effects can thus illuminate basic receptor mechanisms in brain as well as provide support for empiric clinical therapies. The discovery of alterations in gene expression appears to indicate a novel, and potentially important, effect of long-term benzodiazepine administration.

ACKNOWLEDGEMENTS

The author thanks his colleagues, Drs. David J. Greenblatt and Richard I. Shader, and other laboratory colleagues including Drs. Jamie Barnhill, Fred Lopez and Gary Pritchard, and Beth Roy, Wendy Galpern, Andrew Schatzki, Monica Lumpkin and Jack Heller. Supported in part by grant DA-05258 from the U.S. Public Health Service and by a Faculty Development Award in Clinical Pharmacology from the Pharmaceutical Manufacturers Association Foundation.

REFERENCES

Galpern, W. R., M. Lumpkin, D. J. Greenblatt, R. I. Shader, and L. G. Miller (1992). Chronic benzodiazepine administration: VII. Behavioral tolerance and withdrawal and receptor alterations associated with clonazepam adminstration. Psychopharmacology, 104, 225-230.

Galpern, W. R., L. G. Miller, D. J. Greenblatt, and R. I. Shader (1990). Differential effects of chronic lorazepam and alprazolam on benzodiazepine binding and GABA receptor function. Brit. J. Pharmacol., 101, 839-842.

Galpern, W. R., L. G. Miller, D. J. Greenblatt, G. K. Szabo, T. R. Browne, and R. I. Shader (1991). Chronic benzodiazepine administration. IX. Attenuation of alprazolam discontinuation effects by carbamazapine. Biochem. Pharmacol., 42, s99-s104.

Greenblatt, D. J., and R. I. Shader (1978). Dependence, tolerance, and addiction to benzodiazepines. Drug Metab. Dispos., 8, 13-28.

Greenblatt, D. J., L. G. Miller, and R. I. Shader (1990). Neurochemical and pharmacokinetic correlates of the clinical action of benzodiazepine hypnotic drugs. Amer. J. Med., 88, 18s-24s.

Haefely, W. (1988). Partial agonists of the benzodiazepine receptor: from animal data to results in patients. Adv. Biochem. Psychopharmacol., 45, 275-292.

Heninger, C., N. Saito, J. F. Tallman, K. M. Garrett, M. P. Vitek, R. S. Duman, and D. W. Gallager (1990). Effects of continuous diazepam administration of GABA$_A$ subunit mRNA in rat brain. J. Mol. Neurosci., 2, 101-107.

Kang, I., and L. G. Miller (1991). Decreased GABA$_A$ receptor subunit mRNA concentrations following chronic lorazepam administration. Brit. J. Pharmacol., 103, 1285-1287.

Klein, E., T. W. Uhde, and R. M. Post (1986). Preliminary evidence for the utility of carbamazepine in alprazolam withdrawal. Amer. J. Psychiatr., 143, 235-240.

Lopez, F., L. G. Miller, D. J. Greenblatt, S. Chesley, A. Schatzki, and R. I. Shader (1990). Chronic administration of benzodiazepines: V. rapid onset of behavioral and neurochemical alterations after alprazolam discontinuation. Neuropharmacology, 29, 237-241.

Marley, R. J., and D. W. Gallager (1989). Chronic diazepam treatment produces regionally specific changes in GABA-stimulated chloride influx. Eur. J. Pharmacol., 159, 217-223.

Miller, L. G. (1991). Chronic benzodiazepine administration: From the patient to the gene. J. Clin. Pharmacol., 31, 492-495.

Miller, L. G., M. Lumpkin, W. R. Galpern, D. J. Greenblatt, and R. I. Shader (1991a). Modification of gamma-aminobutyric acid$_A$ receptor binding and function by N-ethoxycarbonyl-2-ethoxy-1, 2- dihydroquineline in vitro and in vivo: effects of aging. J. Neurochem., 56, 1241-1247.

Miller, L. G., W. R. Galpern, D. J. Greenblatt, M. Lumpkin, and R. I. Shader (1990). Chronic benzodiazepine administration: VI. A partial agonist produces behavioral effects without tolerance or receptor alterations. J. Pharmacol. Exp. Ther., 254, 33-38.

Miller, L. G., D. J. Greenblatt, J. G. Barnhill, and R. I. Shader (1988a). Chronic benzodiazepine administration: I. Tolerance is associated with benzodiazepine receptor binding downregulation and decreased gamma- aminobutyric acid A receptor function. J. Pharmacol. Exp. Ther., 246, 170- 176.

Miller, L. G., D. J. Greenblatt, R. B. Roy, A. Gaver, F. Lopez, and R. I. Shader (1989a). Chronic benzodiazepine administration: III. Upregulation of gamma-aminobutyric acid$_A$ receptor binding and function associated with chronic benzodiazepine antagonist administration. J. Pharmacol. Exp. Ther., 248, 1096-1101.

Miller, L. G., D. J. Greenblatt, W. R. Summer and R. I. Shader (1988b). Chronic benzodiazepine administration: II. Discontinuation syndrome is associated with upregulation of gamma-aminobutyric acid$_A$ receptor complex binding and function. J. Pharmacol. Exp. Ther., 246, 177-182.

Miller, L. G., M. Lumpkin, D. J. Greenblatt, and R. I. Shader (1991b). Accelerated benzodiazepine receptor recovery after lorazepam discontinuation. FASEB J., 5, 93-97.

Miller, L. G., S. Woolverton, D. J. Greenblatt, F. Lopez, and R. I. Shader (1989b). Chronic benzodiazepine administration: IV. Rapid development of tolerance and receptor downregulation associated with alprazolam administration. Biochem. Pharmacol., 38, 3773-3777.

Olsen, R. W., and A. J. Tobin (1990). Molecular biology of GABA$_A$ receptors. FASEB J., 4, 1469-1480.

Pritchard, G. A., W. R. Galpern, M. Lumpkin, and L. G. Miller (1991). Chronic benzodiazepine administration: VIII. Receptor upregulation produced by chronic exposure to the inverse agonist FG-7142. J. Pharmacol. Exp. Ther., 258, 280-285.

Rickels, K., W. G. Case, E. Schweizer, F. Garcia-Espana, and R. Fridman (1990). Long-term benzodiazepine users 3 years after participation in a discontinuation program. Psychopharmacol. Bull., 26, 63-66.

Roy-Byrne, P.P., and D. Hommer (1988). Benzodiazepine withdrawal: overview and implications for treatment of anxiety. Amer. J. Med., 84, 1041-1045.

Schweizer, E., K. Rickels, W. G. Case, and D.J. Greenblatt (1991). Carbamazepine treatment in patients discontinuing long-term benzodiazepine therapy. Effects on withdrawal severity and outcome. Arch. Gen. Psychiatry, 48, 448-452.

Tietz, E. I., H. C. Rosenberg, and T. H. Chiu (1986). Autoradiographic localization of benzodiazepine receptor downregulation. J. Pharmacol. Exp. Ther., 236, 284-291.

GUIDELINES FOR DEVELOPMENT OF A NEW DIURETIC AGENT

D. Craig Brater
Indiana University School of Medicine
Department of Medicine
Clinical Pharmacology Division
Indianapolis, IN 46202-2879

INTRODUCTION

Preclinical assessment of a diuretic agent is straightforward with dual goals of identifying the active substance and its site of activity. In addition, one must determine whether the diuretic gains access to its site of action from the blood as opposed to the urine, and depending upon those findings, assess mechanisms by which access to the active site occurs. Both in vivo and in vitro studies are required to assess the specific nephron segment at which the diuretic has activity. These studies are important for predictions as to efficacy and side effects. Knowledge that a diuretic has its effects at a particular nephron site allows prediction of the degree of natriuresis that will occur and also the concomitant excretion of other electrolytes which may impact on adverse effects (e.g., potassium or magnesium).

PRECLINICAL STUDIES

Source of Activity - Parent Drug or Metabolite

In the earliest studies it is very important to determine whether activity resides in the parent drug or instead occurs via a metabolite. To assess this question, one must perform pharmacokinetic and drug metabolism studies in order to determine pathways of elimination and identify metabolites. Metabolites can then be either isolated or synthesized de novo for use in studies to assess their activity. Determination of metabolic pathways will additionally provide insight into the potential influence of different phenotypes of drug metabolism and/or disease states on the disposition of the new diuretic agent. For example, if it is found that the compound is predominantly excreted in the urine unchanged (about 70% or more) then there

Integration of Pharmacokinetics, Pharmacodynamics, and Toxicokinetics in Rational Drug Development, Edited by A. Yacobi *et al.*, Plenum Press, New York, 1993

is little need to be concerned about metabolites. Similarly, if a compound is eliminated mainly by glucuronidation, one would predict that hepatic dysfunction or phenotypic poor metabolizers would be no different in their kinetics compared to control subjects. Moreover, drug interactions of metabolism would be less likely. If the drug is metabolized via cytochrome P450, then hepatic disease might be predicted to influence metabolic capacity; in addition, one would need to explore the cytochrome P450 isoenzyme through which metabolism occurs to derive insight into whether or not there may be substantial numbers of patients with the phenotype of poor metabolism of the new drug and potential drug interactions of metabolism.

An example of the importance of delineating whether activity resides in the parent drug or a metabolite is the recent diuretic muzolimine. This drug was found to be quite effective in a variety of edematous disorders and was hypothesized to reach its site of action from the blood as opposed to the urine side of the nephron because of the fact that negligible amounts of unchanged drug were excreted into the urine (Dal Canton and co-workers, 1981; Faedda and co-workers, 1985). This mode of access to the site of action was presumed to be unique to this agent and thereby potentially imply a therapeutic advantage. In reality, nephron site of action studies found that the parent drug itself had no activity from either the blood or the urine side of the nephron (Graven and Kolling, 1983; Greger and Schlatter, 1983). As such, activity must reside in a metabolite. When muzolimine was introduced into broader clinical trials, an alarming incidence of severe neurologic toxicity occurred and the drug was withdrawn from development. It is conceivable that toxicity was associated solely with the parent drug and that it might have been avoided if preclinical work had demonstrated that activity resided in a metabolite such that the metabolite itself was developed as the diuretic agent as opposed to the prodrug muzolimine.

Nephron Site of Action

Several methods can be used to determine the nephron site of activity of a new diuretic. Whole animal studies should be performed using clearance techniques (Seldin and Rector, 1973). Two separate studies should be performed: one under water loading conditions in which a maximal water diuresis is induced by administering hypotonic fluids to the animal; the other experimental paradigm should be during hydropenia in which exogenous infusions of antidiuretic hormone are given so that a maximal antidiuretic effect is assured. Collation of results from administering the diuretic in each of these two conditions can provide considerable insight into the site at which a diuretic has its effects. This can be ascertained by examining the pattern of electrolyte and free water excretion under the influence of the diuretic, as shown in Table 1. Blockade of reabsorption in the proximal tubule can be detected in several fashions, perhaps the most sensitive of which is by assessment of effects on the fractional excretion of lithium (FE_{Li}) (Thomsen et al., 1969; Kirchner, 1987; Koomans et al., 1989). A slow-release lithium preparation can be administered to the animal (or man) prior to study. Since most lithium is reabsorbed in the proximal tubule, an increase in its fractional excretion offers indirect evidence that the compound has its effects proximally. In addition, since the majority of sodium bicarbonate is reabsorbed in the proximal tubule, an increase in urinary bicarbonate would also imply a proximal site of activity. Phosphate is similarly reabsorbed predominantly in the proximal tubule, and an increase in its excretion offers further

TABLE 1. Markers of Specific Nephron Sites of Diuretic Activity

Proximal tubule	FE_{Li}
	urinary bicarbonate
	urinary phosphate
	C_{H_2O}
	$C_{H_2O}/[C_{Cl} + C_{H_2O}]$
Thick ascending limb	$T^{C_{H_2O}}$
of the loop of Henle	$FE_{Na} = 20\%$
Distal tubule —	
Diluting segment	$C_{H_2O}/[C_{Cl} + C_{H_2O}]$
Collecting duct	FE_K

indirect evidence. Lastly, during water diuresis conditions, inhibition of solute reabsorption at the proximal tubule results in increased delivery of solute to the diluting segment of the nephron so that greater free water clearance C_{H_2O} occurs (Seldin and Rector, 1973; Thomsen et al., 1969; Kirchner, 1987; Koomans et al., 1989; Rosin et al., 1970).Since the clearance of chloride plus that of free water $(C_{Cl} + C_{H_2O})$ quantifies delivery of solute to the diluting segment in water diuretic conditions, one would predict that a diuretic affecting the proximal tubule would result in no change in the clearance of free water relative to this delivery term. Thus, a collation of several indirect markers can provide insight into whether or not the diuretic has a proximal tubular effect.

To assess whether or not the diuretic inhibits solute reabsorption at the thick ascending limb of the loop of Henle, insights can be gained from the absolute magnitude of sodium excretion. Diuretics that have effects at this nephron segment are the most efficacious and can result in a maximal fractional excretion of sodium of approximately 20%. Thus, any new diuretic agent that results in sodium excretion of this magnitude can be assumed to have effects at the thick ascending limb of the loop of Henle. Since this segment of the nephron is critical for maximizing the ability to concentrate the urine in hydropenic conditions, one can also gain inferences that a diuretic works in this segment by observing a decrease in free water reabsorption $T^C_{H_2O}$ during hydropenic conditions (Seldin and Rector, 1973).

The distal tubule generates free water since solute is reabsorbed but no reabsorption of water occurs at this nephron segment. As such, inhibition of solute reabsorption at this site results in a decreased ability to generate free water during water diuretic conditions. Since free water generation is also dependent upon delivery of solute to this segment, one must assess free water clearance relative to solute delivery. In doing so, if one observes a decrease in free water formation, an effect at the diluting segment or distal tubule can be inferred (Seldin and Rector, 1973).

At the collecting duct, sodium is reabsorbed in exchange for potassium, in contrast to more proximal portions of the nephron wherein sodium and potassium are reabsorbed in parallel. As such, a diuretic with effects at the collecting duct will decrease potassium excretion concomitantly with an increase in sodium excretion. This pattern of electrolyte excretion in and of itself indicates an effect of a new diuretic agent at the collecting duct (Seldin and Rector, 1973).

Whole animal clearance studies should be coupled with other methods for discerning the nephron site of effect of a new diuretic agent. Micropuncture techniques can be utilized as well as in vivo microperfusion. Since these techniques cannot gain access to all nephron sites, a somewhat better method is to employ microperfusion of isolated nephron segments. This procedure entails rapid dissection of the kidney to obtain small segments of a nephron that can then be perfused in vitro. Use of this technique also allows determination as to whether or not the new diuretic has its effects from the blood or the urine side of the nephron as will be discussed subsequently. By performing studies on different nephron segments throughout the kidney, one can determine the site at which the new agent has its effects.

Peritubular vs Luminal Site of Action

Most current diuretics have their effects from the lumen as opposed to the peritubular side of the nephron. In the intact animal, this means that it is diuretic that reaches the urine that is important for effect as opposed to the amount of diuretic in the blood. Microperfusion of isolated nephron segments is an ideal in vitro method for determining whether a new diuretic has its effects from the lumen or the peritubular surface. One can perfuse the lumen of the isolated segment with the diuretic and if inhibition of solute reabsorption is observed, one can conclude that the diuretic has its effects from the luminal side of the nephron. In contrast, if there is no effect from the lumen but administration of the compound into the bathing solution results in inhibition of solute reabsorption, one can conclude that the diuretic has its effects from the peritubular or blood side of the nephron. Such data can then be confirmed by additional studies in animals or man.

If one discovers that the diuretic exerts its effect from the lumen side of the nephron, one must then delineate how the compound gains access to this compartment. So doing could occur by filtration at the glomerulus. This component of access to the urine can be quantified by simply assessing the degree of protein binding of the compound. From this information, one can calculate the amount of unbound drug in the plasma, and knowing glomerular filtration rate, the amount of drug that appears in the urine via filtration. In general, for drugs that are highly protein bound, only trivial amounts of diuretic reach the urine via filtration and they instead gain their access to this compartment by being actively secreted at the proximal tubule (Odlind, 1979; Odlind and Beermann, 1980). If it is discovered that secretion is the main mechanism for entry to the active site, then one must discern whether the drug is secreted through an organic acid pathway or an organic base pathway; if the former, one would predict that probenecid would diminish secretion, and if the latter, secretion would be inhibited by cimetidine. Studies as to the secretory pathway can be performed in whole animals, in isolated perfused kidneys, or by using vesicles of isolated renal tubular plasma membranes.

Pharmacokinetics/Pharmacodynamics

Whole animal studies should be employed to delineate the pharmacokinetics of the new diuretic and to assess the relationship between concentrations of the drug and response. Such studies will help in designing dosing regimens for studies in man. Pharmacodynamic assessment should incorporate knowledge gained from prior studies as to the mechanism by which the compound reaches the active site. As such, if the drug exerts its effect from the lumen of the nephron, then pharmacodynamic assessment should relate amounts of diuretic in the urine to response. In contrast, if a drug exerts its effects from the blood side of the nephron, then one should assess the relationship between blood concentrations and response.

CLINICAL STUDIES

Studies similar to those performed in animals must also be performed in man, though one is obviously more limited in their scope in that renal tissue cannot be obtained. As such, site of action studies must employ clearance techniques using the same methodology and the same markers for site of activity as described previously (Seldin and Rector, 1973).

To determine whether the drug is effective from the peritubular as opposed to the luminal side of the nephron, one can use information gleaned from animal studies to explore this question efficiently. As such, for example, if animal studies demonstrate a luminal site of activity and that access is gained by active secretion via the organic acid pathway, one can perform a two-part crossover study in which the subject receives on one occasion the diuretic itself and on another occasion the diuretic after pre-treatment with probenecid. Because probenecid will disrupt the relationship between concentrations of the diuretic in blood and in urine, one would observe that relating serum concentrations of the drug to response would demonstrate that probenecid causes a rightward shift in the pharmacodynamic profile. In contrast, if the drug exerts its effects from the lumen surface of the nephron, the relationship between urine amounts of drug and response would reveal no effect of probenecid pretreatment (Chennavasin and co-workers, 1979).

Pharmacokinetic and pharmacodynamic studies should also be performed in human subjects and these studies should be guided by prior data in animals that identify elimination pathways. Since many patients who receive diuretics are elderly, all development programs should include studies in this cohort. In addition, if one discovers in preclinical testing that a drug is eliminated predominantly by metabolism, one should pursue assessment of the influence of phenotypes of drug metabolism, of the influence of hepatic disease on kinetics and response, and of the influence of inhibitors of hepatic metabolism on kinetics and response.

Pharmacokinetic/pharmacodynamic studies should be performed in the different clinical conditions in which the diuretic might be used, including congestive heart failure, renal insufficiency, and cirrhosis. Other studies might be conducted to assess hemodynamic effects of the drug, both acutely and chronically. Results of the latter might influence exploration of possible use as an antihypertensive agent.

Efficacy studies should then be performed using doses derived from the pharmacokinetic/pharmacodynamic data. Such studies should be performed in all potential clinical conditions where the new diuretic might be used, including studies of patients with hypertension and with a variety of edematous disorders.

CONCLUSIONS

Development of a diuretic agent can proceed through a logical series of studies that allow one to be efficient in evaluating the new compound. Critical to efficient development is the early delineation of the activity of the parent compound itself, assessment of the nephron segment at which activity occurs, and the route by which the agent gains access to its active site. This fundamental data can be used to design additional preclinical and clinical studies that should maximize the amount of useful information gleaned from each study performed. Though orderly progression from one set of studies to the other might incur a cost in terms of time of development, the savings associated with a higher percentage of meaningful studies being performed results in an overall more cost effective strategy for development.

ACKNOWLEDGEMENTS

Supported by grants AG07631 and DK33794 from the National Institutes of Health.

REFERENCES

Chennavasin, P., R. Seiwell, D. C. Brater, and W. M. M. Liang (1979). Pharmacodynamic analysis of the furosemide-probenecid interaction in man. Kidney Int., 16, 187-195.

Dal Canton, A., D. Russo, R. Gallo, G. Conte, and V. E. Andreucci (1981). Muzolimine: a high-ceiling diuretic suitable for patients with advanced renal failure. Br. Med. J., 282, 595-598.

Faedda, R. S., G. F. Branca, B. Contu, and E. Bartoli (1985). Demonstration of action of muzolimine on the serosal side of the Henle's loop cells. Z. Kardiol., 74 (suppl 2), 166-170.

Graven, J., and B. Kolling (1983). Effects of muzolimine in microperfusion studies of loops of Henle in rats. In V. E. Andreucci (Ed.), Recent Advances in Diuretic Therapy. Excerpta Medica, Amsterdam. pp. 37-45.

Greger, R., and E. Schlatter (1983). Cellular mechanism of the action of loop diuretics on the thick ascending limb of Henle's loop. Klin. Worchenschr., 61, 1019-1027.

Kirchner, K. A. (1987). Lithium as a marker for proximal tubular delivery during low salt intake and diuretic infusion. Am. J. Physiol., 253, F188- F196.

Koomans, H. A., W. H. Boer, and E. J. D. Mees (1989). Evaluation of lithium clearance as a marker of proximal tubule sodium handling. Kidney Int., 36, 2-12.

Odlind B. (1979). Relationship between tubular secretion of furosemide and its saluretic effect. J. Pharmacol. Exp. Ther., 208, 515-521.

Odlind, B., and B. Beermann (1980). Renal tubular secretion and effects of furosemide. <u>Clin. Pharmacol. Ther.</u>, <u>27</u>, 784-790.

Rosin, J. M., M. A. Katz, F. C. Rector, and D. W. Seldin (1970). Acetazolamide in studying sodium reabsorption in diluting segment. <u>Am. J. Physiol.</u>, <u>219</u>, 1731-1738.

Seldin, D. W., and F. C. Rector (1973). Evaluation of clearance methods for localization of site of action of diuretics. In A. F. Lant and G. M. Wilson (Eds.), <u>Modern Diuretic Therapy in the Treatment of Cardiovascular and Renal Disease</u>. Excerpta Medica, Amsterdam. pp. 97-111.

Thomsen, T., M. Schou, I. Steiness, and H. E. Hansen (1969). Lithium as an indicator of proximal sodium reabsorption. <u>Pflügers Arch.</u>, <u>308</u>, 180-184.

PRECLINICAL PHARMACODYNAMICS OF ANTI-INFLAMMATORY DRUGS.

Asoke Mukherjee, Conrad Chen, Lucy Jean, and Claude B. Coutinho
Center for Drug Evaluation and Research
Food and Drug Administration, Rockville, Md 20857

ABSTRACT

During the past three decades research into the development of anti-inflammatory (AI) drugs has given rise in the main to the cyclooxygenase inhibitors. More recent efforts, based on a better understanding of the pathophysiology of the inflammatory process, have led to the development of unique and novel molecular entities as potential candidates for use in the treatment of inflammation. However, lack of suitable animal models that mimic the human disease and specific markers to follow immunological response that might possibly be associated with the disease process have made the selection of which new drug to take into clinical trials more difficult. This review discusses some of the advantages and disadvantages of animal models used routinely for the evaluation of AI agents and includes some suggestions as to how one might approach the development of newer models that may help identify novel AI drugs with varying mechanisms of therapeutic action.

INTRODUCTION

Inflammatory diseases are the manifestation of host reactions to self and non-self constituents of living organisms whereas inflammation is a process which results from injury and terminates with healing. The quest for a better understanding of the inflammatory process has gone on from the era of Hippocrates and continues to the present day. During this period, both scientists and physicians have indeed increased their understanding of the pathophysiology, diagnosis and prognosis of inflammatory diseases. However, progress in the search for novel therapeutic agents to treat inflammatory disease has been limited by both the lack of suitable animal models to identify such agents and our lack of understanding of the "precise" pathophysiology of different inflammatory diseases.

Integration of Pharmacokinetics, Pharmacodynamics, and Toxicokinetics in Rational Drug Development, Edited by A. Yacobi *et al.,* Plenum Press, New York, 1993

ANTI-INFLAMMATORY AGENTS

The available AI drugs for the treatment of rheumatoid arthritis include the corticos-teroids, cyclooxygenase inhibitors, slow acting disease-modifying agents and cytotoxic drugs. The AI drugs used clinically and those under development are presented in Table 1. They represent several chemical classes of compounds which exert their effects by one or more mechanisms of action.

The corticosteroids are an important class of compounds introduced to clinical practice in the middle of this century (Arthritis Foundation, 1985; Hench and co-workers, 1949) for the treatment of a variety of allergic and inflammatory conditions. Approximately eight corticosteroids identified by generic names are available.

Prostaglandin cyclooxygenase inhibitors represent another important group of AI agents. With advancement in our knowledge of cyclooxygenase mediated lipid metabolism (Vane, 1971) and the effect of salicylates on this pathway, a number of such inhibitors have been made available to the clinician. Currently, about seventeen cyclooxygenase inhibitors,

TABLE 1. Anti-Inflammatory Drugs

1.	Corticosteroids
2.	PG cyclooxygenase inhibitors
3.	Antimalarials, D-Penicillamine, gold salts, 5-aminosalicylic acid, sulfasalazine
4.	Thromboxane receptor or synthetase inhibitors
5.	5-Lipoxygenase inhibitors and leukotriene antagonists
6.	Inhibitors of cytokines e.g., IL-1, IL-2, IL-4
7.	Antimetabolites, e.g., purine and pyrimidine synthesis inhibitors
8.	Growth factors to promote healing (biotechnology products) e.g., PDGF, FGF, TNF, TGF-beta
9.	Others, e.g., immunomodulators and inhibitors of superoxides.

commonly referred to as non-steroidal anti-inflammatory drugs (NSAID'S), are available in the U.S. for treating pain associated with a variety of disorders and inflammatory conditions. Efforts continue to develop additional cyclooxygenase inhibitors having fewer side effects and greater selectivity towards alleviating fever, pain or inflammation. These agents have contributed to our understanding of the existence of distinct differences in the role of lipid mediators in the pathogenesis of fever, pain and inflammation. In addition to the corticos-teroids and cyclooxygenase inhibitors, a number of compounds with unrelated structures and mechanisms of action are available to treat rheumatoid arthritis. Examples of this group are the anti-malarials, D-penicillamine, gold salts, 5-aminosalicylic acid, sulfasalazine, etc. These disease modifying compounds found their way into clinical practice pursuant to follow-up research emanating from a primary clinical observation. They were not a product of what is termed "rational drug development".

More recently, research into alternate pathways of lipid metabolism, for example, through lipoxygenase and thromboxane synthetase (Samuelsson, 1983; Hamberg, Svensson and Samuelsson, 1975; Needleman, Minkes and Raz, 1976), has led to the development of inhibitors to these enzymes. Several such inhibitors are currently being evaluated for use in the treatment of a variety of diseases including those associated with inflammation.

Early in this century, the concept that chemical mediators link several organs to orchestrate specialized functions led to the discovery of adrenergic and cholinergic agents (Cannon and Uridil, 1921; Loewi and Navratil, 1926). In similar fashion, the immunologic concept that inflammatory cells communicate with each other (Dinarello, 1984; Mizel, 1989) has given rise to the cytokines, inhibitors of which are of continuing interest with respect to their potential as AI agents. Additionally, a number of inhibitors of adhesion between endothelial or antigen presenting cells and T-helper lymphocytes are under evaluation as anti-inflammatory agents (Dustin et al., 1986; Springer et al., 1987).

Following the use of methotrexate in psoriatic arthritis, research into the usefulness of cytotoxic agents for the treatment of arthritis continues. Recent observations (Martin and Gelfand, 1981) that certain enzyme deficiency states may play a role in precipitating opportunistic infections and immunodeficiency disease have led to the development of several inhibitors of these enzymes that inhibit T-lymphocyte function (Sircar and Gilbertsen, 1988; Gilbertsen and Sircar, 1990). These inhibitors may be useful in the treatment of rheumatoid arthritis. Additionally, several growth factors (PDGF, FGF, EGF, TNF, TGF-beta) are being investigated for their role in the treatment of inflammation, particularly to augment the wound healing process (Folkman and Klagsbrum, 1987). The role of hypoxic reperfusion injury on synovial inflammation has been revisited. A recent review by Merry et al. (1990) suggests that inflammatory changes in joints result from the generation of toxic free radicals, a phenomenon suggested for hypoxic cardiac injury. Based on this concept, efforts are being directed to the development of anti-oxidants and free radical scavengers for use in the treatment of inflammatory joint disease (Halliwell, Hoult and Blake, 1988).

The research and development effort required for the discovery of novel AI agents is both complex and competitive. In general the aforementioned agents and approaches are the product of our ever increasing understanding of the inflammatory process. This must be supported by the development of appropriate in vivo and in vitro animal models to evaluate potential AI drugs if we are to add significantly to the currently available armamentarium of AI agents.

IN VIVO ANIMAL MODELS

Table 2 lists some of the animal models frequently used to evaluate compounds that may be useful for treating inflammation and observing or measuring effects on systemic autoimmune diseases. These models represent both non-immunogenic and immunogenic stimuli for the induction of inflammation.

The carrageenin-induced acute paw edema model in rats (CARR), introduced by Winter et al. (1962), has been a handy tool to screen numerous potential AI drugs, some of which, following clinical evaluation, are currently being used in clinical practice. Recently, Otterness and Gans (1988) examined the results of four commonly used models to determine which was the best predictor of the human clinical dose of NSAIDs. They concluded that the CARR model showed the best dose proportionality between laboratory test dose and clinical dose. Dose was found to scale as body surface area for CARR. Thus, the measurement of plasma levels associated with pharmacologic response to drug over an appropriate period of time in this model could provide early insights into whether or not a pharmacokinetic-pharmacodynamic relationship might be useful in the clinical development of the drug along the lines suggested by Lieberman et al. (1991).

TABLE 2. In Vivo Animal Models

1.	Carrageenin-induced paw edema in rats
2.	Adjuvant-induced arthritis in rats
3.	Type II collagen-induced arthritis in rat and mouse models
4.	Spontaneous autoimmune model in mice.

The autoimmune models, e.g., adjuvant-induced and collagen-induced polyarthritis as well as allergic encephalomyelitis in rats, are extensively used for the preclinical evaluation of potential AI agents. Each of these models has specific advantages. Recently, it has been recognized that the adjuvant-induced model does not induce synovial change but rather represents a model of human periostitis (Billingham, 1990). When the clinical and pathological characteristics of rheumatoid arthritis and Reiter's syndrome in man are compared to adjuvant arthritis in rats it will be noticed that the rat model lacks rheumatoid factors. Therefore, use of this model to screen potential drugs that might modify the role of these factors may not be appropriate (Rainsford, 1982).

The Type II collagen-induced arthritic model described by Trentham et al. (1977) has several advantages over the adjuvant-induced model. Type II collagen-induced arthritis in rats or mice show both periostitis, synovitis (Billingham, 1990; Caufield et al., 1982; Stuart, Townes and Kang, 1982) and humoral immunity thus permitting a potential AI agent to be evaluated for its effectiveness in the presence of these conditions in two rodent species including rheumatoid factors.

The use of specific strains of mice, for example, MRL mice, to evaluate compounds for use in the treatment of systemic autoimmune disease has gained popularity as a model for screening potential immunomodulators or immunosuppressants (Popovic and Barlett, 1986; Rordorf-Adam and co-workers, 1986).

NEWER EXPERIMENTAL MODELS AND METHODS

Several published reviews (Billingham, 1990;Rainsford, 1982) on the development of AI drugs have focused on the inadequacy of existing models. It is important therefore to

TABLE 3. Newer Models and Methods

1. Development of Mycoplasma-induced arthritis in rabbits and swine
2. Transgenic animal model of arthritis
3. Models in which functional parameters can be measured.

address the need for developing newer models. Some suggestions based on literature findings over the last three decades are presented in Table 3 for consideration.

Mycoplasma-induced arthritis in rabbits and swine is a model we believe could be further explored. Although clinical evidence on the cause and effect relation between Myco- plasma infection and rheumatoid arthritis is unclear, there are reports in the veterinary literature (Cole and Cassell, 1979; Barden and Deeker, 1971) to suggest that one could use this model with a fair degree of reproducibility. The model could also provide help in selecting the animal species most susceptible to a selective class of compounds. For example, inhibitors of 5-lipoxygenase that are currently under development have shown inhibition of 5-HETE release in rats. However, these compounds do not appear efficacious when tested in the rat adjuvant model. Perhaps because the rat is not susceptible to 5-lipoxygenase catalyzed products. Thus, it might be worthwhile to test such compounds in another animal species, such as the rabbit, using the Mycoplasma-induced arthritic model. Apart from this, as proposed by several researchers (Cole and Cassell, 1979; Phillips, 1986) one can gain further knowledge from the mycoplasma model on the role of infectious agents in the pathogenesis of rheumatoid arthritis and other autoimmune diseases. Recent reports on the mechanisms of autoimmunity (Phillips, 1986; Friedman and co-workers, 1991) suggest that constituents of microorganisms may trigger autoimmune disease. Therefore, screening constituents of bacteria, fungi and viruses for their potential capability of inducing experimental arthritis in various species may be a worthwhile research endeavor.

With the advancement of methods related to recombinant DNA techniques and our knowledge of the genetic basis of autoimmune disease another worthwhile endeavor might involve exploring the usefulness of a transgenic animal model. The development of transgenic animal models that mimic the human arthritic condition may serve as a useful tool in the evaluation of potential AI compounds. Several laboratories are presently engaged in the development of transgenic mice which express major histocompatibility antigens (HLA-B27 and HLA-DQW6) to probe autoimmune responses leading to Type I diabetes, ankylosing spondylitis, thyroid disease and myasthenia gravis (Biotard, 1990; Campbell and Harrison, 1990; Chritadoss et al., 1990; Nickerson et al., 1990; Shinagawa, 1990, Taurog et al., 1988).

Improvement of the methods used for measuring the effects of potential AI compounds should also be considered a worthwhile endeavor. For the past two decades, measurement of the volume of the inflamed paws or joints has been the focus of drug efficacy determinations in preclinical screening procedures. However, such efficacy parameters do not reflect any functional improvement that may be related to treatment. If our goal is to develop AI agents that improve an arthritic patient's ability to function better, as opposed to an improvement of the pathological condition, the development and use of animal models that permit an evaluation of relevant functional parameters would be a worthwhile goal. For example, the development of a functional model based on the ability of an arthritic animal to walk a measurable distance or perform a certain task, following treatment with a potential AI drug candidate may be useful. Such an assessment in arthritic animals has been described by van Arman et al. (1970).

NEED FOR MARKERS

Recent research trends in the anti-inflammatory field have led to the synthesis and development of novel AI drugs that affect immunological responses associated with the inflammatory process. Thus, based on our knowledge of the expected mode of action of such drugs, it would be important to identify specific markers; for example: for macrophages, helper and suppressor T-lymphocytes, acute phase proteins, etc. that would be helpful in assessing the immunological usefulness of a compound to the anti-inflammatory process and to its clinical development.

IN VITRO MODELS

Some in vitro tests which may be used to confirm and optimize structure-activity relationships of any series of new molecular entities, designed on the basis of computerized modeling are given in Table 4. Since these tests may be conducted on both animal or human cells or cultured cell lines involved in the inflammatory process, they could confirm and establish in vitro species differences or similarites in the activity of the test compounds.

TABLE 4. In Vitro Models

1.	Platelet and neutrophil aggregation
2.	Lymphocyte proliferation assays
3.	Mixed lymphocyte reaction assays
4.	Mitogen-induced proliferation of T and B-lymphocytes, Molt-4 and MGL cell lines
5.	Assay for B, T_4 and T_8 lymphocyte markers.

PHARMACOKINETIC, PHARMACODYNAMIC AND TOXICITY RELATIONSHIPS

It is important to establish the existence, if any, of a relationship between the pharmacologic or toxicologic effect of a drug and/or its metabolites and its plasma and/or tissue concentration. Such information, generated during the preclinical stages of drug development or in early clinical trials, would be useful in the design of concentration controlled clinical trials and in assessing possible target organ toxicity of many drugs, including AI compounds under investigation.

Information on the physicochemical properties of a drug, for example: pK_a and plasma protein binding characteristics, is also useful. Brune et al. (1976) have suggested that pK_a and plasma protein binding characteristics may predict AI activity for cyclooxygenase inhibitors. Although a clear-cut reason for this phenomenon is not known, it can be speculated that highly bound AI drugs reach inflamed tissue sites to exert their pharmacologic effect through the extravasation of proteins resulting from a change in capillary permeability at the site of inflammation.

CONCLUSION

In the early 1960's a concerted effort was made to develop animal models for screening potential AI agents. This effort gave rise to several screening procedures which are being used today. We would like to encourage those engaged in anti-inflammatory drug discovery programs in the 1990's to revive the effort made in the 1960's and address once again the need: (1) for developing newer in vitro and in vivo animal models for screening potential new drug entities, (2) to develop specific immunologic markers that would be useful in evaluating novel compounds whose mechanism of action might affect immunologic responses involved in the disease process and, (3) to consider generating pharmacokinetic-pharmacodynamic (PK-PD) data early in the course of the drug development process together with information on drug plasma and tissue levels associated with possible adverse reactions observed during preclinical toxicity studies. These efforts would more than likely not only contribute to the discovery of AI drugs but also aid in a more rapid clinical evaluation of such drugs.

ACKNOWLEDGEMENTS

Authors are thankful to Dr. John G. Harter, Director, Pilot Drug Evaluation Staff for his suggestions towards the preparation of this review. We are also thankful to Ms. Karen Milbourne, Ms. Megen Beall, Ms. Jenny Veach and Mr. Clint Perez for typing the manuscript.

REFERENCES

Arthritis Foundation (1985). History of Rheumatology in the United States., pp. 115-142.

Barden, J. A., and J. L. Deeker (1971). Mycoplasma hyorhinis swine arthritis. 1. clinical and microbiological features. Arth. Rheum., 14, 193- 201.

Billingham, M. E. J. (1990). Models of arthritis and the search for antiarthritic drugs. In M. C. L. E. Orme (Ed.), Anti-rheumatic Drugs, Pergamon Press, New York. pp.1-47.

Biotard, C. (1990). Pathophysiology of the autoimmune diseases. Klin. Wochenschr, 68, 1 -9.

Brune, K., P. Graf, and M. Glatt (1976). Inhibition of prostaglandin synthesis in vivo by nonsteroidal anti-inflammatory drugs: evidence for the importance of pharmacokinetics. Agents and Actions, 6, 159-164.

Campbell, I. L., and L. C. Harrison (1990). Molecular pathology of type I diabetes. Mol. Biol., 7, 299-309.

Cannon, W. B., and J.E. Uridil (1921). Studies on the condition of activity in endocrine glands. VIII. Some effects on the denervated heart of stimulating the nerves of the liver. Am. J. Physiol., 58, 353-354.

Caufield, J. P., A. Hein, R. Dynesius-Trentham, and D. Trentham (1982). Morphologic demonstration of two stages in the development of type II collagen-induced arthritis. Lab. Invest., 46, 321-343.

Chritadoss, P., C. S. David, M. Shenoy, and S. Keve (1990). Alpha transgene in B10 mice suppresses the development of myasthenia gravis. Immunogenetics, 31, 241-244.

Cole, B. C. and G. H. Cassell (1979). Mycoplasma infections as models of chronic joint inflammation. Arth. Rheum., 22, 1375-1381.

Dinarello, C. A. (1984). Interleukin-1., Rev. Infec. Dis., 6, 51-95.

Dustin, M. L., R. Rothlein, A. K. Bhan, C. A. Dinarello, and T. A. Springer (1986). Induction by IL-1 and interferon-gamma: Tissue distribution, biochemistry, and function of natural adherence molecule (ICAM-1). J. Immunol., 137, 245-254.

Folkman, J., and M. Klagsbrum (1987). Angiogenic factors. Science, 235, 442-447.

Friedman, S. M., D. N. Posnett, J. R. Tumang, B. C. Cole, and M. K. Crow (1991). A potential role for microbial superantigens in the pathogenesis of systemic autoimmune disease. Arth. Rheum., 34, 468-480.

Gilbertsen, R. B., and J. C. Sircar (1990). Enzyme cascades: Purine metabolism and immunosuppression. In C. Hansch (Ed.), Comprehensive Medicinal Chemistry, Vol. 2, Pergamon Press, New York. pp. 443-480.

Halliwell, B., J. R. Hoult, and D. R. Blake (1988) Oxidants, inflammation, and anti-inflammatory drugs. FASEB J., 2, 2867-2873.

Hamberg, M., J. Svensson, and B. Samuelsson (1975). Thromboxanes: A new group of biologically active compounds derived from prostaglandin endoperoxides. Proc. Natl. Acad. Sci., 72, 2994-2998.

Hench, P. S., E. C. Kendall, C. H. Slocumb, and H. F. Polley (1949). Effect of a hormone of the adrenal cortex (17 hydroxy-11 dehydrocorticosterone), compound E and of pituitary adrenocortico-tropic hormone on rheumatoid arthritis: Preliminary report. Proc. Staff Meet. Mayo Clin., 24, 181.

Lieberman, R., M. Katzper, M.Cooper, C. Myers, G. Burke, L. Sanathanan, and C. Peck (1991). Bayesian PK concentration controlled trials of suramin anticancer therapy. Clin. Pharmacol. Ther., 49, 155.

Loewi, O., and E. Navratil (1926). Uber humorale Ubertragbarkeit der Herznervenwirkung. X. Mitteilung Uber das Schicksal des Vagusstoff. Pflugers Arch. Gesamte Physiol., 214, 678-688.

Marry, P., M. Grootveld, and D.R. Blake (1990). Free radicals and hypoxic reperfusion injury. A mechanism producing persistent synovitis. Topical Reviews, Arthritis Rheumatism Council, London.

Martin, D. A., and E. W. Gelfand (1981). Biochemistry of diseases of immunodevelopment. Ann. Rev. Biochem., 50, 845-877.

Mizel, S. B. (1989). The interleukins. FASEB.J., 3, 2379-2388.

Needleman, P., M. Minkes, and A. Raz (1976). Thromboxanes: Selective biosynthesis and distinct biological properties. Science, 193, 163-165.

Nickerson, C. L., K. L. Hogen, H. S. Luthra, and C. S. David (1990). Effect of H-2 genes on expression of HLA-B27 and Yersinia-induced arthritis. Scan. J. Rheum. Suppl., 87, 85-90.

Otterness, I. G., and D. J. Gans (1988). Nonsteroidal anti-inflammatory drugs: an analysis of the relationship between laboratory animal and clinical doses, including species scaling. J. Pharm. Sci., 77, 790-794.

Phillips, P. E. (1986). Infectious agents in the pathogenesis of rheumatoid arthritis. Seminars in Arth. Rheum., 16, 1-10.

Popovic, S., and R. R. Barlett (1986). Disease modifying activity of HWA 486 on the development of SLE in MRL/1-mice. Agents and Actions, 19, 313-314.

Rainsford, K. D. (1982). Adjuvant polyarthritis in rats: Is this a satisfactory model for screening antiarthritic drugs? Agents and Actions, 12, 452-458.

Rordorf-Adam, C., B. Rordorf, D. Serban, and A. Pataki (1986): The effects of anti-inflammatory agents on the serology and arthritis of the MRL 1pr/1pr mouse. Agents and Actions, 19, 309-310.

Samuelsson, B. (1983). Leukotrienes: Hypersensitivity reactions and inflammation. Science, 220, 568-575.

Shinagawa, H. (1990). The effects of HLA class II genes on the susceptability to autoimmune thyroid diseases. Fukuoka Igaku Zasshi. Fukuoka Acta Medica, 81, 97-111.

Sircar, J. C., and R. B. Gilbertsen (1988). Purine nucleoside phosphorylase (PNP) inhibitors: Potentially selective immunosuppressive agents. Drugs of the Future, 13, 653-668.

Springer, T. A., M. A. Dustin, T. K. Kishimoto, and S. D. Marlin (1987). The lymphocyte function-associated LFA-1, CD 2, and LFA-3 molecules: Cell adhesion receptors of the immune system. Ann. Rev. Immunol., 5, 223-252.

Stuart, J. M., A. S. Townes and A. H. Kang (1982). The role of collagen autoimmunity in animal models and human disease. J. Invest. Derm., 79, 121S-127S.

Taurog, J. D., J. P. Durand, F. A. el-Zaatari, and R. E. Hammer (1988). Studies of HLA-B27 associated disease. Am. J. Med., 85, 59-60.

Trentham, D. E., A. S. Townes, and A. H. Kang (1977). Autoimmunity to type II collagen: an experimental model of arthritis. J. Expt. Med., 146, 857-868.

van Arman, C. G., R. P. Carlson, E. A. Risley, R. H. Thomas, and G. W. Nuss (1970). Inhibitory effects of indomethacin, aspirin and certain other drugs on inflammation induced in rat and dog by carrageenin, sodium urate and ellagic acid. J. Pharmacol. Exp. Ther., 175, 459-468.

Vane, J. R. (1971). Inhibition of prostaglandin synthesis as a mechanism of action for aspirin like drugs. Nature (New Biol.), 231, 232-235.

Winter, C. A., E. A. Risley, and C. W. Nuss (1962). Carrageenin induced edema in hind paw of the rat as an assay for anti-inflammatory drugs. Proc. Soc. Expt. Biol. Med., 111, 544-547.

THE ROLE OF PHARMACOKINETICS IN THE DRUG DEVELOPMENT PROCESS

Leslie Z. Benet
Department of Pharmacy, University of California
San Francisco, CA 94143-0446

ABSTRACT

Ten critical pharmacokinetic and pharmacodynamic parameters should be determined for each new drug, both in test animal species and in man. These ten parameters, listed in order of importance, are: 1) clearance, 2) effective concentrations, 3) extent of availability, 4) fraction of the available dose excreted unchanged, 5) the blood/plasma concentration ratio, 6) half-life, 7) toxic concentrations, 8) protein binding, 9) volume of distribution, and 10) rate of availability.

INTRODUCTION

Pharmacokinetics serves as a useful tool in the drug development process both in terms of therapeutics and in defining the drug's disposition characteristics. Ten critical pharmacokinetic and pharmacodynamic parameters should be determined for each new drug both in test animal species and in man. These 10 parameters, in what I believe to be their order of importance in the drug development process are listed in Table 1.

The first three parameters are necessary to define the appropriate dosing rate (amount/day) of a drug by a particular route of administration. Most drugs are given as multiple doses achieving a particular steady-state relationship in each patient. Under those conditions, the following relationships hold:

$$Rate\ In = Rate\ Out \qquad\qquad (Eq.\ 1)$$

$$Availability \cdot Dosing\ Rate = Clearance \cdot Average\ Concentration \qquad (Eq.\ 2)$$

$$F \cdot Dose / \tau = CL \cdot Target\ Concentration \qquad\qquad (Eq.\ 3)$$

Integration of Pharmacokinetics, Pharmacodynamics, and Toxicokinetics in Rational Drug Development, Edited by A. Yacobi *et al.*, Plenum Press, New York, 1993

TABLE 1. The Critical Pharmacokinetic and Pharmacodynamic Parameters in Drug Development (in order of importance)

1.	Clearance
2.	Effective Concentration Range
3.	Extent of Availability
4.	Fraction of the Available Dose Excreted Unchanged
5.	Blood/Plasma Concentration Ratio
6.	Half-Life
7.	Toxic Concentrations
8.	Extent of Protein Binding
9.	Volume of Distribution
10.	Rate of Availability

The rate of drug input into the systemic circulation will be the availability (F) multiplied by the dose divided by the dosing interval (τ). At steady state, this rate of input will equal the rate of elimination of drug from the body which is defined as clearance (CL) multiplied by the measured concentration. For defining the appropriate dosing rate, then, the first three parameters in Table 1 are necessary. Equation 3 has particular usefulness in therapeutics where the appropriate dosing rate may be determined with knowledge of the effective concentrations of a drug for a particular disease state, the bioavailability of the drug via a particular route of administration and the systemic clearance of the drug in the patient. Such parameters are available for a number of drugs where average population estimates are presented, as well as the effect of particular disease conditions on these parameters. For example, see Benet and Williams (1990) where such a compilation for 243 drugs is presented.

Equation 3 may also be useful in the drug development process when one is attempting to evaluate whether a particular route of administration for a drug may be feasible. For example, the question is often asked as to whether a drug may be effectively administered by the transdermal route. Rearrangement of Equation 3 allows estimation of the dose per day that would be necessary to be transported across the skin:

$$Dose\ per\ Day = CL \cdot Target\ Concentration\ /\ F_{topical} \qquad (Eq.\ 4)$$

Data for the antihypertensive drug clonidine from Benet and Williams (1990) suggest that clearance averages 217 ml/min in a 70 kg man, while the effective target concentrations range from 0.2 - 2 ng/ml. Thus, even without knowing the topical bioavailability of such a compound, it is possible to calculate the available dose per day which must be administered by multiplying clearance times the target concentration yielding values of 0.062 - 0.62 mg/day. Obviously, such a delivery rate is achievable with commercial clonidine transdermal preparations labeled to yield 0.1, 0.2, or 0.3 mg/day.

Many readers may be surprised at the high placement I have given parameters 4 and 5 in Table 1. However, these are necessary to make one of the most important judgements in the drug development process. That is, can this drug be successfully marketed as an oral dosage form in man? Knowledge of the fraction of the dose excreted unchanged in urine allows one to estimate nonrenal clearance, which may be assumed to represent hepatic clearance. The blood to plasma concentration ratio allows one to convert the more easily measured plasma concentrations and their derived parameters into blood concentration measurements. Then, the ratio of the hepatic blood clearance to hepatic blood flow in each species subtracted from one, yields an estimate of the maximum oral bioavailability. This is depicted in Equations 5-7.

$$CL = CL_{renal} + CL_{nonrenal} = CL_{renal} + CL_{hepatic} + CL_{other} \qquad (Eq.\ 5)$$

$$CL_{organ} = Q_{organ} \cdot ER \qquad (Eq.\ 6)$$

$$F_{max} = 1 - \frac{CL_{hepatic}}{Q_{hepatic}} \qquad (Eq.\ 7)$$

As noted in Equation 5, nonrenal clearance includes both hepatic and all other clearance mechanisms besides the renal route. However, in most cases CL_{other} may be assumed to be negligible so that an estimate of $CL_{hepatic}$ may be obtained. As indicated in Equation 6, the clearance of any organ is equal to the blood flow to that organ (Q_{organ}) multiplied by the extraction ratio (ER). The maximum oral bioavailability (F_{max}), that is the bioavailability assuming complete dissolution in the GI fluids and complete absorption of the drug into the hepatic portal blood without loss due to degradation mechanisms in the GI fluids or in the gastrointestinal membranes, can be determined as one minus the hepatic extraction ratio as depicted in Equation 7. If the calculated F_{max} is a small number, then no amount of formulation or drug dosage regimen modification can improve the bioavailability of the drug. Furthermore, a small change in $CL_{hepatic}$ or $Q_{hepatic}$ in Equation 7 can yield a relatively large change in F_{max} when this value is quite low.

The importance of the blood/plasma ratio comes into play in attempting to utilize pharmacokinetic parameters determined from plasma concentrations to estimate F_{max}. This may be illustrated using pharmacokinetic parameters for the drug labetalol. For example, the tabulation in Goodman and Gilman (Benet and Williams, 1990) indicates that the oral bioavailability of this drug is 18 ± 5% while the plasma clearance is 1750 ± 700 ml/min/70kg. Urinary excretion of labetalol is less than 5% and elimination may be assumed to be almost exclusively via hepatic metabolism. The high plasma clearance value given above may present conceptual problems since this clearance is significantly greater than hepatic plasma flow which approximates 825 ml/min/70kg and even greater than hepatic blood flow of 1500 ml/min/70kg. Therefore, putting the plasma hepatic clearance and either of these flows into Equation 7 would result in a negative value for bioavailability. However, one must realize that the maximum clearance of an organ of elimination such as the liver is equal to the flow of drug to that organ, that is, the blood flow to the organ. Since drug may distribute into blood cells, when one only considers plasma elimination, a reservoir of drug in the blood cells is available to rapidly distribute back into the plasma. Thus, one must use the hepatic blood clearance and hepatic blood flow in Equation 7. Hepatic blood clearance for labetalol may be determined knowing that the blood to plasma ratio for the drug is 1.4, or alternatively, the blood cell to plasma concentration ratio and the hematocrit, the fraction of the blood made up of blood cells. The relationship between blood and plasma clearance, the blood to plasma ratio, or the blood cell to plasma ratio is given in Equation 8, where the subscripts b, p and bc indicate blood, plasma and blood cells, respectively.

$$\frac{CL_p}{CL_b} = \frac{C_b}{C_p} = 1 + H \left\{ \frac{C_{bc}}{C_p} - 1 \right\} \qquad (Eq.\ 8)$$

Utilizing the plasma clearance given above and the blood to plasma ratio for labetalol of 1.4, an average blood clearance of 1250 ml/min/70kg may now be determined. When this value is inserted into Equation 7 together with the hepatic blood flow of 1500 ml/min/70kg, then one calculates a predicted maximum bioavailability of 0.17, almost identical to the average 0.18 value listed above, determined experimentally.

As stated above, the maximum bioavailability should be calculated in each animal species evaluated, as well as in man, early in the drug development process to make a rational decision about the potential for further development of the drug in an oral dosage form. Drugs which exhibit very high first-pass hepatic metabolism should only be pursued in the drug development process when the chemical compound exhibits unique pharmacodynamic characteristics which justify development of a compound which will be expected to show high variability and low bioavailability in the patient population. Drug companies can save significant amounts of money in the drug development process by making a realistic assessment of the potential of achieving a marketable oral dosage form early in the development process. Too often in the past, statements such as "I don't care what the blood levels are, only the levels at the site of action" have led companies to pursue development of compounds exhibiting significant pharmacodynamic effects following intravenous administration in animals, eventually leading to "killing" the compound after significant investments in Phase III studies when it is then realized that if the drug does not yield blood levels following oral dosing, there is little chance that significant reproducible efficacy can be achieved via this route of administration.

To carry out such first pass analyses in animals, one must have an estimate of hepatic blood flow. Table 2, modified from Boxenbaum (1984), lists approximate values for hepatic blood flow in the species usually employed in pharmacokinetic studies during drug development.

Since initial studies will be carried out in animals, one may ask: Will a high hepatic clearance, low oral bioavailability drug in animals also exhibit similar characteristics in man? At this point in the development of correlations between animal and human drug metabolism, it is not possible to answer this question positively. Often drugs exhibiting high hepatic clearance, low first-pass bioavailability in animals will also show similar characteristics in man. However, at this stage in our understanding of the various metabolic isozymes, it is necessary to actually carry out studies in man to ascertain that what is observed in the animal models is relevant to man. In my experience, when the small and large animal species tested

TABLE 2. Hepatic Blood Flow (modified from Boxenbaum, 1984)

Species	ml/min/kg	L/hr/kg
mouse	86	5.2
rat	69	4.1
monkey	52	3.1
rabbit	44	2.7
dog	30	1.8
man	21.4	1.3

in preclinical drug evaluation both yield low first-pass bioavailability, this most likely will occur in man. However, this is not always true and decisions concerning potential bioavailability and variability in man must await actual studies in human volunteers.

Since the pioneering discussions of clearance in the early 1970s (Rowland and co-workers, 1973; Wilkinson and Shand, 1975), much has been made of the differences between high clearance (extraction ratio) and low clearance drugs and the interpretation of the effect of pathological and physiologic changes on drug kinetics. (See chapter 12 in Rowland and Tozer (1989) for an excellent discussion of these points.) Utilizing the venous equilibration, or well-stirred model, the relevant equations are presented in Figure 1.

The clearance equation in terms of a particular organ is presented at the top middle of the figure as Equation 9. For high extraction ratio drugs, clearance becomes almost exclusively

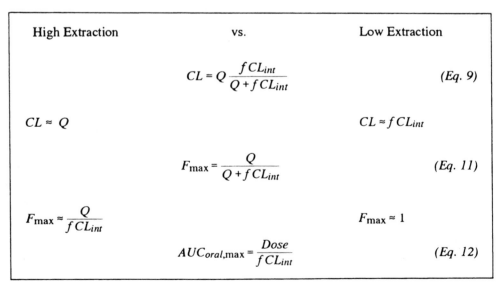

High Extraction   vs.   Low Extraction

$$CL = Q \frac{f CL_{int}}{Q + f CL_{int}} \qquad (Eq.\ 9)$$

$$CL \approx Q \qquad\qquad CL \approx f CL_{int}$$

$$F_{max} = \frac{Q}{Q + f CL_{int}} \qquad (Eq.\ 11)$$

$$F_{max} \approx \frac{Q}{f CL_{int}} \qquad\qquad F_{max} \approx 1$$

$$AUC_{oral,max} = \frac{Dose}{f CL_{int}} \qquad (Eq.\ 12)$$

Fig. 1. Critical equations utilizing the well-stirred model to define clearance, maximum oral bioavailability and maximum area under the curve following an oral dose for high extraction and low extraction ratio drugs.

dependent on organ blood flow, whereas for low extraction ratio drugs, clearance depends upon the fraction unbound in blood (f) and the intrinsic ability of the organ to remove drug independent of flow parameters, that is clearance intrinsic (CL_{int}). For example, for hepatic enzymatic elimination, clearance intrinsic would be a measure of the enzyme's ability to clear drug when the reaction is carried out in a beaker. In fact, it is now well recognized that the product of $f CL_{int}$ is the parameter best related to the Michaelis-Menten enzymatic saturability parameters of maximum velocity (V_{max}) and the Michaelis constant (K_m) as given in Equation 10, where C_{organ} is the concentration of drug in the organ of elimination.

$$f CL_{int} = \frac{V_{max}}{K_m + C_{organ}} \qquad (Eq.\ 10)$$

Thus, it is obvious from Figure 1 that high extraction ratio drugs will not exhibit saturable elimination kinetics or be affected by changes in protein binding or by stimulation or inhibition of the elimination process. Likewise, low extraction ratio drugs will not be affected by changes in blood flow to the organ. However, when the maximum bioavailability is predicted utilizing Equation 11 in the middle of Figure 1, then it can be seen that the oral bioavailability of a high extraction ratio drug will be affected by all three of the parameters defining clearance, whereas low extraction ratio drugs are unaffected by these changes since first-pass metabolism is essentially negligible. As mentioned above, much has been made of the comparison of clearance and bioavailability for low and high extraction ratio compounds. However, both in therapeutics and in drug development, the primary concern will be with actual area under the curve following the oral dose since this will be a measure of how much drug becomes available by the most popular route of administration. Equation 12 at the bottom of Figure 1 indicates that the area under the curve for an oral dose, independent of the magnitude of the extraction ratio, will be inversely related to the fraction of drug unbound in the blood and the clearance intrinsic of the organ, and independent of blood flow to the organ. Thus, in patients where a change may occur due to a pathological condition or when we are comparing one subset of patients with another, for example elderly versus children, it is important to realize that Equation 12 will always be useful in interpreting the effects of pathological and physiological variables.

Returning to Table 1, half-life and toxic concentrations are listed as the next critical parameters to be considered. Half-life is a very important parameter in therapeutics, since half-life defines the dosing interval. After determining the extent of oral drug bioavailability and the other parameters necessary to define it, half-life is probably the next most important parameter in terms of deciding the appropriateness of a drug for further development. Drugs with very short half-lives create problems in maintaining steady-state concentrations in the therapeutic range and a successful drug product will require a dosage form which allows a relatively constant prolonged input . Drugs with a very long half-life are favored in terms of efficacy considerations, however, this long half-life may be a negative in terms of toxicity considerations. Figure 2 illustrates the importance of half-life in defining the dosing interval.

The figure depicts the relationship between the frequency of theophylline dosing and the plasma concentration time course when a steady-state theophylline plasma level of 15 µg/ml is desired. The smoothly rising curve shows the plasma concentrations achieved with an intravenous infusion of 0.667 mg/min or 40 mg/h to a 68 kg woman exhibiting an average theophylline clearance of 0.65 ml/min/kg. The steady-state theophylline plasma level achieved is midway within the therapeutic concentration range of 10-20 μg/ml. The figure also depicts the time course for eight hourly administration of 320 mg and 24 hourly administration of 960 mg. In each case the mean steady-state concentration is 15 μg/ml. However, the peak to trough ratio and the concentrations achieved with the once daily dosing of a rapidly released formulation would result in concentrations in the toxic range, exceeding 20 μg/ml for certain periods of time, as well as concentrations expected to not yield efficacy, i.e. less than 10 μg/ml, for significant periods during each dosing interval. In contrast, the eight hourly dosing, which is approximately equivalent to the half-life of theophylline, shows a two-fold range in peak to trough which stays within the therapeutic plasma concentration range.

Although half-life is a very important parameter in therapeutics, defining the dosing interval, half-life can be a very misleading parameter when one is attempting to use pharmacokinetics as a tool in defining drug disposition. As depicted in Equation 13, half-life may vary as a function of both of the two physiologic-related parameters, volume and clearance.

$$t \, ^1\!/_2 = \frac{0.693 \cdot V}{CL} \qquad\qquad (Eq. \ 13)$$

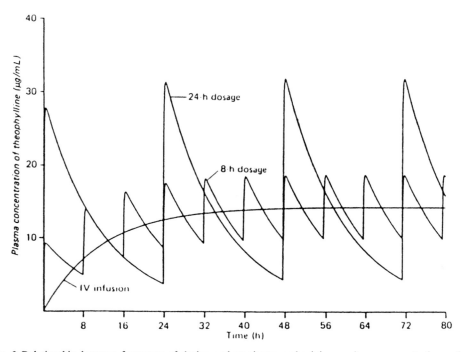

Fig. 2 Relationship between frequency of dosing and maximum and minimum plasma concentrations when a steady-state theophylline plasma level of 15 μg/ml is desired. The time course of plasma concentrations for a 0.667 mg/ml infusion, an 8 hourly 320 mg oral dose and a 960 mg, 24 hourly dose are depicted. Reproduced from Benet (1992) with permission.

For example, as Klotz and co-workers (1975) have shown, the increase in half-life of diazepam with age does not result from a decrease in clearance but rather due to an increase in volume as the patient ages. Clearance, a measure of the body's ability to eliminate the drug, does not significantly decrease with age. However, when volume increases, less drug is in the blood flowing to the liver, the major organ of elimination, and thus the time that the drug remains in the body is increased.

Yet half-life is an important parameter in therapeutics, since this parameter defines the dosing interval at which drugs should be administered. Half-life also describes the time required to attain steady-state or to decay from steady-state conditions after a change in the dosage regimen. Equation 13 describes the half-life relationship for a drug that appears to follow one-compartment body kinetics. However, many drugs appear to exhibit multiple half-lives and these are reported in the literature usually designated as "distribution" and "terminal elimination" half-lives. Defining the "relevant" half-life in such situations has been addressed by Benet and co-workers (Benet, 1984; Ferraiolo and Benet, 1985; Gloff and Benet, 1990). More recently, Benet has described so-called multiple dosing half-lives, the half-life for a drug which is equivalent to the dosing interval to choose so that plasma concentrations (Equation 14) or amounts of drug in the body (Equation 15) will show a 50% drop during a dosing interval at steady-state. These parameters are defined in terms of the mean residence time in the central compartment (MRTC) and the mean residence time in the body (MRT).

$$t_{\frac{1}{2}_{MD}}^{plasma} = 0.693 MRTC \qquad (Eq.\ 14)$$

$$t_{\frac{1}{2}_{MD}}^{amount} = 0.693 MRTC \qquad (Eq.\ 15)$$

The eighth parameter listed in Table 1, the extent of protein binding, has already been discussed in terms of Figure 1. The ninth parameter, volume of distribution, has been a subject of controversy since a number of volume parameters may be calculated in pharmacokinetics. It is probably worthwhile to enumerate why we want to know volume of distribution. First, volume allows us to predict steady-state concentrations, particularly maximum and trough values. In addition, knowledge of volume allows one to predict the ability of dialysis to remove drug from the body. Drugs exhibiting large volumes of distribution are characterized by little drug in the blood, and therefore dialysis cannot be very successful in removing a significant quantity of drug from the body since the dialyzer, like an organ of elimination, can only remove drug in the blood flowing through it. Of most importance is the use of volume to determine whether disease states affect drug distribution rather than clearance (while could lead to half-life changes independent of changes in organs of elimination). The diazepam example given above reflects this use. The volume of distribution steady-state (V_{ss}) is the most appropriate volume to consider when determining this parameter. V_{ss} is the value which relates concentrations of drug in the systemic circulation to the amount of drug in the body during multiple dosing.

I consider the rate of availability the least important of the critical parameters listed in Table 1, since it is most amenable to investigator modification in the drug development process. Note that I have not listed pharmacokinetic model parameters as critically important, since in most cases, particularly at steady-state, the one-compartment body model, defined by parameters 1, 6, 9 and 10 will suffice for what I believe is the critical need for data modeling, that is, for use in developing pharmacokinetic /pharmacodynamic models, the major subject of this book.

REFERENCES

Benet, L. Z. (1984). Pharmacokinetic parameters: which are necessary to define a drug substance?. Eur. J. Resp. Dis., 65, Suppl. 134, 45-61.

Benet, L. Z., and R.L. Williams (1990). Design and optimization of dosage regimens: pharmacokinetic data. In A. G. Gilman, T. W. Rall, A. S. Nies and P. Taylor (Eds.), The Pharmacological Basis of Therapeutics, 8th ed. Pergamon Press, New York. pp. 1650-1735.

Benet, L.Z. (1992). Pharmacokinetics: absorption, distribution and elimination. In B.G. Katzung (Ed.), Basic and Clinical Pharmacology, 5th ed. Appleton and Lange, Norwalk, Connecticut. pp. 35-48.

Boxenbaum, H. (1980). Interspecies variation in liver weight, hepatic blood flow, and antipyrine intrinsic clearance: extrapolation of data to benzodiazepines and phenytoin. J. Pharmacokinet. Biopharm., 8, 165-176.

Ferraiolo, B. L., and L. Z. Benet (1985). Pharmacodynamic considerations in the development of new drug delivery concepts. In R. T. Borchardt, A. J. Repta, and V. J. Stella (Eds.), Directed DrugDelivery: The Multi- disciplinary Problem, The Humana Press, Clifton, New Jersey. pp. 13-33.

Gloff, C. A., and L. Z. Benet (1990). Pharmacokinetics and protein therapeutics. Advanced Drug Delivery Reviews, 4, 359-386.

Klotz, U., G. R. Avant, A. Hoyumpa, S. Schenker, and G. R. Wilkinson (1975). The effects of age and liver disease on the disposition and elimination of diazepam in adult man. J. Clin Invest., 55, 347-359.

Rowland, M., L. Z. Benet, and G. G. Graham (1973). Clearance concepts in pharmacokinetics. J.Pharmacokinet. Biopharm., 1, 123-135.

Wilkinson, G., and D.G. Shand (1975). The physiological approach to hepatic blood clearance. Clin. Pharmacol. Ther., 18, 377-390.

IMPLEMENTATION OF AN EFFECTIVE PHARMACOKINETICS RESEARCH PROGRAM IN INDUSTRY

Avraham Yacobi, Vijay K. Batra, Robert E. Desjardins,
Robert D. Faulkner, Gabriela Nicolau, William R. Pool,
Anita Shah and Alfred P. Tonelli
American Cyanamid Company
Medical Research Division, Pearl River, NY 10965

ABSTRACT

Over the past decade the application of pharmacokinetic data in drug development has gradually increased. Today it is well recognized that successful drug development programs include meaningful supportive pharmacokinetic data. An effective pharmacokinetic program begins at the preclinical phase with well defined objectives to support pharmacology/toxicology programs, to determine effective/toxic blood concentration ranges and to help in expediting early phase I studies in man. The clinical pharmacokinetic program may be classified as follows: i) pharmacokinetics during safety and tolerance studies in man to determine key pharmacokinetic parameters including linearity over the utilized dose range, and related effective and toxic blood concentrations; ii) pivotal pharmacokinetic studies to determine metabolism profile and major active/inactive metabolite(s) in man, extent of first-pass metabolism, absolute and/or relative bioavailability, effect of food on absorption, dose proportionality, route and mechanism of elimination, bioequivalency of final dosage forms and to establish therapeutic dosing regimens; and iii) studies supporting labeling to determine pharmacokinetics in special populations, effect of disease states and interactions with concomitantly administered drugs. A successful pharmacokinetic program is done prospectively to support the design of safety evaluation studies, to assist in expediting the Phase I/II programs, and to facilitate the Phase III trials in patients.

INTRODUCTION

The development of a new chemical entity (NCE) from discovery to therapeutic use is a long, complex and very costly process which may consume $100-200 million over a period

Integration of Pharmacokinetics, Pharmacodynamics, and Toxicokinetics in Rational Drug Development, Edited by A. Yacobi *et al.*, Plenum Press, New York, 1993

of 5-10 years. The seemingly unrealistic cost is attributed largely to regulatory demands and partially to the industry's uncertainty relative to what is actually needed to prove safety and efficacy of a NCE. Further, the failure to plan prospectively and lack of a systematic approach to drug development has compounded the complexity and cost of drug development.

During the past two years, the FDA has proposed the effective use of pharmacodynamics and pharmacokinetics in drug development with the primary focus to reduce the time and cost of developing a NCE (see pages 1-5). In fact, advanced new drug development programs utilize pharmacokinetic, pharmacodynamic and metabolism studies to support early new molecule screening and safety and efficacy studies of NCEs in animals and man.

The application of pharmacokinetics in the preclinical stages of drug development is as important as that for clinical development. For instance, critical to the proposed expedited dosing escalation strategy in Phase I clinical oncology trials is the availability of pharmacokinetic and pharmacodynamic data in animals (Collins, pages 49-53; Collins et al., 1986 and 1990; Gianni et al., 1990).

As the NCE enters the development stage, the availability of essential toxicokinetic data can be instrumental in the conduct of safety evaluation testings and in the understanding of the toxicity data (Barry and Yacobi, 1984; Yacobi, Krasula and Lai, 1984; Batra and Yacobi, 1989; de la Iglesia and Greaves, 1989). Although the basic principles and needs for pharmacokinetic data may apply to all NCEs, the development of a definitive pharmacokinetic program must consider the type and class of NCEs. The objectives of the pharmacokinetic program should be defined accordingly.

An effective pharmacokinetic program needs to be prospectively planned with clear objectives. Each study should be conducted to generate definitive information. It is equally important to avoid studies which are not needed and may fall under the category of: nice to do; may be needed; may be required by the regulatory bodies; or, may be nothing more than "icing on the cake." Non-definitive studies can cause unnecessary clutter and become a significant budget drain on an already very complex program. Any additional studies with clear-cut academic values should be treated accordingly and contracted out at a later time to academic programs.

The purpose of this presentation is to discuss the key elements of an effective pharmacokinetics research program to support the development of a new drug.

II. Discovery Support Pharmacokinetics

By definition, the pharmacologic effect exerted by a drug is related to its concentration in the body. Therefore, to be effective, a chemical entity commonly intended for oral use should demonstrate: a) favorable physicochemical properties for absorption; b) a structure which does not lend itself to extensive first-pass metabolism; c) favorable elimination and stability characteristics in the body to allow it to reach the blood circulation in sufficient concentration at the site of action; and, d) receptor affinity to exert a specific pharmacologic action.

Early pharmacokinetic evaluation of potential NCEs from a given class of compounds can provide pivotal information to select a more successful candidate. A basic requirement in these pharmacokinetic studies is the availability of a suitable analytical procedure to quantitate the concentrations of drug in biologic fluids. Once available, the analytical method supports the characterization of the initial pharmacokinetic profile of NCE candidates. For example, basic pharmacokinetic data of two potential NCE analogs with a similar pharmacologic spectrum, were compared in rats and dogs using the same dose and under similar conditions. One of the compounds produced higher blood concentrations than the other with a bioavailability of 82 vs 21% in rats and 87 vs 10% in dogs (approximately four- and eight-fold difference, respectively), and a longer half-life of 1 hour vs 0.5 hour.

The NCE with the more favorable pharmacokinetic characteristics was recommended for further development. Interestingly, in the initial ascending dose clinical trials in normal subjects, pharmacokinetic profiles, similar to those observed in animals, were found for the two NCEs.

III. Preclinical Pharmacokinetics

i. **Bioanalytical Considerations** Once a NCE is selected as a clinical lead, a preclinical program is developed to prepare an "Investigational New Drug (IND)" application. Among the highest priority items is a commitment to establish rugged analytical methodologies. From the beginning, it is very likely that sample analyses may potentially become rate-limiting throughout the development of the drug, thereby complicating the conduct of pharmacokinetic, pharmacodynamic, metabolism and key safety and efficacy studies. Also, if the analytical methods do not provide accurate quantitation of the drug and metabolites, all results and derived conclusions will be questionable.

To avoid these pitfalls, the following analytical factors need careful consideration: a) availability of specific methodologies and the source of procedures for estimating the drug and its metabolite(s); b) quality assurance and methods validation which will assure the ruggedness of the assay; c) re-validation at each drug analysis site prior to methods utilization; d) feedback and adjustments when needed on the assay's sensitivity requirements during different stages of drug development; e) fine tuning and modification due to interfering endogenous and exogenous compounds in different populations, drug interaction studies and disease states, (these situations may require further improvement to assure adequate sensitivity or the specificity of the assay); f) unanticipated problems or breakdown in quantitation; and, g) timing of drug analysis turnaround which may determine the pace of drug development.

Close bioanalytical interaction with clinical and the project development team will keep all aware of possible pitfalls and will allow for expeditious adjustments in analytical and development strategy when needed.

ii. **Supporting Pharmacodynamics in Animal Models** Pharmacokinetics offers a unique opportunity to support early pharmacology studies in animal models. Its use allows the characterization of the pharmacologic effect versus blood drug concentration profiles which can serve as a common basis for safety evaluation studies in animals and in early Phase I safety-tolerance studies in man. The variability associated with the quantitation of pharmacologic action is often greater than that seen for blood concentrations.

127

Thus, development of pharmacodynamic models would require appropriate methodologies to quantitate an effect or a surrogate parameter using reproducible mathematical models to relate effect to blood concentrations of drug and/or active metabolite(s). The measured effect should be related to the intended indications for which the drug is developed. Also, these methodologies developed in animal models may assist in evaluating procedures to measure effect and to prospectively validate the methodologies in man.

iii. Absorption, Distribution, Metabolism and Excretion (ADME) Several key parameters, which directly influence the drug behavior in the body, must be characterized to support the safety evaluation studies in animals:

a) Oral Bioavailability from Toxicology Delivery Systems - The drug is usually administered in suspension or solution, in diet or in a solid dosage form. In safety evaluation studies, relatively large doses are administered to test species. It is essential to know the extent of bioavailability for all doses. Since absorption process(es) may become saturated at higher doses, it is critical to ascertain that extent of bioavailability is proportional to the increase in dose. Duration and extent of drug exposure depends on the extent and rate of absorption.

b) Tissue Distribution - It is important to determine drug disposition in the body, in target organs and tissues, particularly those which are the sites of pharmacologic/toxicologic action, excretion and metabolism. Also, the use of a radiolabelled compound becomes extremely helpful to determine persistence and potential accumulation of the NCE in tissues. This information will be used to determine dosimetry to support potential metabolism studies in man.

c) Mass Balance and Elimination Pathways - It is critical to determine both the metabolic fate and elimination pathway(s) of a NCE. The pathway of excretion (e.g. in urine or in bile), as unchanged compound or after biotransformation, and the relative amounts in the excreta will provide basic information on the excretion behavior of the NCE in vivo. This information is useful in evaluating if the elimination pathways in man and toxicology species are qualitatively similar.

d) Metabolism - Biotransformation can be a major pathway of elimination. The knowledge of individual metabolites, particularly those that are active, can be very helpful. The pharmacologic action of the metabolites should be characterized as early as possible. More importantly, the safety profile of the major metabolites should be evaluated rapidly. Metabolism studies in toxicology species have become of major importance in drug development. Preferably, the metabolism profiles in these species are comparable to that in man. During the course of metabolism studies, several scenarios may be possible:

1) the drug may be converted to active metabolites in which case, the relative potency and the pharmacokinetics of the metabolites need to be determined. For instance, a prodrug is quantitatively converted to an active metabolite;

2) a major pharmacologically inactive metabolite is formed in which case, its pharmacokinetics in disease state (i.e., renal and/or hepatic impairment) may become important;
3) a major inactive metabolites might compete with endogenous and/or exogenous
   compounds for protein binding sites or receptor binding. As a result, its safety in
   toxicology species to support clinical studies needs to be determined;
4) minor active metabolites may be formed in which case, the importance of characterizing their pharmacokinetics will depend on the relative potency and the effect
   elicited on the body;
5) minor inactive metabolites do not require any additional work;
6) first-pass metabolism is often saturable and largely depends on the rate of absorption (characterization of its impact on bioavailability will have important consequences for development of oral sustained release formulations which by design
   have a slower rate of release and the absorption resulting in a greater extent of metabolism); and
7) for racemic drugs, stereoselective metabolism will help establish the ratio of enantiomers in the body; this is important when one enantiomer is much more active
   than the other and when there is a significant difference in their rate of metabolism and elimination (Eichelbaum and Somogyi, 1984; Eichelbaum, Mikus and
   Vogelgesang, 1984; Echizen and co-workers, 1985a and 1985b).

e) Protein Binding - The free drug concentration (unbound to plasma proteins) in blood
is responsible for eliciting pharmacologic/toxicologic action and for elimination of the
drug from the body. The relationships between body clearance and free fraction in
plasma and between pharmacologic action and free blood concentrations of the drug
are well established. When plasma protein binding is relatively low, the total plasma
concentrations will adequately describe the pharmacokinetics and pharmacodynamics
of drugs. For extensively bound drugs, however, it may be more realistic to use as a
guide, effective/toxic free drug concentrations rather than total levels (free and bound
to proteins) in blood. For example, pharmacokinetic data were obtained for a cardiovascular drug given intravenously in rats (5 mg/kg), dogs (3 mg/kg), and man (0.5
mg/kg). The respective drug protein binding was 70, 85 and 95% corresponding with
free fractions of 30, 15 and 5%. At these dose levels, there was about a two-fold
difference in total Cmax between man (0.2 mcg/ml) and rats and dogs (0.4 mcg/ml).
Calculations of the free Cmax of the drug, however, showed a twelve-fold difference
between rats and man (0.12 vs 0.01 mcg/ml) and a seven-fold difference between dogs
and man (0.07 vs 0.01 mcg/ml). These free concentration data demonstrate that at a
given total plasma concentration, the drug will elicit a much higher effect in rats and
dogs than in man. Furthermore, the relative exposure to the drug is much greater when
the active moeity, i.e. the free concentration, is taken into account.

f) Enzyme Induction - the knowledge of potential enzyme induction is important for a
number of reasons. Most importantly, it may help in the interpretation of safety data
when the blood concentrations of the NCE unexpectedly diminish or the blood concen-

trations of metabolite(s) uncharacteristically elevate. Liver enzyme induction may also result in proliferation of the smooth endoplasmic reticulum systems and in an increase in liver weight and possible hepatic toxicity. Enzyme induction is usually dependent on the size of the dose and duration of dosing.

IV. Supporting Safety Evaluation Studies

Safety evaluation studies are typically conducted in two different animal species, utilizing at least three different dose levels (high, intermediate and low) and a control group. A key to the success of any toxicology program is the selection of the appropriate dose levels following the initial dose range-finding study.

Toxicokinetic data assists in the selection of a dosing regimen based on both achieved toxicity and estimated blood levels from earlier pharmacodynamic studies. Equally important is to determine the maximum blood levels (Cmax) and area under the blood concentration vs time curve (AUC) values of the drug that are associated with the highest no-effect dose and to a dose which produces the desired pharmacologic action. Determination of blood and/or tissue levels at toxic doses following dose-escalation provides basic information which may be used as a reference in future studies. This approach may be of particular interest in the evaluation of target organ toxicity.

In safety evaluation studies, where eliciting severe toxicity and mortality is not the intended end point, monitoring blood concentrations may be useful to avoid accumulation of excessive levels in the body.

As discussed earlier, the rate and extent of absorption of the drug plays a major role in the extent and duration of body exposure. At high doses, where absorption may be limited by solubility or saturable process(es), lack of dose proportionality or dose-dependent absorption may limit systemic exposure.

An important factor in the safety study design is defining a dosing frequency which does not result in excessive drug and/or metabolite accumulation. Ideally, dosing frequency should mimic that intended in man. However, due to physical and practical limitations, this may not always be possible. Knowledge of toxicokinetic parameters should allow a dosing regimen and dosing frequency which will produce the most reliable safety evaluation data under the desired study conditions.

Prior awareness of drug disposition and biotransformation also allows a better understanding of dose-response or blood concentration-response of the drug and its metabolite(s), particularly, if the latter is active.

Other pivotal toxicokinetic information is related to placental transfer and excretion in milk which will directly support reproduction as well as age related studies. The absorption and clearance of most drugs can be both dose- and age-dependent. In neonates and young animals, the elimination rate from the body may be significantly less than that in adult animals. Similarly, in old animals, age-related changes in physiologic parameters may result in significant alteration in toxicokinetic parameters. An early evaluation of key parameters will help in the development of dosing regimen for safety evaluation studies at different ages. This information, together with the knowledge of effective/toxic blood levels, would also allow one to monitor blood concentrations during long-term safety evaluation studies and to properly adjust doses to avoid excessive toxicity.

V. Species Differences

Key to the success of the initial clinical program are the early estimates of safe and potentially effective doses based on extrapolation from preclinical safety and efficacy data. In reality, this process is quite complicated due to large interspecies differences in the ADME of a NCE, which in turn may result in large differences in the response among the animals. From the anatomical, physiological and biochemical standpoint, mammals are remarkably similar. The major difference among the species is the body size, which may affect the size and performance of the internal organs. The exploitation of the similarities and differences has allowed interspecies scaling of some pharmacokinetic parameters with significant findings which might allow a more successful transition from the preclinical to the clinical stages of drug development (Boxenbaum, 1984; Campbell and Ings, 1988; Mordenti and Chappel, 1989).

The allometric analysis of the pharmacokinetic parameters require definitive ADME studies in several animal species (at least three) which are used in pharmacology and safety evaluation studies.

These studies may include mice, rats, rabbits, dogs and monkeys, which allow several orders of magnitude difference in body weight. Estimates of pharmacokinetic parameters such as elimination rate constants, volume of distribution, total body clearance and AUC values, may facilitate the development of dosing regimens in man.

Another key component in preclinical safety evaluation studies is the interspecies comparison of the metabolism profiles (Rahmani et al., 1988; Fabre et al., 1990). Early in-vitro metabolism studies would allow qualitative comparison between man and animal species used in toxicology studies. Further, as early as possible in development, in-vivo metabolism studies in man will provide for invaluable and timely information for the toxicologist to re-evaluate safety studies in animals with respect to adequate safety and ADME data to reconcile and compliment any differences in metabolite(s) blood concentrations between man and toxicology species.

Species differences in protein binding should be carefully evaluated for highly protein bound NCEs. It is critical that in any extrapolation of effective/toxic blood concentrations proper adjustments are made for the protein bound fractions.

Overall, teamwork and joint effort among toxicology, clinical and pharmacokinetic/pharmacodynamic scientists is essential for a systematic approach to drug development. This has a potential to reduce the scope and the number of preclinical and clinical studies, which in turn will result in significant cost reduction during the drug development program.

VI. Clinical Pharmacokinetic Program

Depending on the purpose of the program, in many cases, pharmacokinetics is referred to as either Phase I or Phase IV studies. This classification, however, does not adequately describe the utilization of pharmacokinetics in the overall clinical development program. In this presentation, the clinical pharmacokinetic program in support of Phases I-III are divided as follows: a) pharmacokinetics during safety and tolerance studies; b) pivotal pharmacokinetic studies; and (c) studies supporting labeling. The pharmacokinetic program to support Phase IV clinical trials and ANDA's is not discussed here.

a) Pharmacokinetics During Safety and Tolerance Studies - Pharmacokinetics of a NCE is characterized as part of the Phase I safety studies (single and multiple dose) in which for the first time, the NCE is given to a small population of normal subjects (with the exception of cytotoxic NCEs which are tested in patients). Based on preclinical data, a small starting dose, usually subtherapeutic, is administered and then carefully escalated until some clinically significant adverse reaction is observed, the desired clinical endpoint is achieved, or predefined values of peak blood concentration and/or AUC is attained.

In addition to the safety assessment, the following pharmacokinetic objectives may be met during the Phase I studies: 1) to characterize the pharmacokinetics of the NCE in man; 2) to facilitate dosing escalation in man utilizing preclinical effective/toxic blood concentrations as the target endpoint and the observed pharmacokinetic profile in the subjects; 3) to assess linearity of pharmacokinetics in subjects (in the absence of a significant deviation from linearity this study may adequately describe dose-proportionality over a broad range of doses); 4) to determine accumulation potential of the NCE and/or its metabolite(s) during multiple dose tolerance studies; 5) to estimate the projected maximum tolerated blood concentration which is associated with the highest dose in man after single and multiple dosing; and 6) to use the pharmacokinetic and safety profiles in man together with pharmacodynamic data in animals to select dosing regimen for Phase II studies.

b) Pivotal Pharmacokinetic Studies - These studies are designed to fully characterize the pharmacokinetics of a NCE and to develop basic information described below which will help facilitate the safety and efficacy trials in man. These studies are:

1) Absolute and/or relative bioavailability (as compared to a rapidly absorbed formulation) of a NCE should be determined as early as possible. This basic information is useful in dosing selection. The bioavailability data will provide information on the magnitude of the first pass metabolism, if any, which is critical in developing optimal delivery systems. Also, it will help in the design of oral controlled release dosage forms, if necessary.

2) Effect of food on absorption may be critical to the timing of drug administration. Drugs, which are primarily absorbed from the upper regions of the gastrointestinal tract, may be affected by food which commonly delays gastric emptying and alters both gastric motility and gastric pH. Poorly water soluble drugs which are poorly absorbed from the gastrointestinal tract, may be most influenced by food. Furthermore, food may indirectly influence drug absorption by affecting release of the drug from the formulation in the stomach.

3) Metabolism issues were described earlier in the preclinical section of this chapter. The basic principles also apply in man. Determination of mass balance, the metabolism pathways and the identification of metabolite(s) in man serves the following key purposes: i) if a metabolite(s) is active, the relative contribution to the overall effect will be assessed and a decision will be made to characterize the pharmacokinetics and pharmacodynamics of the metabolite in man; ii) for safety evaluation purposes, by virtue of metabolism of the NCE in-vivo, the metabolite will be evaluated for toxicity findings. As stated before, it is preferable, therefore, that the metabolism profiles in the toxicology species are comparable to that in man; iii) inactive major metabolite(s) may interact with concomitantly administered drugs or may accumulate in the body due to a disease condition (e.g. renal impairment). This will necessitate a decision relative to the quantitation of the major inactive metabolite in relevant pharmacokinetic studies; and iv) these data will serve as a guide in developing analytical procedures to support the pharmacokinetics and pharmacodynamics of the metabolite(s) in man and animals.

4) Pharmacokinetics and pharmacodynamics as part of the Phase II program will provide basic information in the design of effective dosing regimens for safety and efficacy trials in patients. These studies will assess the blood concentrations associated with drug response and potential adverse reactions. Depending on the extent of protein binding, these blood concentrations may be expressed as total (free and bound to proteins) or free (unbound fraction of the total concentrations). The effective and toxic blood concentration ranges, together with the pharmacokinetic parameters of the NCE, will facilitate dosing selection and adjustments in individual patients.

c) Pharmacokinetic Studies Supporting Labeling - These studies are conducted to collect important data which may help in dosing adjustments in different populations and in disease states. Upon approval of the drug, the data are also documented in the package insert for the practitioner and ultimately the patient's benefit. Some of these studies may be needed to support the Phase III programs; others should be considered as part of Phase IV. These studies are:

1. Age-dependent pharmacokinetics (elderly and pediatric population). The studies which are commonly conducted in a normal elderly population may not produce any meaningful data. Any differences from a younger population may be related to some factors including impairment of renal, hepatic or cardiac functions. In such cases, it may be prudent to conduct pharmacokinetic studies in an elderly group as part of other studies specifically designed for a disease state. For example, pharmacokinetic parameters for an antibiotic drug which is primarily excreted unchanged by the kidneys was compared between young and elderly volunteers. Some insignificant changes in various pharmacokinetic parameters were observed and were related to renal function. For other drugs, significant alteration in pharmacokinetics have been observed in which case, a study in an appropriate elderly population will be needed. In the normal pediatric population, however, where the excretory organs have not reached maturity, pharmacokinet-

ics of most drugs will differ with age and pivotal pharmacokinetic parameters will be helpful in individualization of effective doses. In the case of an antibiotic in pediatric patients, there were significant differences in the clearance of the drug in different age groups. Therefore, the clearance values were used in dosing selection.

2. Effect of disease state, particularly hepatic and renal impairment which are primary routes of metabolism and excretion, respectively, need to be studied. These studies are critical depending on the pathway of the drug elimination from the body. If the drug is primarily excreted unchanged in urine, the hepatic impairment study may not add any significant pharmacokinetic information. Also, if the drug undergoes extensive metabolism and the metabolite(s) are eliminated in the bile, the renal impairment study should not be considered critical. If the metabolite(s) is eliminated by the kidneys, a renal impairment/failure study may be needed to ascertain metabolite elimination from the body.

3. Other studies such as population kinetics, gender effect, drug interactions, tissue levels (antibiotic), polymorphic metabolism, etc. should be considered on a case-by-case basis and may not be necessary as part of early drug development but should be considered in the Phase IV program.

VII. Cost Effective Pharmacokinetic Program

Before addressing the key components, it may be prudent to reflect on the cost-benefit aspects of an effective pharmacokinetic program. Principally, all pharmacokinetic studies should have clear cut objectives. Otherwise, there will be a needless use of resource. A successful pharmacokinetic program is launched to support: a) NCE screening in discovery stages to assist in identifying a more successful lead; b) to assist in identifying dosing regimens for safety studies in animals and in reducing the number of studies; c) metabolism characterization in different species and determining potentially active metabolite(s); d) supporting early clinical studies in man, determining effective dosing regimens; e) supporting safety and efficacy studies in patients and reducing the number of clinical trials; and f) supporting rational drug delivery systems development.

An expanded pharmacokinetic program from discovery to regulatory registration may seldom approach 5% of the total cost for the development of a NCE. The return, however, may be measured by either a reduction in time or a decrease in cost of drug development. The reduction in the time of development and approval by world-wide regulatory agencies may be measured by the return over the expedited period.

REFERENCES

Barry, H., and A. Yacobi (1984). Preclinical toxicokinetics. In A. Yacobi and H. Barry, III, (Eds.), Experimental and Clinical Toxicokinetics. American Pharmaceutical Association, APS, Washington, pp. 1-7.

Batra, V. K., and A. Yacobi (1989). An overview of toxicokinetics. In A. Yacobi, J. P. Skelly and V. K. Batra, (Eds.), Toxicokinetics and New Drug Development, Pergamon Press, New York, pp. 1-20.

Boxenbaum, H. (1984). Interspecies scaling, allometry, physiological time and ground plan of pharmacokinetics. J. Pharmacokinet. Biopharm., 10, 201- 227.

Campbell, D. B., and R. M. Ings (1988). New approaches to the use of pharmacokinetics in toxicology and drug development. Human Toxicol., 7, 469- 479.

Collins, J. M., C. K. Grieshaber, B. A. Grieshaber, and B. A. Chadner (1990). Pharmacologically guided Phase I clinical trials based upon preclinical drug development. J. Natl. Cancer Inst., 82, 1321-1326.

Collins, J. M., D. S. Zaharko, R. L. Dedrick, and B. A. Chabner (1986). Potential roles for preclinical pharmacology in Phase I clinical trials. Cancer Treatment Reports, 70, 73-80.

de la Iglesia, F. A., and P. Greaves (1989). Role of toxicokinetics in drug safety evaluations. In A. Yacobi, J. P. Skelly and V. K. Batra, (Eds.) Toxicokinetics and New Drug Development. Pergamon Press, New York, pp. 21- 32.

Echizen, H., B. Vogelgesang, and M. Eichelbaum (1985a). Effects of d,l- verapamil on atrioventricular conduction in relation to its stereoselective first-pass metabolism. Clin. Pharmacol. Ther., 38, 71-76.

Echizen, H., T. Brecht, S. Niedergasass, B. Vogelgesang, and M. Eichelbaum (1985b). The effect of dextro-, levo-, and racemic verapamil on atrioventricular conduction in humans. Amer. Heart J., 109, 210-217.

Eichelbaum, M., and A. Somogyi (1984). Inter- and intra-subject variation in the first-pass elimination of highly cleared drugs during chronic dosing. Eur. J. Clin. Pharmacol., 26, 47-53.

Eichelbaum, M., G. Mikus, and B. Vogelgesang (1984). Pharmacokinetics of (+)-, (-)- and (+)-verapamil after intravenous administration. Br. J. Clin. Pharmacol., 17, 453-458.

Fabre, G., J. Combalbert, Y. Berger, and J. P. Cano (1990). Human hepatocytes as a key in-vitro model to improve preclinical drug development. Eur. J. Drug Metab. Pharmacokinet., 15, 165-171.

Gianni, L., L. Vigano, A. Surbone, D. Ballinari, P. Casali, C. Tarella, J. M. Collins, and G. Bonadonna (1990). Pharmacology and clinical toxicity of 4'-iodo-4'- deoxydoxorubicin: an example of successful application of pharmacokinetics to dose escalation in Phase I trials. J. Natl. Cancer Inst., 82, 469-477.

Mordenti, J., and W. Chappel (1989). The use of interspecies scaling in toxicokinetics. In A. Yacobi, J.P. Skelly, and V.K. Batra (Eds.), Toxicokinetics and New Drug Development, Pergamon Press, New York, pp. 42- 96.

Rahmani, R., B. Richard, G. Fabre, and J. P. Cano (1988). Extrapolation of preclinical pharmacokinetic data to therapeutic drug use. Xenobiotica, 18 (Suppl.), 71-88.

Yacobi, A., R. W. Krasula, and C. M. Lai (1984). Selective disposition studies in drug safety evaluation. In A. Yacobi and H. Barry, III, (Eds.), Experimental and Clinical Toxicokinetics. American Pharmaceutical Association, APS, Washington, pp. 47-73.

PHARMACOEPIDEMIOLOGY, POPULATION PHARMACOKINETICS AND NEW DRUG DEVELOPMENT

Thaddeus H. Grasela, Jr.
Department of Pharmacy and Social and Preventive Medicine
Schools of Pharmacy and Medicine
State University of New York at Buffalo
Buffalo, NY 14260

Edward J. Antal
Director, Clinical Pharmacokinetics
The Upjohn Company, Kalamazoo, MI 49001

INTRODUCTION

It is important to recognize that the new drug development process, which begins with the identification of a potential therapeutic compound, continues well into the post-marketing period. The responsibility of regulators, scientists, physicians, and the pharmaceutical industry to pursue knowledge about drug safety and efficacy extends well beyond the time when sufficient information is available to suggest that a drug is safe and efficacious, and warrants marketing. The ultimate uses of newly marketed medications and the clinical milieu into which it will be interposed is extremely dynamic and complex. It is during the early marketing period that a number of drugs approved for marketing were discovered to have serious, unanticipated adverse events requiring at best a change in labeling; and at worst removal from the market at great cost, in terms of credibility and dollars, to both FDA and the pharmaceutical industry (FDA Drug Review, 1990).

Recently, the Food and Drug Administration has been insisting that pharmaceutical companies determine the magnitude of variability in the pharmacokinetics and pharmacodynamics of experimental medications and investigate the sources of this variability in order to ensure an optimal therapeutic response. One approach to this task is to combine the techniques of pharmacoepidemiology and population pharmacokinetic/pharmacodynamic analysis. The goals of this presentation are to examine the drug development process from the perspective of pharmacoepidemiology, discuss the application of innovative data analysis approaches to

Integration of Pharmacokinetics, Pharmacodynamics, and Toxicokinetics in Rational Drug Development, Edited by A. Yacobi *et al.*, Plenum Press, New York, 1993

clinical trial data and observational data obtained in the post- marketing period, and point out some reasons for the value of a close collaboration between pharmacoepidemiology and pharmacokinetics in order to meet the challenges of adequately assessing drug safety and efficacy.

Epidemiology has been defined as the study of the distribution and determinants of disease frequency (MacMahon and Pugh, 1970). A body of knowledge and methodologic techniques has been developed around the notion of collecting and analyzing observational data to test hypotheses that for practical or ethical reasons cannot be investigated using the gold standard of randomized controlled clinical trials. Pharmacoepidemiology is a relatively new subspecialty of this discipline that seeks to blend aspects of epidemiology and pharmacology in order to study the determinants of drug safety and efficacy (Strom, 1989). Nearly all pharmaceutical companies have established departments or divisions of scientists trained in pharmacokinetics in order to perform pharmacokinetic studies for the New Drug Approval package. Many companies have also established programs in pharmacoepidemiology in order to meet regulatory requirements for reporting adverse drug events and to continue the study of drug safety and efficacy in the post-marketing period. Unfortunately, there has been relatively little collaboration across these departments and rarely do post- marketing surveillance studies include the measurement of drug concentrations as a covariate. This collaboration could yield important benefits to the development of new drugs and in some cases provide insight into the nature of adverse events reported for a new drug.

The three phases of the drug development process established in 1962 by the Harris Kefauver amendment represent a rigorous gauntlet for the evaluation of drug safety and efficacy prior to approval for marketing. In the past 30 years, this process has been both staunchly defended and vigorously criticized for perceived strengths and/or limitations, depending on one's perspective. It has long been recognized that this extensive evaluation is not without its costs. It is not unusual for a new clinical entity to take up to 10 years of clinical evaluation before it is allowed on the market, and it has been estimated that it costs approximately $125 to $200 million to bring a new chemical entity from laboratory to clinic. Although these costs seemed defensible in an earlier time, in the current political and patient care environment a number of important events have helped to shape, and support, mounting criticism of the drug development process. Patients with serious diseases have demanded rapid access to potentially life- saving medication. This has resulted in extreme pressure on FDA to abbreviate the approval process particularly for life-threatening diseases, such as AIDS and Alzheimer's disease. It must be recognized, however, that this approach is not without hazard. An abbreviated evaluation, particularly when the total number of patients exposed to the drug prior to marketing is reduced, necessarily means that less will be known about a drug at the time of approval. There are numerous examples of FDA approved medications that were subsequently discovered to have unexpected adverse events detected in the post-marketing period. In spite of the time and money expended to assess drug safety and efficacy there are important limitations in the knowledge of drug safety and efficacy obtained from pre-marketing studies. In general, studies are too small, the study population is too narrowly defined, the evaluation covers a narrowly defined indication, and studies are of relatively short duration. As a result, the total experience with a drug at the time of marketing is small, relative to the breadth and depth of patient exposure that will occur after marketing. These short comings will only be magnified in the face of expedited approval and this necessarily means that post-marketing surveillance studies are going to become an integral part of the drug approval cycle.

A recent report by the U.S. General Accounting Office has reported that of the 198 drugs approved by the FDA and marketed by pharmaceutical companies between 1976 and 1985, 102 (51.5%) had serious post-approval risks as evidenced by significant labeling changes or withdrawal from the market (FDA Drug Review, 1990). There are a broad range of reasons for the appearance of these adverse drug events in the post-marketing period. In some cases, the adverse events represent rare idiosyncratic events which are not predictable and which are not discovered in pre-approval trials simply because the number of patients studied relative to the incidence of the event is small. In other cases, the appearance of adverse events in the post-marketing period may occur because of an alteration in pharmacokinetics that occurs in a heretofore unstudied patient population which leads to disproportionately high drug concentrations and augmentation of drug effect, or an alteration in pharmacodynamics which results in enhanced sensitivity to a given drug concentration, or both. For the purposes of illustration, we briefly discuss three examples in which altered pharmacokinetics may represent a component of the mechanism for the adverse event. Midazolam is a water-soluble benzodiazepine marketed for preoperative sedation and for conscious sedation prior to short diagnostic or endoscopic procedures. Shortly after marketing, there were reports of sudden death, particularly in elderly patients undergoing conscious sedation. As a consequence, the product labeling was amended and a black box warning was added warning about respiratory depression and arrest, and the need for dosage individualization, particularly in the elderly. As another example, imipenem, a combination product containing a thienamycin antibiotic and cilastatin sodium, an inhibitor of renal dipeptidase, is a potent broad spectrum antibacterial agent. Post-marketing experience with the antibiotic prompted changes to the precautions section warning that CNS adverse experiences, including seizures, occur especially when recommended dosages were exceeded and that they have occurred in patients without compromised renal function or previous history of an underlying CNS disorder. This precaution was previously limited to those with underlying CNS disorder and/or compromised renal function. In addition, it was observed that seizures occurred at a higher rate in those with severe or marked impairment of renal function.

A final example is the post-marketing experience with the ciprofloxacin-theophylline interaction. During the initial clinical studies it was recognized that ciprofloxacin reduced theophylline clearance by approximately 30% in normal volunteers and stable patients. A review of adverse events reported to the FDA's spontaneous reporting system as of April, 1990 revealed 39 reports of theophylline toxicity and/or increased theophylline levels in patients who were initially receiving theophylline and subsequently prescribed concomitant ciprofloxacin therapy (Grasela and Dreis, 1992). The mean age of these patients was 72 years and they ranged from 31 to 94 years. It is interesting to note that of the 17 patients in whom theophylline concentrations were reported both before and after the addition of ciprofloxacin the mean change in theophylline levels was 114% and ranged from 32% to 308%. Significantly, 14 (36%) of these patients experienced a seizure and there were 3 deaths; one death as a result of the seizure. The mean theophylline concentration at the time of the seizure was 24.8 mg/L with a range of 15.4 to 34.1 mg/L. Although the effect of ciprofloxacin on theophylline metabolism was appreciated prior to marketing, the magnitude of the interaction and the variability in the extent of the interaction was not appreciated from the information obtained from studies of normal volunteers and relatively healthy patients.

These examples highlight the fact that clinicians often observe a higher frequency of adverse events in the post-marketing period than during clinical trials; in many cases because of variability in the pharmacokinetics of the drug in patient populations. These examples also serve to emphasize the fact that the acquisition and analysis of drug experience data, in the form of patient outcome and pharmacokinetic information from patients treated under actual clinical conditions, is essential to the process of ensuring the safe and efficacious use of medications. The collection of this information must continue beyond the traditional phase I to phase III periods and well into phase IV, the post-marketing period. In particular, we must come to appreciate that it is not adequate to focus our efforts only on determining the pharmacokinetics of a drug in traditional patient populations, such as liver failure, or renal failure; nor is it adequate to study only homogenous patient populations with mild degrees of illness. Drug safety and efficacy must be studied in the context of how the drug will be actually used in clinical practice. This is a challenge that can only be met if pharmacokineticists and pharmacoepidemiologists are prepared to collaborate and incorporate a population approach to pharmacokinetics and pharmacodynamics in pre-marketing and post-marketing studies (Sheiner and Benet, 1985).

CHANGING PRIORITIES OF DRUG APPROVAL PROCESS

It is important to recognize that there are major shifts in the priorities of scientists, regulators, and clinicians as a drug progresses through the approval process. These changes in priorities serve to create a database that grows in size and complexity over the course of drug evaluation, particularly if one is willing to include data collected during post-marketing studies. This database can be extremely valuable in answering many questions about drug safety and can be used to improve the design and implementation of subsequent drug studies. Unfortunately, with respect to pharmacokinetic information, we often do not take full advantage of drug concentrations measured during clinical trials.

In the pre-approval period, studies are designed to address key regulatory requirements for approval. Pharmaceutical scientists seek to sufficiently define the safety and efficacy of a drug and gain sufficient knowledge of its pharmacokinetic profile so as to permit regulatory evaluation and obtain subsequent approval of the drug for marketing. This is primarily accomplished by performing randomized double-blind clinical trials to assess drug safety and efficacy. Formal hypothesis testing using standard statistical methods is performed to determine if there is a benefit of the drug relative to placebo or other comparative agents. Pharmacokinetic studies are generally performed in normal, or otherwise healthy patients and standard approaches are used for data reduction and summary.

Once a drug is marketed, the clinical aspects of therapeutic use assume a greater priority. In the post-approval period clinicians seek to understand the safety and efficacy profile of a drug and identify patient risk factors that can result in variability in the desired patient response. The risk factors for adverse events may include altered pharmacokinetics and/or pharmacodynamics in specific patient populations. Pharmacoepidemiologists have utilized epidemiologic methodologies, such as the prospective cohort study or case-control studies, to identify risk factors for adverse events. Although much of this work is often performed using computerized databases which do not lend themselves to the collection of pharmacokinetic data, pharmacokineticists can provide valuable input when prospective data collection studies are initiated as described below.

The acquisition of pharmacokinetic data from patient populations in post marketing surveillance studies is generally not performed, perhaps because of concerns that only intensive pharmacokinetic studies can yield the necessary information or because of the complexity of the analyses required in this setting. The traditional approach to pharmacokinetics is prohibitively expensive if applied to a large population and there are often logistical and ethical problems which arise when attempting to study fragile patient populations, such as the seriously-ill or critical care patient. This problem can be solved by using data analysis methodologies which allow the use of fragmentary clinical and pharmacokinetic data to determine population pharmacokinetic and pharmacodynamic parameters.

THE ROLE OF POPULATION PHARMACOKINETICS

Recent developments in data analysis methodologies, including a mixed effect modeling approach as implemented in the computer program NONMEM, have made it possible to determine the population pharmacokinetic parameter of a drug from limited number of drug concentrations obtained from a large patient population (Beal and Sheiner, 1982). Population pharmacokinetic parameters include the typical values of parameters in a population, i.e., the mean clearance of a drug or the mean shift in clearance associated with a concurrent illness; the magnitude of interindividual variability, i.e., the variability in pharmacokinetic parameters not explained by observable patient factors; and the magnitude of residual variability, i.e., the variability in observed drug concentrations over time within a given individual caused by intraindividual variability in pharmacokinetic, assay error, pharmacokinetic model misspecification, and so forth (Ludden, 1988). The ability to estimate these parameters using only fragmentary drug concentrations greatly compliments the traditional approach to pharmacokinetics by allowing the study of patients in the clinical setting without the artificial constraints frequently necessary for traditional studies.

These tools, and the changing milieu of drug development, have the potential to markedly transform the way in which knowledge of drug pharmacokinetics and drug safety is accumulated. Random blood samples obtained during clinical trials might be used to identify reasons for variability in response, and the incorporation of these methodologies into expanded access programs would permit the early evaluation of patients ineligible for clinical trials. These patients represent an important opportunity to assess drug safety, efficacy, and pharmacokinetics in a population more representative of the patients who will receive a new drug after marketing.

Within the context of the shifting priorities occurring during drug development a variety of different types of data become available during the life history of a drug. It is arguably desirable, but unfortunately infrequently implemented, for this information to be accumulated into a database to facilitate the exploratory analysis of the total experience with a new drug in order to continually update the population pharmacokinetic and pharmacodynamic profile of a drug. From the earliest phase I studies in normal volunteers, to the phase III clinical trials and expanded access programs, and into phase IV, information regarding patient outcome, in conjunction with measured drug concentrations, can and should be collected, pooled and analyzed. This database would facilitate the accumulation of patients from various protocols with infrequently occurring concurrent illnesses or concomitant medications so that in the final database sufficient numbers might be available to evaluate whether a particular clinical condition or concomitant medication is associated with significant alterations in pharmacokinetic parameters. Furthermore, by collecting information about the drug dosing history, the times of sampling and the measured drug concentrations in a patient, one can use the population pharmacokinetic parameters to perform a bayesian analysis in order to obtain estimates of an individual's pharmacokinetic parameters (Peck and Rodman, 1986). In the clinic, these individual pharmacokinetic parameter estimates can then be used in a target drug concentration strategy in order to develop individualized dosing regimens for patients. Although dosage individualization has been performed in this way in the clinical setting for more than a decade, it has been infrequently applied in the clinical trial setting. This process will be necessary, however, if and when randomized concentration controlled trials are performed. The individual pharmacokinetic parameter estimates can also be used in conjunction with the patient's dosing history to generate individualized measures of drug exposure, such as the steady-state average plasma concentration, or the steady-state average area under the plasma concentration curve (AUC), or the total AUC for the duration of drug administration during the clinical trial. This would permit the determination of patient-specific measures of drug exposure for use in the evaluation of efficacy or toxicity that might prove more appropriate than simply the dose.

The incorporation of pharmacokinetic information into the evaluation of drug safety and efficacy will mean that pharmaceutical scientists, in collaboration with pharmacoepidemiologists, must come to grips with the analysis and handling of observational data. The presence of bias is always a consideration when dealing with observational data and evaluating the effect of confounding variables is essential for proper interpretation of findings. There are also important considerations in determining patient compliance with the study protocol and obtaining an accurate dosing history. In addition, physician cooperation with the primary study requirements is essential and any additional data collection must be justifiable and be as non-obtrusive as possible so as to not interfere with the primary study objectives. With proper care and attention to detail this can be accomplished and the remainder of this chapter will focus on an example of the application of a population pharmacokinetic approach in clinical trials, and an example in which drug pharmacokinetics were used in exploring variability in drug efficacy and safety.

POPULATION PHARMACOKINETICS IN CLINICAL TRIALS

The collection of population pharmacokinetic data and use of mixed effect modeling raise important logistic issues regarding the quality of data attainable from clinical trials, the effort required to ensure acceptable data quality, and the impact on clinician compliance with the primary objectives of the study protocol. The specific problems encountered during a study will depend upon the drug under study, the nature of the clinical trial, and the nature of the patient population. An early attempt to address some of these issues was performed using data obtained from two multicenter clinical trials evaluating the efficacy of alprazolam in the treatment of panic related disorders (Antal, Grasela and Smith, 1989). In one study, data collected during the Cross-National Panic study were assembled retrospectively from study files for a NONMEM analysis. In a second study, modifications to the protocol and case report form were made prior to study initiation to allow for prospective collection of accurate information on alprazolam administration times and the times of blood sampling for determination of alprazolam concentrations. A comparison of the results of a population pharmacokinetic analysis of the data from these two trials yields interesting insight into what is possible if there is sufficient interest and effort made in educating investigators regarding the need for collecting high quality data.

In the retrospectively assembled data set, NONMEM analysis was performed on data previously collected from a flexible dose study to evaluate the safety and efficacy of alprazolam versus placebo in patients with panic related disorders. A total of 248 patients were enrolled from 8 study centers and a total of 445 alprazolam plasma concentrations were obtained. Patients ranged in age from 18 to 64 years of age with a mean (SD) of 36.6 (10.7) years. Blood samples were obtained during two clinic visits over the course of the trial. The study protocol directed that these samples were to be collected immediately prior to the administration of the morning dose of alprazolam. Only the patient's total daily dose was recorded during the clinic visit; no information regarding the time of sampling, times of drug administration, or the interval from the last dose to time of sampling was recorded. Medications were dispensed in a vial at the time of each weekly clinic visit and pill counts were performed to encourage patient compliance. Because of the lack of information on the specific timing of critical events, the drug dosing history was recreated for the purposes of the NONMEM analysis by assuming that patients had exactly followed protocol specifications for times of dosing and times of sampling for blood concentrations.

Data for the prospective analysis was collected during the performance of a multicenter clinical efficacy and safety trial of fixed doses of alprazolam in the treatment of panic attacks. Patients were treated for a total of six weeks and weekly clinic visits were scheduled for evaluation of safety and efficacy. A blood sample for determination of alprazolam was obtained at convenient times during the clinic visit. No attempt was made to control the time of blood sampling relative to the previous dose of alprazolam, but the patient was queried regarding the times of alprazolam administration during the day before and the day of sampling. The alprazolam dosing history and time of blood sampling was recorded on a form specifically designed to capture this information. Medication was dispensed in unit dose blister packs and weekly pill counts were performed to encourage patient compliance. A total of 249 alprazolam plasma concentrations were measured in 61 patients at three study centers. The age of these patients ranged from 19 to 60 years of age with a mean (SD) of 37.6 (9.3). Patients in the two study populations were similar in terms of demographic characteristics, diagnoses, and concomitant drug administration.

The alprazolam plasma concentration time data collected from each study were analyzed separately using a one compartment open model with first order absorption and elimination. A proportional error model was used for both interindividual variability and residual variability. Data analysis was performed with the double precision NONMEM program using the PredPP package (Beal and Sheiner, 1983).

The population mean clearance, volume of distribution, and absorption rate constant obtain from the prospective analysis were 0.054 L/hr/kg, 0.76 l/kg, and 1.07 hr^{-1}, respectively. The estimates of the coefficient of variation of the interindividual variability in clearance and volume of distribution were 43% and 66%, respectively, and the residual variability was 27%, also expressed as a coefficient of variation. These estimates of population pharmacokinetic parameters for alprazolam were similar to parameter values obtained from traditional pharmacokinetic studies.

The results of the retrospective data analysis yielded markedly different estimates of the pharmacokinetic parameters. The estimate of the mean clearance was lower than previously reported, 0.042 L/hr/kg, and the estimates of volume of distribution and the absorption rate constant were much smaller than previously were reported, 0.183 L/kg and 0.06 hr^{-1}, respectively. The coefficient of variation of interindividual variability in clearance was 40%, and the variability in volume was unable to be estimated. The estimate of the coefficient of variation in residual variability was 59%.

Comparison of these results indicates, as expected, that there were serious problems with the retrospective data set. This primarily arises from the two-fold increase in the magnitude of residual variability, i.e., 59% versus 27% for the prospective data, and the inability to obtain estimates of some of the parameters of the model. The residual variability is a collection of sources of variability including intraindividual variability in pharmacokinetics, pharmacokinetic model misspecification, assay variability, and variability in patient compliance to the protocol specifications. In the prospective data set, variability in patient compliance was accounted for by capturing information about the times of dosing and the times of blood sampling. Because the retrospective data set was assembled after the trial was completed and no information was available about the times of dosing nor the times of blood sampling, strict compliance of the patient to the protocol was necessarily assumed. It is well recognized that patients will modify their treatment regimens, and the high residual variability reflects the extent to which patients did not take doses at times prescribed by the regimen nor have blood concentrations measured as a trough level prior to the morning dose. In support of this explanation, six patients enrolled in the retrospective study maintained a diary of drug administration times and times of sampling. The recorded times of sampling ranged from 1 to 10 hours after the previous dose and none of the samples were obtained as a morning trough (Antal, Grasela and Smith, 1989).

In order to capture information about drug administration in the prospective study, dosing information was requested for the day prior to and the day of blood sampling. In the case of alprazolam, the drug has a half-life of 8 to 12 hours and this strategy proved to be reasonable since the doses taken by the patient prior to the day before sampling would have little impact on the drug concentration measured on the day of clinic. Based on the results obtained for this study, patient recall for this period of time appears to be reasonable. Important logistical problems would arise, however, in the event that a drug under study had either a much longer or a much shorter half-life than alprazolam. In the case where a drug has a much longer half-life, adjustments in the drug data collection process would be necessary and long term recording of patient dosing information using patient diaries, or the use of medication event monitoring systems would be necessary. At the other end of the spectrum are drugs with a very short half-life and, in this case, timing errors become critical; the times of dosing and sampling for drug concentrations must be recorded accurately. In this setting, it may be necessary to require that the patient come to clinic for supervised drug dosing, followed by the collection of two or three drug concentrations over the next several hours, which for a short half-life drug would represent several half-lives.

In the case of the prospective study described above, the additional requirements for collection of the patients dosing history did not represent an unacceptable burden to research personnel. All blood samples were accompanied by completed dosing information and the primary objectives of this study were satisfied. In addition, the need for random blood sampling was communicated to the investigators and their staff and good variation in collection times were achieved with minimal disruption in the scheduling of clinic visits. The distribution of collection times over the dosing interval is important for estimating all pharmacokinetic parameters relevant to the selected pharmacokinetic model, and is much more informative that the common restriction of measuring only trough levels (Sheiner and Beal, 1983). The use of excessively restrictive sampling strategies represents an unnecessary burden in the collection of population pharmacokinetic data because specific sampling times do not allow for variability in patient schedules and clinic schedules. The results of our analyses suggest that by allowing events to occur as they naturally would, the variability in times of sampling will be sufficient to allow accurate and precise estimates of pharmacokinetic parameters.

THE RELATIONSHIP BETWEEN PHARMACOKINETICS AND DRUG THERAPY OUTCOME

In the prospective data set described above, an additional analysis was performed to determine if there were differences in the apparent oral clearance of alprazolam in patients who responded to drug therapy as compared to the non-responders (Antal, Grasela and Smith, 1989). For the purposes of this analysis, a responder was defined by a 25% or greater reduction in the total number of panic attacks per week during the course of the study. In the non-responders the total clearance was 0.083 L/hr/kg (95% confidence interval of 0.07 to 0.096) and the clearance of alprazolam in patients who responded to therapy was 60% of this value (95% confidence interval 50% to 70%, log likelihood difference 17.3, $p<0.001$). The lower clearance value associated with a responding patient would suggest that these patients had higher alprazolam blood concentrations for a given dosing regimen leading to a greater response. Other patient attributes not associated with drug levels could not be ruled out based on this analysis, however, and further examination of this finding in future studies is warranted. However, this evaluation can have an important impact on the interpretation of the safety and efficacy findings of a study, and may provide a pharmacokinetic explanation for the variability in patient response. Explaining this variability may allow for improvements in the design of clinical trials to improve the overall performance of a drug.

In the example above, we have demonstrated one method for assessing the influence of pharmacokinetics on patient outcomes. There can also be variability in patient response because of variability in the severity of disease, or sensitivity of the patient to drug therapy. To the extent that these sources of variability can be identified, it is desirable to quantify their impact on drug therapy outcome so that the information might be used in prospectively selecting drug therapy for patients and in designing optimal dosing regimens.

Pharmacologists are familiar with pharmacodynamic models such as the E-max model as a method for quantifying the relationship between drug dose, or drug concentration, and patient response when the response to therapy is measured as a continuous variable (Holford and Sheiner, 1981). For many diseases, however, there is no easily quantifiable continuous measurement that can be used to quantify drug therapy outcome and in many cases one must deal with whether or not the patient responded to therapy, where response is defined as a categorical variable, often based on an ad hoc definition. Statisticians working in epidemiology have developed a number of multivariable data analysis approaches, such as logistic regression and survival analysis, for identifying covariates which serve as determinants of response when the outcome variable is dichotomous (Hosmer and Lemeshow, 1989; Lee, 1980). In the case of logistic regression, the probability of being a responder can be determined as a function of patient demographic characteristics, such as age or gender, and pharmacokinetic information, such as the area under the concentration-time curve, steady-state average drug concentrations, peak concentrations, and so forth. There have been few published studies which have used pharmacokinetic information in this way, but the use of multivariable data analysis techniques in conjunction with pharmacokinetic data will undoubtedly increase as we continue to search for explanations for the variability in patient outcomes to drug therapy.

One example of this type of analysis was recently reported by Antal et al. (1988), who studied the relationship between the probability of patients with panic related disorders to respond to alprazolam as a function of alprazolam plasma concentrations. In order to study the relationship between clinical response and alprazolam plasma concentration, Antal et al. (1988), analyzed data from a double-blind, parallel, placebo controlled study with fixed dosages of alprazolam, 2 and 6 mg/day, in panic-related disorders using logistic regression. The dosages were based on pharmacokinetic information that suggested that the steady-state plasma concentration ranges from these two doses would overlap somewhat and result in a wide range of steady-state concentrations for evaluation. It was also expected that the majority of patients in the 2 mg treatment plan would not be adequately controlled whereas patients in the 6 mg group would experience a satisfactory response. A number of outcome measures were used in the initial analysis, but for the purposes of this discussion the focus will be on a classification scheme in which the treatment to baseline ratio of the number of panic attacks was calculated by dividing the number of panic attacks during the final week of treatment by the number of attacks at baseline. Patients were then classified as major, moderate, or non-responders if they had >75%, 25%-75%, or < 25% reduction in panic atacks, respectively. An initial evaluation of the response showed that the mean alprazolam concentrations increased as the proportion of responders increased indicating a positive relationship between alprazolam plasma concentrations and response. The mean alprazolam concentrations for major, moderate, and nonresponders were 39,24, and 8 ng/ml, respectively (p=0.0003). There was considerable overlap, however, in the range of concentrations for each group.

Logistic regression analysis was then performed for patients with a major response and a moderate response to determine the corresponding relationship with alprazolam plasma concentrations. Results of this analysis suggest that the probability of being classified as a major responder starts at approximately 33%, perhaps representing a placebo effect, and asymptotically increased to 90% as alprazolam concentrations increase from 0 to 150 ng/ml. Thus, a 50% and 75% probability of being classified as a major responder was associated with steady-state alprazolam plasma concentrations of 15 and 48 ng/ml, respectively. Likewise, there was a relationship between the probability of developing sedation as a side effect and alprazolam concentrations. At the concentration necessary to produce a 75% probability of a major response, the chance of having treatment associated sedation was <50%.

Although not reported by the authors of this study, logistic regression analysis can also incorporate patient covariates such as age, gender and severity of disease states in order to identify other explanatory variables affecting the success of drug therapy. These factors could then be used in the selection of drug therapy for specific patients, clinical decision making, and so forth.

SUMMARY

The drug approval process is continuing to evolve and the use of observational data and innovative data analysis methodologies is certain to play an increasingly important role in assessing drug safety and efficacy. Pharmaceutical scientists, clinicians and regulatory agencies must cope with the problems of making new life-saving medications available to physicians and patients as expeditiously as possible, without compromising knowledge of drug safety. The changing nature of new drug development requires that we utilize all data available for a drug from the earliest phase I studies to post-marketing surveillance in order to ensure the safe and efficacious use of drugs. A close collaboration between pharma-coepidemiologists and pharmacokineticists trained in population approaches to pharmacokinetics and pharmacodynamics represents an innovative mechanism for identifying patient factors producing variability in outcome from drug therapy and improving the overall safety and efficacy profile of newly developed medications.

REFERENCES

Antal, E. J., T. H. Grasela, and R. B. Smith (1989). An evaluation of population pharmacokinetics in therapeutic trials Part III. Prospective data collection versus retrospective data assembly. Clin. Pharmacol. Ther., 46, 552-559.

Antal, E. J., D. A. Pyne, K. E. Starz, and R. B. Smith (1988). Probability models in pharmacodynamic analysis of clinical trials. In P. Kroboth and R. B. Smith (Eds.), Current Problem and Potential Solutions. Vol. 2. Harvey Whitney Books, Cincinnati. pp. 220-231.

Beal, S. L., and L. B. Sheiner (1982). Estimating population kinetics. CRC Crit. Rev. Biomed. Engineering, 8, 195-222.

Beal, S. L., and L. B. Sheiner (Eds.), (1983). NONMEM Users Guide - Part VI: PREDPP Guide. NONMEM Project Group, University of California at San Francisco, San Francisco, CA.

FDA Drug Review (1990). Post-approval risks 1976-85. United States General Accounting Office, Report to the Chairman, subcommittee on Human Resources and Intergovernmental Relations, Committee on Government Operations, House of Representatives. PEMD - 90 - 15.

Grasela, T. H., and M. W. Dreis (1992). An evaluation of the quinolone- theophylline interaction using the FDA Spontaneous Reporting System. Arch. Intern. Med., 152, 617-621.

Holford, N. H. G., and L. B. Sheiner (1981). Understanding the dose-effect relationship: clinical application of pharmacokinetic-pharmacodynamic models. Clin. Pharmacokinet., 6, 429-453.

Hosmer, D. W., and S. Lemeshow (Eds.), (1989). Applied Logistic Regression. John Wiley and Sons. New York.

Lee, E. T. (1980). Statistical Methods for Survival Data Analysis. Lifetime Learning Publication, Belmont, CA.

Ludden, T. M. (1988). Population pharmacokinetics. J. Clin. Pharmacol., 28, 1059-1063.

MacMahon, B., and T. F. Pugh (Eds.), (1970), Epidemiology, Principles and Methods, Little, Brown and Company, Boston.

Peck, C. C., and J. H. Rodman (1986). Analysis of clinical pharmacokinetic data for individualizing drug dosage regimens. In W. E. Evans, J. J. Schentag, and W. J. Jusko (Eds.), Applied Pharmacokinetics, 2nd edition, Applied Therapeutics, Inc., Spokane, WA, pp. 55-82.

Sheiner, L. B., and S. L. Beal (1983). Evaluation of methods for estimating population pharmacokinetic parameters. III. Monoexponential model: Routine clinical pharmacokinetic data. J. Pharmacokinet. Biopharm., 3, 303-319.

Sheiner, L. B., and L. Z. Benet (1985). Premarketing observational studies of population pharmacokinetics of new drugs. Clin. Pharmacol. Ther., 38, 481-487.

Strom, B. L. (Ed.), (1989). Pharmacoepidemiology. Churchill Livingstone, New York.

ASSESSMENT OF PHARMACOKINETIC DRUG INTERACTIONS IN CLINICAL DRUG DEVELOPMENT

Jerome J. Schentag
Center for Clinical Pharmacy Research and
Department of Pharmaceutics, School of Pharmacy
State University of New York at Buffalo
and The Clinical Pharmacokinetics Laboratory
Millard Fillmore Hospital, Buffalo, NY 14209

ABSTRACT

Drug interactions of a minor nature occur commonly. They are often of little clinical consequence because one or both interacting drugs have wide therapeutic margins for both efficacy and safety. However, clinically significant adverse events do occur as a consequence of drug interactions in small subsets of patients, chiefly older patients with pre-existing organ dysfunction receiving interactants having narrow therapeutic windows. Although clinically rare, these few significant drug interactions have major impact on modern drug development and drug labeling stategies. In the course of registering a new drug, the pharmaceutical industry conducts many drug-drug interaction studies in normal volunteers, and even occasionally in patients. The first layer of these volunteer trials is part of late Phase II, and examines the kinetic interactions which would be anticipated from known relationships of the chemical classes or metabolic pathways. A "Check-list" approach is often followed. More and more frequently, these studies serve several purposes including molecular modification to produce new compounds without the potential for interaction, and competitive marketing. One major issue, seldom addressed, is whether the interactions tested in normal volunteers are subsequently found in patients. There is no assurance that a statistically significant pharmacokinetic interaction in volunteers will reliably predict a clinically significant interaction in patients. This observation led us to examine the degree of pharmacokinetic alteration which might predict a clinically detectable interaction. With a narrow therapeutic index drug like theophylline, we have found that clinical interactions are rarely detectable until the interacting

Integration of Pharmacokinetics, Pharmacodynamics, and Toxicokinetics in Rational Drug Development, Edited by A. Yacobi *et al.*, Plenum Press, New York, 1993

149

agent reduces theophylline clearance by 40-50%. The magnitude of pharmacokinetic change may need to be even greater in order to anticipate clinical interactions between drugs with wider safety margins than theophylline.

INTRODUCTION

Drug interactions have gained attention in drug development largely because of adverse drug reactions which can be traced back to one drug changing the clearance or distribution volume of another. The resulting elevation in serum concentration then causes augmented toxicity bringing the interaction to the attention of the patient and physician. For most of these interactions, the rapidity of detection is directly related to both the magnitude of the interaction, and the toxicity of the interactants.

Patients are surviving longer, with multiple chronic diseases. The number of drugs taken per patient is continually rising. As drugs are used evermore widely in combinations, new interactions are continually being discovered. Fewer and fewer of these are first discovered in phase IV after the drug is marketed, but as recently as 12 years ago, the drug cimetidine was marketed with its initial package insert claiming no drug-drug interactions. Cimetidine was not tested for interactions using the current methods. Furthermore, all of its clinical testing involved relatively healthy young patients with duodenal ulcer disease, so few patients were given concomittant interactants in phase III. Because there was no reason to suspect them, interactions only became clinically apparent after wide use of the drug. Detection of these events required the concomitant use of cimetidine in patients already taking warfarin, theophylline and phenytoin. All the interactions discovered in the postmarketing period were pharmacokinetic, virtually all a result of cimetidine's capacity for inhibition of P-450 dependent microsomal drug metabolism (Sorkin and Davey, 1983; Somogyi and Gugler, 1982).

Perhaps of greatest interest to students of the history of drug interactions, the order of discovery of these cimetidine interactions was directly related to the narrowness of the therapeutic window of the interactants. Thus, the interaction with warfarin was discovered first (Toon and colleagues, 1986; Silver and Bell, 1979) then theophylline (Reitberg, Bernhard and Schentag, 1981; Hsu and colleagues, 1984) followed by wider therapeutic window compounds like benzodiazepines, tricyclic antidepressants, and lidocaine, among others (Klotz and Reimann, 1980; Galbraith and Michnovicz, 1989; Henauer and Hollister, 1984; Bauer and colleagues, 1984).

In retrospect, the pattern of drug interaction discovery displayed by cimetidine in the post marketing phase was the typical one. The markers of drug interaction which reveal the interaction earliest were the very narrow therapeutic window compounds most sensitive to the type of interaction. In the case of cimetidine it was metabolic inhibition. Table 1 provides other examples of drug-drug interactions, in order to demonstrate that the clinically significant interactants are usually the narrow therapeutic window compounds. The drugs causing the interactions are usually members of about five classes of compounds, all of which inhibit metabolism (Toon and colleagues, 1986; Silver and Bell, 1979; Reitberg, Bernhard and

Table 1. Drug Interactions Yielding Increased (Clinically Detectable) Effects[1]

Site	Drug A	Increased Conc. of Drug B[2]	Detectable Endpoint
Hepatic:	Omeprazole Cimetidine Fluoroquinolones Chloramphenicol Azole Antifungals	Cyclosporin Theophylline Phenytoin Warfarin Quinidine	Metabolic Inhibition and Augmented Clinical Effects
Renal:	Gentamicin Cis-Platinum Probenecid Aspirin Quinidine Amphotericin B	Digoxin Lithium Methotrexate Gentamicin 5-Flucytosine	Decreased Renal Elimination and Augmented Clinical Effects

1 Statistically detectable interaction in 12 volunteers = 10% change in B
Clinically recognizable interaction in patients = 40-50% change in B

2 Many more statistically significant interactions escape clinical detection because the Drug B has a wide safety margin.

Schentag, 1981; Hsu and colleagues, 1984; Gugler and Jenson, 1985; Rogge and colleagues, 1988; Peloquin and colleagues, 1989; Rose and colleagues, 1977; Blum and colleagues, 1991; Hardy and colleagues, 1983), inhibit renal excretion (Leigler, Henderson and Hahn, 1969; Mandel, 1976; Schentag, 1980), or rarely, both.

In contrast to the general increase in drug effects noted after the interactions in Table 1, there are also interactions which cause loss of effect. Table 2 provides a listing of compounds which cause clinically detectable decreases in drug effect. Most of these are gastrointestinal complexation reactions which virtually abolish absorption of the interactant (Grasela and colleagues, 1989; Nix and colleagues, 1989; Sorgel and colleagues, 1989; Nguyen and colleagues, 1989; Binnion, 1973; Blum and colleagues, 1991; Powell and Cate, 1985).

The interactant drugs listed as Drug B in Tables 1 and 2 have become the components of the typical checklist for interactions during Industry or FDA driven drug development. The pre-clinical data regarding the new drug's clearance mechanisms, pre-clinical screening of its effects on hepatic microsomes (Pelkonen and Puurunen, 1980), its effect on renal function, the interaction caused by analogues previously studied, and its toxicokinetic data are used to select the first interactants for study in normal volunteers. The likelihood of encountering these drugs together in patient trials often dictates the order of these studies, or once again, the most narrow therapeutic window interactant is the one chosen first for study in volunteers. The exception is warfarin, which is either not studied in volunteers because of its narrow therapeutic window, or studied as one dose with metabolite measurement (O'Reilly, 1984). Warfarin also could be studied in patients already taking the drug for therapeutic purposes, but this design destabilizes the warfarin control of stable patients, and may add risk to the use of warfarin.

Table 2. Drug-Drug Interactions Resulting in Partial to Complete Loss of Effect —Clinically Detectable Cases

Site	Drug A	Decreased Conc. of Drug B	Detectable Endpoint
GI:	Antacids Cholestyramine Charcoal Cimetidine	Fluoroquinolones Tetracyclines Digoxin Ketoconazole	Loss of B Effect (Malabsorption)
Hepatic:	Rifampin	Most Metabolized Compounds	Loss of B Effect (Increased Clearance)

STUDY DESIGN ISSUES FOR DRUG-DRUG INTERACTIONS

Issues of study design to detect and quantitate drug interactions have been extensively reviewed (Browne and colleagues, 1989) and will not be repeated here. Interaction studies typically begin in phase II, and proceed steadily during phase III. Unexpected new findings may create the need for additional studies. Most studies are designed as a two way crossover single dose administration of the interactant. The second administration of the interactant usually follows pre-treatment with the new drug for one dose to as long as one week (steady state exposure). The pre-treatment period must often be longer if the new drug is suspected to be an enzyme inducer.

While the above study design works well (it identifies most interactions significant to patient care, and rarely misses important interactions) there are a few problems. A common problem arises from the fact that interaction studies are performed in early phase II, before the dose of the new drug is known. As many drugs end up with higher doses in labeling, there are problems created when the agency views the interaction data, then notes the company's claim that there is no interaction with the new drug at its subclinical dose. As most of the interactions in Table 1 are dose dependent, these interaction studies often must be repeated, and many do demonstrate interactions at the higher dose. A recent example was observed with fluconazole - a fast track drug approved at four times the dosage that the first interaction studies employed. Recently, it has been used in patients at 8 to 12 times the first dose used in interaction studies. There are clear dose-related interactions with fluconazole, apparent primarily at the higher doses, but missed at lower doses.

Cimetidine also followed this pattern (Bartle, Walker and Shapero, 1983), although fewer studies were done. These types of situations will become fewer as industry places greater emphasis on dose finding in late phase I and early phase II, and as a direct result, industry will conduct more of these interaction studies using a clinically relevant dosage.

SUITABILITY OF NORMAL VOLUNTEERS FOR STUDY OF PHARMACOKINETIC DRUG INTERACTIONS

The normal male volunteer has been the traditional subject of human drug-drug interaction studies. There have been few organized efforts to conduct these studies in any other population. Advantages include standardization, ease of study conduct, and rapid study completion. A drug interaction study in normal volunteers can be executed in a two to four week period. Moreover, if there is a change in the pharmacokinetics of the interactant, it is detectable in a very sensitive manner. A 10% decline in clearance of theophylline can be detected with statistical significance in as little as 12-15 subjects (Gregoire and colleagues, 1987).

It is common for investigators to point out that normal volunteer models may suffer from their lack of relevance to patient care situations. I feel this to be a lesser problem in the study of drug-drug interactions. Few (if any) drug interactions of major significance are undetectable in normal volunteers. Rather, the major problem is that many statistically significant drug interactions are found, all of which produce small changes in the clearance of the interactant. Changes of this magnitude are too small to create a risk to the patients who take the drugs together for therapeutic purposes. Textbooks of drug interactions and computer programs based on these texts have long ago discovered that true statistically significant drug interactions in normal volunteers do not always create detectable adverse consequences in the patient. In fact, virtually all of the clinically detectable drug interactions occur with warfarin, theophylline, and phenytoin. These three drugs share the dual characteristics of narrow therapeutic range and significant susceptibility to metabolic inhibitors. The inhibitors most often responsible for toxicity with these drugs include cimetidine, certain fluoroquinolones, and azole antifungals like ketoconazole. In our experience, a drug must change the clearance of theophylline at least 40% to cause clinical problems. This is the average decline in theophylline clearance which results from cimetidine (Reitberg, Bernhard and Schentag, 1981). In spite of causing an average 40% decline in theophylline clearance, cimetidine-theophylline drug interactions are not common in the patient care arena (Sax, 1987). In fact they are not always found even when directly sought in direct comparison with other H2 antagonists which are supposedly devoid of the metabolic inhibitor characteristic.

There is one agent, enoxacin, which causes about 60 percent decline in theophylline clearance (Rogge and colleagues, 1988). This agent also affects caffeine to a similar degree (Peloquin and colleagues, 1989). Enoxacin causes clinically detectable theophylline toxicity, as would be expected from this magnitude of normal volunteer interaction (Maesen and colleagues, 1984). In contrast, ciprofloxacin causes a statistically significant 25% decline in theophylline clearance (Nix and colleagues, 1987; Wijnands, Vree and Van Herwaarden, 1986), but is rarely associated with theophylline toxicity even in the face of extensive concomitant use (Grasela and colleagues, 1991). Ofloxacin causes 10% decline in theophylline clearance (Gregoire and colleagues, 1987), but this is clearly devoid of clinical significance.

We concluded from our experiences in the post-cimetidine period that narrow therapeutic window interactants like theophylline, warfarin and phenytoin serve as statistically significant markers of drug interaction in normal volunteers, but that at least a 40% decline in their clearance should be documented. Otherwise, it would not be expected that the interaction would have clinical impact. If the number of study subjects is targeted based on the decline in clearance necessary to cause clinical impact (rather than statistically significant differences) then these normal volunteer studies can be conducted at about a quarter of their current cost. As the wide therapeutic margin drug would need even more than 40% change in clearance to see an effect, it is relatively easy to appreciate why many statistically significant normal volunteer interactions will never be seen as patient problems. This would probably remain true even if patients have baseline hepatic disease with associated defects in baseline drug clearance. However, there are few studies conducted as yet in this arena.

We do not argue that these studies not be done. Rather, they should have sample size selected to detect clinically important effects. A power calculation might be done to statistically explore both a clinically significant interaction and a statistically significant interaction, assessing the number of study subjects needed to demonstrate each.

THE CLINICAL IMPACT OF PHARMACOKINETIC DRUG-DRUG INTERACTIONS

The drug development procedures designed to detect and study drug interactions are neither irrational nor haphazard. Rather, they have evolved out of a progressive problem detection and solving process which arose within industry and the agency shortly after marketing cimetidine, and the associated discovery of all the cimetidine interactions in phase IV.

If the system is flawed, this is a consequence of its focus on detection of statistically significant interactions rather than clinically significant problems. Even this focus, for reasons illustrated, is more a misdirection of scarce time and drug development funds, because the system currently in place detects virtually all drug interactions with potential to have clinical impact.

Statisticians could approach the determination of sample size for normal volunteer studies using clearance changes which would demonstrate clinical relevance. This would markedly decrease the cost and effort of performing the typical "checklist" drug-drug interaction studies in normal volunteers, and would facilitate labeling of members of drug classes commonly observed to have drug interactions.

In the future, there should be greater emphasis on detecting clinical adverse events caused by drug- drug interactions. This is an area for population kinetics modeling (Grasela and colleagues, 1991). These results could further serve to identify the degree of interaction necessary to produce significant adverse events, and could eventually lead to the abandonment of certain drugs with high interaction potential.

We still know too little about the patient factors which predispose patients to severe adverse effects by potentiating the interacting drug. Additional research should focus on study of the patients who experience severe drug-drug interactions, to elucidate these potentiating factors.

REFERENCES

Bartle, W. R., S. E. Walker, and T. Shapero (1983). Dose dependent effect of cimetidine on phenytoin kinetics. Clin. Pharmacol. Ther., 33, 649-655.

Bauer, L. A., W. A. Edwards, F. P. Randolph, and R. A. Blouin (1984). Cimetidine induced decrease in lidocaine metabolism. Am. Heart J., 108, 413-415.

Binnion, P. F (1973). Absorption of digoxin and the influence of antacid, antidiarrheal, and ion exchange agents. In O. Storstein (Ed.), Symposium on Digitalis. Gyldendal Norsk Forlag Oslo, pp. 216-223.

Blum, R. A., D. T. D'Andrea, J. H. Wilton, D. M. Hilligoss, M. J. Gardner, E. B. Chin, H. A. Goldstein, and J. J. Schentag (1991). The effect of increased gastric pH on the relative bioavailability of fluconazole and ketoconazole. Ann. Intern. Med., 114, 755-757.

Blum, R. A., J. H. Wilton, D. M. Hilligoss, M. J. Gardner, E. B. Chin, N. J. Harrison, and J. J. Schentag (1991). The effect of fluconazole on the disposition of IV phenytoin. Clin. Pharmacol. Ther., 49, 420-425.

Browne, T. R., D. J. Greenblatt, G. E. Schumacher, G. K. Szabo, J. E. Evans, B. E. Evans, R. J. Perchalski, and R. J. Pylilo (1989). Comparison of methods for determination of pharmacokinetic drug interactions and proposals for new methods. In W. H. Pitlick (Ed.), Antiepileptic Drug Interactions, Demos Publications, New York, pp. 3-38.

Galbraith, R. A., and J. J. Michnovicz (1989). The effects of cimetidine on the oxidative metabolism of estrodiol. N. Engl. J. Med., 321, 269-274.

Grasela, T. H., J. A. Paladino, J. J. Schentag, D. Huepenbecker, J. Rybacki, J. Purcell, and J. B. Fiedler (1991). The clinical and economic impact of oral ciprofloxacin as follow up to parenteral antibiotics. DICP, Ann. Pharmacother., in press.

Grasela, T. H., J. J. Schentag, A. J. Sedman, J. H. Wilton, D. J. Thomas, R. W. Schultz, and A. W. Kinkel (1989). Inhibition of enoxacin absorption by antacids or ranitidine. Antimicrob. Agents. Chemother., 33, 615-617.

Gregoire, S. L., T. H. Grasela, J. P. Freer, K. J. Tack, and J. J. Schentag (1987). Inhibition of theophylline clearance by coadministered ofloxacin without alteration of theophylline effects. Antimicrob. Agents Chemother., 31, 375-378.

Gugler, R., and J. C. Jenson (1985). Omeprazole inhibits oxidative drug metabolism. Gastroenterology, 89, 1235-1241.

Hardy B. G., I. T. Zador, L. H. Golden, D. Lalka, and J. J. Schentag (1983). The effect of cimetidine on the pharmacokinetics and pharmacodynamics of quinidine. Am. J. Cardiol., 52, 172-175.

Henauer, S. A., and L. E. Hollister (1984). Cimetidine interaction with imipramine and nortriptyline. Clin. Pharmacol. Ther., 35, 183-187.

Hsu, K., A. Garton, B. J. Sproule, Y. K. Tam, D. Legatt, and F. A. Herbert (1984). The influence of orally administered cimetidine and theophylline on the elimination of each drug in patients with COPD. Am. Rev. Resp. Dis., 130, 740-743.

Klotz, U. and I. Reimann (1980). Delayed clearance of diazepam due to cimetidine. N. Engl. J. Med., 302, 1012-1014.

Liegler, D. G., E. S. Henderson, and M. A. Hahn (1969). The effect of organic acids on renal clearance of methotrexate in man. Clin. Pharmacol. Ther., 10, 849-857.

Maesen, F. P. V., J. P. Teengs, C. Baur, and B. I. Davies (1984). Enoxacin raises plasma theophylline levels. Lancet, 2, 530.

Mandel, M. S (1976). The synergistic effect of salicylates on methotrexate toxicity. Plast. Reconstr. Surgery, 57, 733-737.

Nguyen, V. X., D. E. Nix, S. Gillikin, and J. J. Schentag (1989). The effect of oral antacid administration on the pharmacokinetics of intravenous doxycycline. Antimicrob. Agents Chemother. 33, 434-436.

Nix, D. E., J. M. DeVito, M. A. Whitbread, and J. J. Schentag (1987). Effect of multiple dose oral ciprofloxacin on the pharmacokinetics of theophylline and indocyanine green. J. Antimicrob. Chemother., 19, 263-269.

Nix, D. E., W. A. Watson, M. E. Lener, R. W. Frost, G. Krol, H. Goldstein, J. Letteri, and J. J. Schentag (1989). Effects of aluminum and magnesium antacids and ranitidine on the absorption of cipro-floxacin. Clin. Pharmacol. Ther., 46, 700-705.

O'Reilly, R. A. (1984). Comparative interaction of cimetidine and ranitidine with racemic warfarin in man. Arch. Intern. Med., 144, 989-991.

Pelkonen, O., and J. Puurunen (1980). The effect of cimetidine on in vitro and in vivo microsomal drug metabolism in the rat. Biochem. Pharmacol., 29, 3075-3080.

Peloquin, C. A., D. E. Nix, A. J. Sedman, J. H. Wilton, R. D. Toothaker, N. J. Harrison, and J. J. Schentag (1989). Pharmacokinetics and clinical effects of caffeine alone and in combination with oral enoxacin. Rev Infect Dis, 11(Suppl 5), S1095.

Powell, J. R., and E. W. Cate (1985). Induction and inhibition of drug metabolism. In W. E. Evans, J. J. Schentag, and W. J. Jusko, (Eds.), Applied Pharmacokinetics, Applied Therapeutics Inc, San Francisco, pp. 139-186.

Reitberg, D. P., H. Bernhard, and J. J. Schentag (1981). Alteration of theophylline clearance and half-life by cimetidine in normal volunteers. Ann. Intern. Med., 95, 582-585.

Rogge, M. C., W. R Solomon, A.J. Sedman, P. G. Welling, R. D. Toothaker, and J. G. Wagner (1988). The theophylline-enoxacin interaction: I. Effect of enoxacin dose size on theophylline disposition. Clin. Pharmacol. Ther., 44, 579-587.

Rose, J. Q., H. K. Choi, J. J. Schentag, W. R. Kinkel, and W. J. Jusko (1977). Intoxication caused by interaction of chloramphenicol and phenytoin. J. Am. Med. Assoc., 237, 2630-2631.

Sax, M. J. (1987). Clinically important adverse effects and drug interactions with H2 receptor antagonists: an update. Pharmacotherapy, 7(Suppl), 110-115.

Schentag, J. J. (1980). Aminoglycoside antibiotics. In W. E. Evans, J. J. Schentag, W. J. Jusko (Eds.), Applied Pharmacokinetics, Applied Therapeutics, Inc., San Francisco, pp. 174-209.

Silver, B. A., and W. R. Bell (1979). Cimetidine potentiation of the hypoprothrombinemic effect of warfarin. Ann. Intern. Med., 80, 348-349.

Somogyi, A., and R. Gugler (1982). Drug interactions with cimetidine. Clin. Pharmacokinet, 7, 23-41.

Sorgel, F., K. G. Naber, U. Jaehde, A. Reiter, R. Seelman, and G. Sigl (1989). Brief report: Gastrointestinal secretion of ciprofloxacin. Evaluation of the charcoal model. Am. J. Med., 87(Suppl 5A), 62-65.

Sorkin, E. M., D. L. Davey (1983). Review of cimetidine drug interactions. DICP, 17, 110-20.

Toon, S., K. J. Hopkins, F. M. Garstang, B. Diquet, T. S. Gill, and M. Rowland. (1986). The warfarin-cimetidine interaction: stereochemical considerations. Br. J. Clin. Pharmacol., 21, 245-246.

Wijnands, W. J. A., T. B. Vree, and C. L. A. Van Herwaarden (1986). The influence of quinolone derivatives on theophylline clearance. Br. J. Clin. Pharmacol., 22, 677-682.

PHARMACOKINETIC/PHARMACODYNAMIC MODELS AND METHODS

Davide Verotta [a,b]
Lewis B. Sheiner [a,c]
[a] Department of Pharmacy, School of Pharmacy, University of
California, San Francisco, California, 94143.
[b] Department of Anesthesia, School of Medicine, University of
California, San Francisco, California, 94143.
[c] Department of Laboratory Medicine, School of Medicine,
University of California, San Francisco, California, 94143.

INTRODUCTION

Non-steady-state drug concentrations and concomitant pharmacological effects are an attractive data source for learning about dose-response, because experiments can be done quickly, and hence in available clinical settings. However a potential pitfall of this kind of experiment is clear from a plot of effect and drug observations vs time: often the two resulting curves seem to be "out of phase". To give an example, the upper panels of Figure 1 show simulated data with the maximal value of the effect occurring before the maximal drug concentration. The reverse situation is shown in the lower panels of Figure 1: the maximal value of the effect occurs after the maximal drug concentration. In either case a plot of observed effects (connected in time order) vs observed drug concentration describes a loop. A "literal" interpretation of such a plot suggests that different effect levels occur at the same drug concentration level (at different times).

Suppose that a drug's pharmacology is such that its effect is solely and instantaneously related to drug concentration and that this relationship does not vary with time (i.e. the relationship is always "one to one"). Then, a possible explanation of the phenomenon just described is that the levels of observed drug and drug at the site of action (effect site) are not always the same. Drug concentration at the effect site is "related to" observed drug concentration, but distributional delays put the drug levels "out of phase". The idea underlying most of the methodologies discussed in this chapter is to "align" (or "put in phase") observed drug concentration with drug concentration at the effect site. The end result is that a plot of effect

Integration of Pharmacokinetics, Pharmacodynamics, and Toxicokinetics in Rational Drug Development, Edited by A. Yacobi *et al.*, Plenum Press, New York, 1993

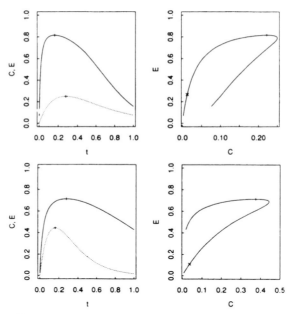

Figure 1. Simulated data. Upper panels: proteresis (see text). Lower panels: hysteresis (see text). Left panels: simulated effect (E) (solid line) and drug concentration (C) (dashed line) vs time; the + sign marks the maximum E and C, respectively. Right panels: simulated E vs C (in time order); the + sign marks the maximum E, the x sign marks the begining (with respect to time) of the loop.

vs "aligned" drug concentration (i.e. drug concentration at the effect site) more closely resembles a one to one relationship.

This chapter describes a general semiparametric model that is used to "align" observed and effect site drug concentration and to estimate the effect vs drug concentration relationship. Extensions of the model dealing with two drugs (agonist and antagonist), and tolerance are also described.

Section 2 is the core of the chapter. It describes the type of pharmacokinetic/pharmacodynamic (PK/PD) data we consider, describes the semiparametric model we propose, and differentiates between what we call parametric and semiparametric models. It also outlines the algorithms needed to compute the models' predictions, together with an efficient general minimization algorithm that can be used to estimate the parameters of the models described in the chapter. Section 3 concentrates on the parameter estimation problem. Section 4 sketches some statistical considerations and hints at possible solutions to the model discrimination, and model order determination problems. A short bibliographical note about semiparametric models ends the chapter.

THE ANALYSIS OF PHARMACOKINETIC/PHARMACODYNAMIC (PK/PD) DATA

2.1 The PK/PD Data

We consider a PK/PD experiment in which drug is given to a subject at a certain site of administration. At different times thereafter drug concentration is observed at a site (v) (e.g.

the venous blood) together with an effect (e.g. heart rate, temperature) which is, in general, related to concentrations at a different site e. Suppose, for simplicity of exposition, that both observed drug concentration and effect vs time curves have a single peak (the peak effect is greater than the baseline effect). If the effect peak occurs *after* the drug concentration peak we will refer to the situation as "hysteresis" (where we use the word in its Greek etymological meaning of "comes late"). If the effect peak occurs *before* the drug concentration peak we will refer to the situation as "proteresis" (where the neologism is meant to mean "comes early" [Campbell, 1990]). In the hysteresis case, a plot of effect vs concentrations (connected in time order) shows an anticlockwise loop (often referred to as anti/counterclockwise hysteresis); in the case of proteresis the same plot shows a clockwise loop (often also referred to as clockwise hysteresis).

To give an example of a PK/PD experiment and of hysteresis, Figure 2, top panel, shows midazolam concentrations (forearm venous plasma), and the effect [total power in the (0.5 - 30.0) Hz interval of the EEG power spectrum, expressed as percentage of baseline (baseline = voltage recorded before start of infusion = 100%)] against time (min). The data come from one healthy male human volunteer given midazolam 5 mg/min by i.v. infusion from time 0 min to time 3 min (Michael Bührer, personal communication). When the effect is plotted vs the plasma concentration (bottom panel), a counterclockwise (hysteresis) loop is seen.

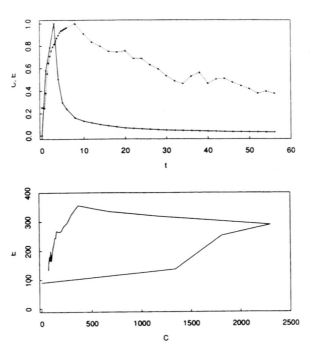

Figure 2. Upper panel: observed midazolam C (ng/ml) (connected by a solid line), and observed E (see text) (connected by a dashed line) vs time t (min); the + sign marks observed E and C. (C and E are scaled to have maximum value 1.) Bottom panel: counterclockwise hysteresis curve of E vs observed midazolam concentration.

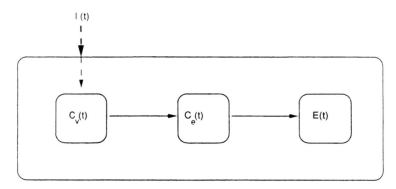

Figure 3. Dose-effect relationship I: drug is input into the system, reaches site v, and from v reaches site e, $C_e(t)$ induces the effect $E(t)$. The dark boxes indicate that only $C_v(t)$ and $E(t)$ are observed.

2.2 A Model for the PK/PD Data

We describe the PK/PD data by means of the following assumed sequence of events: drug is input into the system (where by system we mean the whole organism to which drug is given, for example the human male of the midazolam example of Fig. 2), reaches site v (e.g. the venous blood), and from v reaches site e (e.g. brain blood). Effect results from the presence of drug in e (see Figure 3). The time delay between the appearance of drug in v and in e is responsible for the hysteresis shown in the lower panel of Figure 2.[1]

To obtain a more formal description of the PK/PD model we first introduce some notation, then define the functional form and the assumptions of the model. The mathematical functions considered in this chapter, have arguments time (t, where t is 0 at the start of input), and/or (drug) concentration (C), and some (vector of) parameters. In our notation, we will explicitly indicate all the arguments of a function only as convenient. Vector quantities will be indicated using boldface type. Drug concentration at time t in a site x of the body is indicated by $C_x(t)$ [e.g. drug concentration in v, and e at time t are indicated by $C_v(t)$ and $C_e(t)$, respectively], the effect (E) at time t is indicated by $E(t)$. For an arbitrary function of t [$f(t)$] its "area under the curve" [$\int_0^t f(t)dt$] is indicated by Af.

Suppose, as is often the case, that in a particular experiment the input is through a unique site (e.g. a vein, or the mouth for an oral formulation). To describe the relationship between drug input and measured drug concentration for an arbitrary site x of the system, we define two functions. The first, which we call the residence function [$R_x(t)$], gives the concentration in x for a given arbitrary input to the *system*. [For the particular case that the total input to the system is through site x, this function is equivalent to the so called disposition function of site x (see e.g. Veng-Pedersen and co-workers, 1992).] The second function, which we call the

---

[1] In fact, time delays between drug concentration in e and observed effect are indistinguishable from those between v and e, so that the model is more general than it looks.

transit function [$T_x(t)$], gives the concentration in site x for a given arbitrary input to the site. [This function is often called the "open loop" disposition function of a site. It is the function that would be observed if the site were isolated from the system and a unit bolus dose were given.]

If the system is linear with respect to the input,[2] the concentration in site x can be written as the convolution of $R_x(t)$ with $I(t)$:

$$C_x(t) = I(t) * R_x(t) \tag{1}$$

where $I(t)$ indicates the total input rate (mass/time) to the system at time t, and the asterisk denotes the convolution operator.[3]

If the site x is linear with respect to the input (note that system linearity implies that any site in the system is linear, but not vice versa), the concentration in site x can be written as the convolution of $T_x(t)$ with $I_x(t)$ [the total input rate (mass/time) to site x over time]:

$$C_x(t) = I_x(t) * T_x(t) \tag{2}$$

The functions $R_x(t)$ and $T_x(t)$ both have dimensions of reciprocal volume; some properties of the functions are: $R_x(0) = T_x(0) = 1/V_x$, (where V_x is the volume of site x), $R_x(\infty) = T_x(\infty) = 0$.

Assuming that the functions $R_x(t)$ and $T_x(t)$ are invariant under time translations,[4] Equations 1 and 2 imply:

ASSUMPTION A1: drug distribution in any system site is considered linear and time invariant with respect to the input to the system or to the site.

To compute the predicted drug concentration in v at an arbitrary time t we utilize either its residence function [if $I(t)$ is known], or its transit function [if $I_v(t)$ is known], or simply use the predictions obtained by smoothing C_v data (see below). To compute the predicted drug concentration in e we first make the following additional assumption:

---

[2] Linearity of the response with respect to input is satisfied if: (i) the response to a sum of inputs is equal to the sum of the responses to the individual inputs, and (ii) if the input is multiplied by a constant the response is multiplied by the same constant.

[3] The convolution with respect to time of two functions $f(t)$ and $g(t)$ is the integral:

$\int_{-\infty}^{\infty} f(\tau)g(t-\tau)\,d\tau$, where τ is an integration variable. If, as in all cases considered here

$f(t)$, $g(t) = 0$ for $t < 0$, the convolution is equal to $\int_{0}^{t} f(\tau)g(t-\tau)d\tau$.

[4] Time invariance, with respect to the input, is satisfied if for arbitrary times t_1 and t_2, the response to an input at t_1 is the same as the response to the same input at t_2, just translated in time.

ASSUMPTION A2: the input rate of drug to e at any time is proportional to the current drug concentration in v.

If we know the transit function of e (see below) this last assumption, together with A1, permits the computation of drug concentration in e for arbitrary input once we know $C_v(t)$, or, alternatively, $I(t)$ and $R_v(t)$. Indeed, from the definition of a transit function, it follows that given the input rate to e [which, because of A2, is proportional to $C_v(t)$ or, equivalently, to $I(t)*R_v(t)$] one can compute $C_e(t)$ by convolving $T_e(t)$ with $C_v(t)$, or with $I(t)*R_v(t)$.

To complete a description of the data one need only establish the relationship between $C_e(t)$ and effect. To do so we introduce:

ASSUMPTION A3: the effect at any time t depends only on the concentration of drug in e at time t.

Under this last assumption we need only define a (memoryless, time-invariant) function of $C_e(t)$ [$PD(C_{e,}(t))$] to fully describe the PK/PD relationship.

2.3 Parametric vs Semiparametric Approaches

To estimate the functions $R_v(t)$, $T_e(t)$, and $PD[C_e(t)]$, the first step is to select candidate functions from some specific families of functions. The choice of these familes determines the difference between what we may call parametric and semi-parametric approaches. If the families allow some sort of mechanistic interpretation we call the approach a parametric one. For example consider the approach to modeling the PK/PD system of Figure 2 that was first proposed by Segre (1968). There $R_v(t)$ is a multiexponential, $T_e(t)$ is a monoexponential, $PD[C_e(t)]$ is a hyperbola. In this form (i) $R_v(t)$ is interpretable as describing a compartmental model (Carson and co-workers, 1983); (ii) $T_e(t)$ can be interpreted as the transit function of a compartment with elimination given by a first-order process; and (iii) the hyperbolic PD model can be interpreted in terms of receptor/drug interaction.

In a nonparametric approach the function families do not have a clear mechanistic interpretation. In general, they are chosen for their approximation properties. In a nonpara-metric alternative to Segre's parametric approach one might choose $R_v(t)$, $T_e(t)$, and $PD[C_e(t)]$ to belong to the, e.g., spline family[5] (DeBoor, 1978). We note that the spline family does not

---

[5] A spline function is characterized by a strictly increasing sequence of p real values $(t_1 < \cdots <t_p)$ called knots, and by its order k. In the interval (t_i,t_{i+1}) the spline is a polynomial of order k, and across each t_i, derivatives of order 0 to k–1 are continuous. Qualitatively, a (cubic) spline smoothly interpolates between a set of arbitrary (x,y) points if a knot is placed at each realized value x. A spline function can be represented by a linear combination of so called basis functions. To give an example, consider a straight line (which can be viewed as a linear spline with 2 knots, $t_1 = -\infty$ and $t_2 = \infty$). A straight line can be represented by the linear combination of the constant (1) and identity (t) functions in the following way: $y(t) = a \, 1 + b \, t$, where a and b are coefficients defining the particular linear combination of basis functions (i.e. the particular straight line). Similarly, a more general spline function can be represented using B-spline basis functions [$B_i(t)$] (DeBoor, 1978), in the following way: $y(t) = \sum_i \theta_i \, B_i(t)$ for some values of the coefficients $\theta_1,\ldots,$.

Table 1. The Function Families Considered in This Chapter

Family	Mathematical form
Spline	$\sum_i \theta_i B_i(x)$
Multiexponential	$\sum_i \theta_{2i-1} exp(-\theta_{2i}x), \sum_i \theta_{2i-1} = 1$

where $B_i(x)$ is a, e.g., B-spline basis function (DeBoor, 1978).

allow a meaningful mechanistic interpretation (one can at most say that a spline is a linear filter, but so is every other linear function). Importantly, however, splines have excellent approximation properties. For this last reason the family has enjoyed increasing popularity in a variety of applications (Wegman and Wright, 1983; Buja and co-workers, 1989).

It is traditional in pharmacokinetics and pharmacodynamics to use parametric models that allow mechanistic interpretation. This is appropriate in many circumstances, especially for definitive analyses. In this chapter we suppose that there is little or no prior information on the shape of the models. Once this is recognized, a nonparametric approach may be part of an initial analysis strategy because it imposes few assumptions on the data analysis, and protects the analyst against model misspecification. Accordingly, in this chapter we describe models in which $R_v(t)$ belongs to a nonparametric family (spline), $T_e(t)$ belongs to a parametric family (sum of exponentials), and $PD[C_e(t)]$ belongs to a nonparametric family (spline) (see Table 1). Because of the blend of nonparametric and parametric families, and the use of the convolutions (Eqs. 1 and 2), we call these models semiparametric.

We now detail the form and solution of the semiparametric PK/PD model. The model for $C_v(t)$ and $C_e(t)$ is written as

$$C_v(t) = I(t) * R_v(t, \alpha) \tag{3a}$$

$$C_e(t) = I(t) * R_v(t, \alpha) * \frac{T_e(t, \beta)}{AT_e} \tag{3b}$$

In Equation 3a, $R_v(t, \alpha)$ is a spline function, α is a vector of parameters identifying the particular spline function, and $I(t)$ is known. In Equation 3b, $T_e(t, \beta)$ belongs to the multiexponential family [with $T_e(0, \beta) = 1$], and β is a vector of parameters identifying the function. For example, $T_e(t, \beta) = exp(-\beta_1 t)$ where β_1 is the first order rate of elimination of drug from e.

Note that since $C_e(t)$ is not observed, its units are arbitrary. Equation 3b has the convenient property that at steady-state the concentration in v (C_v^{ss}) equals the concentration in e (C_e^{ss}).[6] Consequently, a concentration-response curve (C_e vs. E) can be viewed as an estimate of the curve C_v^{ss} vs. E, similar to the curve that would be obtained from a series of steady-state experiments. Note that if $R_v(t)$ is of no interest, or $I(t)$ is unknown, one can simply use a spline function to represent $C_v(t)$, and obtain the alternative representation for $C_e(t)$:

$$C_e(t) = C_v(t,\alpha) * \frac{T_e(t,\beta)}{AT_e} \qquad (3c)$$

This last approach, using linear segments (linear interpolating spline) to interpolate drug concentration observations, has proved adequate in past applications (Unadkat and co-workers, 1986). An additional minor advantage of this last approach is that AI above must then be satisfied for site e only.

Finally, the pharmacodynamic model is written

$$E(t,\gamma) = PD[C_e(t),\gamma] = PD[I * R_v * T_e / AT_e,\gamma] \qquad (4)$$

where, $PD[C_e(t),\gamma]$ is a spline function, γ is a vector of parameters identifying the particular spline function, and we omit most of the arguments in the functions for clarity of notation.

Having defined the functions used by the semiparametric approach, and the model for *PK/PD* data (Equations 3 and 4), the solution to the analysis problem is to identify the parameters α, β, and γ from the data. A way of doing so is to minimize some measure of the badness of fit (BOF) of the model defined by Equations 3 and 4 to the PK/PD data (see Section 3, page 174) with respect to the model parameters. In symbols we indicate the minimizing parameters by

$$\hat{\alpha} = arg[min \; BOF \; (C_v,\overline{C}_v)], \qquad (5)$$
$$\alpha$$

$$\hat{\beta},\hat{\gamma} = arg[min \; BOF(PD(C_e),\overline{E})] \qquad (6)$$
$$\beta,\gamma$$

where the notation $\min_{\alpha} f(\alpha)$ indicates the minimum of $f(\alpha)$ with respect to α, *and* $arg[\min_{\alpha} f(\alpha)]$ indicates the particular value of α minimizing $f(\alpha)$; C_v and $PD(C_e)$ are the vectors of predictions for C_v and E, C_e is the vector of predicted concentrations in e, and $\overline{C}_v$, and $\overline{T}$ are the vector of observed C_v and E. Remember that C_v depends on α (Equation 3a), C_e on α and β (see Equation 3b), and $PD(Ce)$ on α, and β (see Equation 4). For given α

---

[6] This can be verified by considering that

$$C_e^{ss} = lim_{t \to \infty} C_e(t) = lim_{t \to \infty} C_v^{ss} * T_e(t)/AT_e = \int_0^\infty C_v^{ss} T_e(t-\tau)/AT_e d\tau = C_v^{ss}/AT_e \int_0^\infty T_e(\tau)d\tau = C_v^{ss}.$$

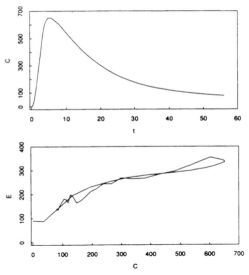

Figure 4. Upper panel: predicted midazolam concentration (ng/ml) in e vs time t (min). Bottom panel: the final counterclockwise hysteresis curve of E vs predicted midazolam concentration in e.

and β the convolutions in Equations 3 are computed analytically, or at worst numerically. The estimate defined in Equation 6 is conditioned on the estimate of α from Equation 5; this is a kind of separation of PK from PD that we consider appropriate especially (but not only) in exploratory analysis.

Figure 4 shows the results of an analysis of the type described above of the data reported in Figure 2, when $T_e(t,\beta) = exp(-\beta_1 t)$. The upper panel shows the estimated $C_e(t)$ vs time curve, the bottom panel shows the estimated $E(t)$ vs $C_e(t)$ plot using the semi-parametric approach. The loop is no longer present. The constant β_1, called k_{eo} in previous articles (e.g. Unadkat and co-workers, 1986), is estimated as 0.125 (min^{-1}). The shape of the curve suggests a complex relationship (note the fast initial portion and the less than hyperbolic rise) between E and C_e suggesting that assuming an arbitrary parametric PD model *a priori* might have introduced bias in the analysis.

2.4 A More General Semiparametric Model

An elaboration of the model associated with Figure 3 can be used to describe both hysteresis and proteresis, and can also include tolerance. This model recognizes that at any time the total input to v and e is proportional to the concentration in a central (unobserved) arterial site (a) (see Figure 5) (Verotta and co-worker, 1989). The semiparametric pharmacokinetic model now takes the form

$$C_a(t) = I(t) * R_a(t,\alpha) \tag{7a}$$

$$C_v(t) = C_a(t,\alpha) * \frac{T_v(t,\beta)}{A\,T_v} \tag{7b}$$

$$C_e(t) = C_a(t,\alpha) * \frac{T_e(t,\beta)}{A T_e} \qquad (7c)$$

In Equations 7 $R_a(t,\alpha)$ belongs to the spline family, $T_e(t,\beta)$ and $T_v(t,\beta)$ belong, in general, to multiexponential families. The mean transit time of drug in a site x (equal, in general, to $AT_x/T_x(0)$, see Verotta and co-workers (1991), and also Covell and co-workers (1984) for general definitions) determines its average rate of equilibration with respect to other sites. For example, suppose $T_e(t)$ and $T_v(t)$ are monoexponential with exponents β_1 and β_2, respectively. When $1/\beta_1$ (the mean transit time of drug in e) is shorter than $1/\beta_2$ (the mean transit time of drug in v), we observe proteresis, while when $1/\beta_2$ is shorter than $1/\beta_1$, we observe hysteresis.

To give an example of the ability of this model to represent both hysteresis and proteresis, we look back at the data reported in Figure 1. These are data simulated using the model described by Equation 7, with $T_e(t)$, $T_v(t)$, and $C_a(t)$ monoexponentials, and $PD(C_e) \equiv C_e/(\gamma_1 + C_e)$, where $\gamma_1 = 0.1$. The exponent in $C_a(t)$ is $\alpha_1 = 5$. The upper left panel shows a plot of E (solid line) and C_v (dashed line) vs time when the exponent of $T_v(t)$ is $\beta_2 = 2.5$, and the exponent of $T_e(t)$ is $\beta_1 = 7.5$ ($1/\beta_2 > 1/\beta_1$: proteresis); note that the maximum PD preceeds the maximum C_v. The upper right panel is a plot of E vs C_v (connected in time order), showing the corresponding clockwise loop. The lower left panel shows a plot of E (solid line) and C_v (dashed line) vs time when $\beta_2 = 7.5$ and $\beta_1 = 2.5$ ($1/\beta_2 < 1/\beta_1$: the more often observed hysteresis case); the maximal PD is after the maximal C_v. The lower right panel shows the corresponding counterclockwise hysteresis loop.

A real example demonstrates the occurrence of proteresis. Nicotine concentration vs heart rate (effect) data are taken from Porchet and co-workers (1989). In this work, a nicotine infusion was given to seven subjects (17.5, 1.75, and 0.35 µg/min/kg from time 0 to 1.5 min, 1.5 to 30 min, and 30 to 180 min, respectively). The mean data are reported. The upper panel of Figure 6 shows nicotine concentrations, and heart rate vs time (min). Proteresis, a

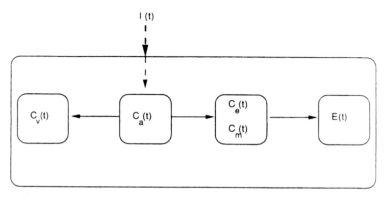

Figure 5. Dose-effect relationship II: drug is input into the system, reaches site a, and from a reaches site v, and e; $C_e(t)$ and $C_m(t)$ induce the effect $E(t)$.

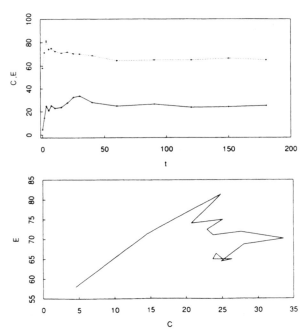

Figure 6. Upper panel: observed venous nicotine concentration (ng/ml) (connected by a solid line) and E (see text (connected by a dashed line) vs time (min); the + sign marks the observations. Bottom panel: clockwise hysteresis curve of E vs observed nicotine concentration. (Porchet and co-workers, 1988).

phenomenon that cannot be explained by the model described in Equations 3 and 4 [Equation 3b can only delay $C_e(t)$ with respect to $C_v(t)$, and consequently can only explain hysteresis] is quite evident from the plot. The lower panel of Figure 6, a plot of heart rate vs plasma concentration, shows the corresponding clockwise loop. The analysis of this data is also complicated by the observation that tolerance develops with time after exposure to nicotine (Porchet and co-workers, 1988). One can notice this phenomenon from the upper panel of Figure 6, where E fails to increase after the second peak of C_v observed at 30-50 min. Before proceeding further, we consider models for the combined action of two active species, an agonist and an antagonist: a particular form of this model will be used to model tolerance.

Let the concentration of the antagonist at time t be denoted $C_m(t)$. Different models can be described taking the clue from standard parametric models. The first one is the noncompetitive antagonist model (Hammes, 1982):

$$PD[C_e(t), C_m(t), \rho, \gamma, \delta] = \rho_1 \frac{C_e(t)}{C_e(t) + \gamma_1} \frac{1}{1 + C_m(t)/\delta_1} \qquad (8)$$

where ρ_1 is the maximum (possible) effect. In this model, $C_m(t)$ can be thought of as reducing ρ_1. We propose the following analogous semiparametric model:

$$PD[C_e(t), C_m(t), \rho, \gamma, \delta] = \rho_1 \, PD[Ce(t), \gamma](1 - PD[C_m(t), \delta]) \qquad (9)$$

where $PD[C_e(t),\gamma]$ and $PD[C_e(t),\delta]$ belong to the spline family, are constrained to be positive and monotonic non decreasing, $PD[0,\gamma]=PD[0,\delta]=0$, $PD[C_e^{max},\gamma]=1$, $PD[C_m^{max},\delta]\leq1$, where C_e^{max}, and C_m^{max} are the maximal concentration achieved by $C_e(t)$ and $C_m(t)$, respectively. (ρ_1 is now the maximum achieved effect.)

The standard competitive antagonist model (Hammes, 1982) takes the form

$$PD[C_e(t),C_m(t),\rho,\gamma,\delta] = \rho_1 \frac{C_e(t)/(1+C_m(t)/\delta_1)}{C_e(t)/(1+C_m(t)/\delta_1)+\gamma_1} \qquad (10)$$

In this model $C_m(t)$ can be thought as "scaling" $C_e(t)$. We propose the following analogous semiparametric extension:

$$PD[C_e(t),C_m(t),\rho,\gamma,\delta] = \rho_1\, PD[C_e(t)\,(1-PD[C_m(t),\delta]),\gamma] \qquad (11)$$

where $PD[C_e(t),\gamma]$ and $PD[C_m,\delta]$ are constrained as in the model described by Equation 9, and if $1-PD\,[C_m(t),\delta]=1/(1+C_m\,(t)/\delta_1)$, and $PD[\cdot,\gamma] = \cdot/(\cdot+\gamma_1)$ then Equation 11 is the same as Equation 10.

The mechanisms of action of models described by Equations 10 and 11 can, of course, be combined, to give the uncompetitive antagonist model (Hammes, 1982):

$$PD[C_e(t),C_m(t),\rho,\gamma,\delta] = \rho_1 \frac{C_e(t)}{C_e(t)+\gamma_1/(1+C_m(t)/\delta_1)} \frac{1}{1+C_m(t)/\delta_1} \qquad (12)$$

A semiparametric analogue is

$$PD[C_e(t),C_m(t),\rho,\gamma,\delta] = \rho_1 PD[C_e(t)/(1-PD[C_m(t),\delta]),\gamma]\,(1-PD[C_m(t),\delta]) \qquad (13)$$

Even more flexible PD models can be obtained using a general multidimensional spline representations of the interaction of C_e and C_m (DeBoor, 1978).

If both C_e and C_m arise from a single drug source (i.e. C_m is an actual or hypothetical metabolite), the models described by Equations 8 through 13 combined with that of Equation 7 provide a means of modeling both tolerance and proteresis, as seen in the nicotine example. Let the concentration $C_m(t)$ (in e) be given by

$$C_m(t) = C_a(t,\alpha) * \frac{T_m(t,\beta)}{AT_m} \qquad (7d)$$

where $T_m(t,\beta)$ belongs to the multiexponential family. For example if $PD[C_m(t),\delta]= 1/(\delta_1/C_m(t)+1)$ in Equation 9, and $PD[C_e(t),\gamma]$ represents the effect expected in the totally non-tolerant state, then δ_1 is the concentration of metabolite ($C_m^{ss} = C_v^{ss}$ see below) at which half tolerance is achieved. As pointed out for Equation 3, Equations 7 imply that at steady-state $C_a^{ss} = C_v^{ss} = C_m^{ss} = C_e^{ss}$. Suppose drug elimination from e, v, and m are first order with rate constants β_1, β_2, and β_3 respectively. Then one notes that in the case of a no-tolerance PD model ($\delta_1 = \infty$ in models described by Equations 8, 10 and 12; $\delta_i = 0$, i=1, ... in the models described by Equations 9, 11 and 13) a plot of (strictly increasing) E vs C_e, describes a clockwise loop (proteresis) when β_1 is greater than β_2, and a counterclockwise one in the opposite case. As far as the assumptions are concerned for the tolerance model, A1 above is required for all sites v, a, e, and m; A2 generalizes to:

ASSUMPTION A2*: the input rate of drug to e, v, and m is proportional to drug concentration in a.

And A3 becomes:

ASSUMPTION A3*: the effect at any time t depends only on the concentration of drug and metabolite in e at time t.

Table 2 lists the assumptions of the models we propose.

Assuming α known (but see below), the remaining unknown parameters of the models described by Equations 7/8 through 13 can be estimated by

$$\hat{\beta},\hat{\rho},\hat{\gamma},\hat{\delta} = arg[\underset{\beta,\rho,\gamma,\delta}{min}\ BOF(PD(C_e,C_m),\overline{E})] \qquad (14)$$

where $PD(C_e,C_m)$ is the vector of predictions for E given by a model of the form of Equations 8-13.

Table 2. The Assumptions of the Models

Pharmacokinetics
    Equations 3
        A1 Drug distribution in the system is linear and time invariant with respect to
            the input to the system
        A2 The input rate of drug to e is proportional to drug concentration in v
    Equations 7
        A1 Unchanged
        A2* The input rate of drug to e, v and m is proportional to drug concentration
            in a
Pharmacodynamics
    Equation 4
        A3 The effect at any time t depends only on the concentration of drug in e at
            time t
    Equations 8 - 13
        A3* The effect at any time t depends only on the concentration of antagonist
            species in e at time t

The minimization of Equation 14 is in terms of β, ρ, γ, and δ, yet $C_e(\beta)$ and $C_m(\beta)$ depend on α through $R_a(t,\alpha)$. To estimate the latter, note that from Equations 7a and b

$$C_v(t) = [I * T_v (\beta)/AT_v]*R_a(\alpha) \qquad (15)$$

where we use the commutative property of convolution. In Equation 15 $I(t)$ is known and, for fixed β, so is $T_v(t,\beta)$.

Using a deconvolution method one can then estimate the vector

$$\hat{\alpha}\,|\,I,\beta = arg[\min_{\alpha} BOF(C_v(I,\alpha,\beta),\overline{C_v})] \qquad (16)$$

where the notation $\hat{\alpha}\,|\,I, \beta$ stresses that this particular vector is obtained conditional on $I(t)$ and β. From Equations 7c and d one may therefore obtain

$$C_e(t) = [I*T_e(\beta) /AT_e]*R_a(\hat{\alpha}\,|\,I,\beta) \qquad (17)$$

$$C_m(t) = [I*T_m(\beta) /AT_m]*R_a(\hat{\alpha}\,|\,I,\beta) \qquad (18)$$

and use these in Equation 14. A more detailed description of the algorithm used to compute $C_e(t)$

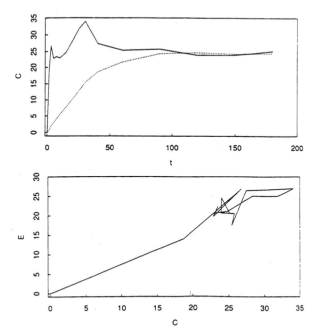

Figure 7. Upper panel: predicted nicotine (solid line) and hypothetical nicotine metabolite (dashed line) concentration (ng/ml) in e vs time (min). Bottom panel: the final counter clockwise hysteresis curve of no-tolerance E vs predicted nicotine concentration in e (see text).

and $C_m(t)$ was described by Verotta and co-workers (1989) where the deconvolution method adopted to estimate $\hat{\alpha}|I, \beta$ constrains $R_a(t,\alpha|I, \beta)$ to be non-negative and non-increasing (see Verotta, 1989).

Suppose for simplicity that ρ_1 is eliminated as a parameter [$PD(C_e^{max},\gamma)$ must then not be constrained to be unity]. If *BOF* is in the form of the usual residual sum of squares (see Section 3, page 174) a simpler algorithm can exploit the fact that $\gamma(\delta)$ appears linearly in the model described by Equation 9 for given β and $\delta(\gamma)$, if $PD[C_e(t),\gamma]$, $PD[C_m(t),\delta]$ are in the spline family.[7] The algorithm is:

> Repeat:
>> For trial β
>>> Estimate α as in Equations 15 and 16
>>> Repeat
>>>> 1. Find $\hat{\gamma}$ given $\hat{\delta}$
>>>> $$\hat{\gamma} = arg[\min_{\gamma} BOF(PD(C_e)(1-PD(C_m)),\overline{E})]$$
>>>>
>>>> 2. Find $\hat{\delta}$ given $\hat{\gamma}$
>>>> $$\hat{\delta} = arg[\min_{\delta} BOF(PD(C_e)(1-PD(C_m)),\overline{E}]$$
>>> Until *BOF* fails to decrease.
> Until *BOF* fails to decrease.

Each inner step of this algorithm is a (constrained) linear least squares problem, which is computationally simpler than a general constrained non-linear least squares problem. Of course a similar algorithm, exploiting the conditional linearity of γ, can be used in the cases of the models described by Equations 11 and 13. Figure 7 shows the results of the analysis of the data reported

---

[7] This can be verified as follows. Using the B-spline basis, and eliminating ρ_1, the model described by Equation 9 can be written

$$PD = [\sum_i \gamma_i \, B_i \, (C_e(t))] \, [1 - \sum_j \delta_j \, B_j(C_m(t))] \tag{19}$$

Fixing δ each γ_i multiplies a known function of $C_m(t)$ and $C_e(t)$. Fixing γ, Equation 19 can be rearranged as follows:

$$PD = [\sum_i \gamma_i B_i(C_e(t))] - \sum_j \delta_j [B_j(C_m(t))(\sum_i \gamma_i B_i(C_e(t)))] \tag{20}$$

where the first term is known, and in the second each δ_j multiplies a known function of $C_m(t)$ and $C_e(t)$, therefore Equation 20 is a linear function of δ. Note that the models described by Equations 11 and 13 are both conditionally linear in γ but not in δ.

in Figure 6, when $T_e(t,\beta) = \exp(-\beta_1 t)$, $T_v(t,\beta) = exp(-\beta_2\ t)$, $T_m(t,\beta) = exp(-\beta_3 t)$, and the model of Equation 9 is used with $PD[C_m(t),\delta] = 1/(1+\delta_1/C_m(t))$. The upper panel shows the estimated $C_e(t)$ vs time curve, superimposed on the estimated $C_m(t)$ vs time curve; the lower panel shows the observed $E(t)$ multiplied by the estimated $1 + C_m(t)/\delta_1$, vs the estimated $C_e(t)$ from the semi-parametric approach (i.e. the 'pure' non-tolerant effect vs C_e plot). The constants β_1, β_2, and β_3 were estimated to be 1.09, 0.73, and 0.027 (min^{-1}), respectively, and δ_1 to be 12.63 (ng/ml). The shape of the curve suggests a linear relationship between non-tolerant E and C_e.

3. ESTIMATION

Although Hull et al. (1978) and we (e.g. Fuseau and Sheiner, 1984; Verotta and Sheiner, 1987) and here in the analyses of the midazolam and nicotine data) first approached the estimation problem by using a *BOF* that penalized for the distance between the upper and lower limbs of the hysteresis loop, a simpler and more general approach is to disregard the loop structure, and simply fit a spline function [S(γ)] (or, more generally, a smooth function, see Buja and co-workers, 1989) to the $\overline{E}$ vs C_e, data. *BOF* is then taken to be the usual sum of squared residuals (RSS) between predictions and observations:

$$BOF = [\overline{E} - S(\gamma)]^2 \qquad (21)$$

Verotta and Sheiner (1991b) have recently used this approach. It has the advantage of simplicity (no special algorithms are needed), and allows simple generalizations to more complex situations (e.g. when metabolites are measured).

To give an example we simulated error free data as follows: $I(t)$ is an infusion with rate 1, lasting .25; $R_v(t) = e^{-\beta_2 t}$, $\beta_2 = 5$; $C_v(t) = R_v(t)*I(t)$; $T_e(t) = e^{-\beta_1 t}$, $C_e(t) = C_v(t)*\beta_1 e^{-\beta_1 t}$, $\beta_1 = 7.5$; and finally $PD(C_e) = C_e /(\delta_1 = C_e)$, $\delta_1 = 0.1$. The left panels of Figure 8 (upper to lower) show $C_v(t)$ (solid line) with superimposed $C_e(t)$ (dashed line) computed for $\beta_1 = 12.5$ (rate "too fast"), $\beta_1 = 7.5$ ("just right"), and $\beta_1 = 2.5$ ("too slow"). Note how the maximal C_e concentration always comes after the maximal C_v concentration. The right panels of Figure 8 (upper to lower) show the corresponding E vs C_e, plots (for β_1 "too fast", "just right", and "too slow", respectively). The values of *BOF* corresponding to the upper right ("too fast") and lower right ("too slow") panels of Figure 8, are 1.39, and 8.25, respectively. BOF is approximately 0 for the "just right" case.

We close this section with the remark that one must impose constraints on the kinetic parameters β. For example, when using the model described by Equations 3 and 4 with $T_e(t) = e^{-\beta_1 t}$, β_1 cannot be so small ("slow") that the loop (E vs C_e) "is opened". Often one can impose these constraints based on the physiology of drug distribution.

4. STATISTICS AND MODEL ORDER DETERMINATION

Assume that the errors in the effect observations have independent normal distributions with zero means and common variance σ^2. If the *BOF* of Equation 21 is used, an estimate of σ^2 might be obtained as: $\hat{\sigma}^2 = RSS/[n - \#(\beta) - \#(\delta) - \#(\gamma)]$, where RSS corresponds to the esti-

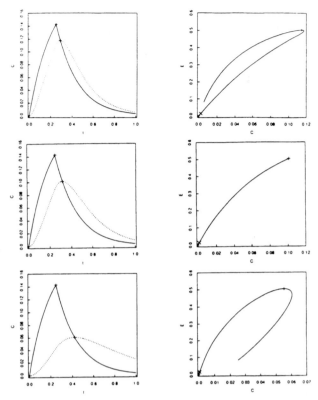

Figure 8. Simulated data. Left panels: simulated C_v (solid line) and (different) C_e (dashed line) vs time (see text). Right panels: simulated E (connected in time order) vs (different) C_e (see text). See legend to Figure 1.

mated $\hat{\beta}$, $\hat{\delta}$, and $\hat{\gamma}$ and # (a) indicates the number of elements in the vector **a** [e.g. #(a) = #(a$_1$, ... a$_m$)^T = m]. Then one might use well known (asymptotic) results to obtain estimates of the standard deviations of the (asymptotically gaussian distributed) parameters (Bates and Watts, 1989). We remark, however, that these asymptotic results are of dubious utility, and/or of problematic interpretation when the parameters are subject to inequality constraints, or to prior information of which no explicit account is taken in the stochastic formulation of the model.

One might also use the Akaike criterion (1974) to choose the number of exponentials in the transit functions in Equation 7, and to choose between different PD models for Equation 6.

5. SHORT BIBLIOGRAPHY OF SEMIPARAMETRIC PK/PD MODELS

To the best of our knowledge, the first attempt to modify the PK/PD model of Segre (1968) to achieve a less parametric representation was reported by Hull and co-workers (1978), and further elaborated by Fuseau and Sheiner (1984). In this last paper $R_v(t)$ is a multiexponential, $T_e(t)$ is a monoexponential, and $PD(t)$ is a linear spline. A similar approach, in which $T_e(t)$ is a multiexponential, has recently been presented by Veng-Pedersen and co-workers (1991). In the work of Unadkat and co-workers (1986) $C_v(t)$ is represented by a linear spline, $T_e(t)$ is a monoexponential, and $PD(t)$ is a linear spline (see also Section 3). Multiexponentials are used to represent $T_e(t)$ in the work of Verotta and Sheiner (1991b).

The no-tolerance version of the model defined by Equations 7-9 was first described in the work of Verotta and co-workers (1989) in the same semiparametric setting described above, but with $T_v(t)$ and $T_e(t)$ monoexponential functions. Tolerance was added in the paper of Sheiner (1989), and elaborated upon by Verotta and Sheiner (1991a). The models for competitive/uncompetitive antagonism are introduced in this chapter. Reviews of the (system theory related) conceptualization underlying the approach can be found (Verotta and Sheiner, 1988; Veng-Pedersen and Gillespie, 1988). A further extension of the approach to include situations where drug concentrations are not observed was recently presented (Verotta and Sheiner, 1991b).

ACKNOWLEGEMENTS

Work supported in part by USDHEW Grants AG03104 and GM26691.

REFERENCES

Akaike, H. (1974). A new look at the statistical model identification. IEEE Trans. Automat.Contr., 19:716-723

Bates, D. M. and D. G. Watts (1988). Nonlinear Regression Analysis and its Applications. John Wiley & Sons, New York.

Buja, A., T. Hastie, and R. Tibshirani (1989). Linear smoothers and additive models (with discussion). Ann. Stat., 17:453-555.

Campbell, D. B. (1990). The use of kinetic-dynamic interactions in the evaluation of drugs, Psychopharmacology,100:433-450.

Carson, E. R., C. Cobelli, and L. Finkelstein (1983). The Mathematical Modeling of Metabolic and Endocrine Systems. John Wiley & Sons, New York.

Covell, D. G., M. Berman, and C.Delisi (1984). Mean residence time-theoretical development, experimental determination, and practical use in tracer analysis. Math. Biosci., 72:213-244.

DeBoor, C. (1978). A Practical Guide to Splines,. Springer-Verlag, New York.

Fuseau, E. and L. B. Sheiner (1984). Simultaneous modelling of pharmacokinetics and pharmacodynamics with a nonparametric pharmacodynamic model. Clin. Pharmacol. Ther., 35:733-741.

Gibaldi, M. and D. Perrier (1982). Pharmacokinetics,2nd edition, Marcel Dekker, New York.

Hammes, G. G. (1982). Enzyme Catalysis and Regulation. Academic Press, New York.

Hull, C. J., B. H. VanBeem, K. McLeod, A. Sibbald, and M. J. Watson (1978). A pharmacokinetic model for pancuronium. Br. J. Anesthes., 50:1113-1123.

Porchet,H. C., N. L. Benowitz, L. B. Sheiner, and J. R. Copeland (1988). Apparent tolerance to the acute effect of nicotine results in part from distribution kinetics. J. Clin. Invest., 244:231-236.

Segre, G. (1968). Kinetics of interaction between drugs and biological systems. Il Farmaco, 23:907-918.

Sheiner, L. B. (1989). Clinical pharmacology and the choice between theory and empiricism. Clin. Pharmacol. Ther., 46:605-615.

Unadkat, J. D., F. Bartha, and L. B. Sheiner (1986). Simultaneous modelling of pharmacokinetics and pharmacodynamics with nonparametric kinetic and dynamic models. Clin. Pharmacol. Ther., 40:86-93.

Veng-Pedersen, P. and W. R. Gillespie (1988). A system approach to pharmacodynamics I: theoretical framework. J. Pharm. Sci.,77:39-47.

Veng-Pedersen, P., J. W. Mandema, and M. Danhof (1991). A system approach to pharmacodynamics III: an algorithm and computer program COLAPS for pharmacodynamic modeling. J Pharm. Sci, 80:488-495.

Verotta, D. (1989). An inequality-constrained least-squares deconvolution method. J. Pharmacokinet. Biopharm., 19:269-289.

Verotta, D. and L. B. Sheiner (1987). Simultaneous modeling of pharmacokinetics and pharmacodynamics IV: an improved algorithm. Comput. Applicat. Biosci., 3:345-349.

Verotta D. and L. B. Sheiner (1988). Parametric and semi-parametric approaches to non-steadystate pharmacokinetic and pharmacodynamic data. Biomedical Measurement Informatics Control, 2:161-169.

Verotta, D. and L. B. Sheiner (1991a). Semiparametric models of the time course of drug action," in C. J. Van-Boxtel, M. Danhof, and N. H. G. Holford, Eds. The In Vivo Study of Drug Action: Principles and Applications of Kinetic Dynamic Modelling. Elsevier Science Publishers, Amsterdam.

Verotta, D. and L. B. Sheiner (1991b). Semiparametric analysis of non-steady-state pharmacodynamic data.J. Pharmacokinet. Biopharm., 19:691-712.

Verotta, D. S. Beal, and L. B. Sheiner (1989). Semiparametric approach to pharmacokinetic pharmacodynamic data. Am. J. Physiol., 256 (Regulatory Integrative Comp. Physiol. 25): R1005-R1010.

Verotta, D., L. B. Sheiner, and S. L. Beal (1991). Mean time parameters for generalized physiological flow models (semi-homogeneous linear systems). J. Pharmacokinet. Biopharm., 19:319-331.

Wegman, E. J., and L. W. Wright (1983). Splines in statistics. J. Am. Stat. Assoc.,78:351-365.

PHARMACOKINETIC AND PHARMACODYNAMIC MODELING APPLIED TO ANESTHETIC DRUGS

Donald R. Stanski
Departments of Anesthesia and Medicine (Clinical Pharmacology)
Stanford University School of Medicine
Stanford, CA 94305, and Palo Alto Veterans Administration Hospital
Palo Alto, CA 94304

ABSTRACT

Several different classes of drugs are used in clinical anesthetic practice. These include muscle paralyzing drugs, potent inhalational anesthetics, intravenous hypnotics and opioids. The measurement of drug effect for each of these classes differs in complexity and resolution. Many concepts of drug pharmacokinetic and pharmacodynamic modeling have been developed with anesthetic drugs. This has occurred because the drug effects are generally profound, can be quantitated in a reasonable manner and are relatively rapid in onset. Understanding anesthetic clinical pharmacology and therapeutics is intimately linked to pharmacokinetic and pharmacodynamic modeling concepts.

INTRODUCTION

The clinical practice of anesthesia involves making a patient insensible to the noxious stimulation that occurs during surgical procedures. The first clinically useful anesthetic was diethyl ether, introduced by Morton in 1846, at which time Oliver Wendel Holmes used the word "anesthesia" to describe the new phenomenon that made surgical procedures possible. While the anesthetic state can be created with a single drug, common clinical practice involves the use of polypharmacy to achieve induction of anesthesia, adequate maintenance during the surgical procedure and finally rapid emergence. The following classes of drugs are used routinely in clinical practice:

Integration of Pharmacokinetics, Pharmacodynamics, and Toxicokinetics in Rational Drug Development, Edited by A. Yacobi *et al.*, Plenum Press, New York, 1993

1) Depolarizing and non-depolarizing muscle paralyzing drugs (ie succinylcholine, pancuronium, vecuronium, atracurium). These drugs cause paralysis of somatic motor muscles and prevent movement.

2) Inhalational anesthetics (ie isoflurane, halothane, enflurane). These drugs are administered as a gas via the lungs. They can cause a complete anesthetic state in adequate concentrations, however they are frequently combined with nitrous oxide (a weak inhalational anesthetic) and opioids. Inhalational anesthetics cause analgesia, unconsciousness, muscle relaxation and amnesia, all characteristics of the anesthetic state.

3) Intravenous anesthetics (ie thiopental, methohexital, etomidate, propofol). These drugs are given intravenously to rapidly induce unconsciousness. They are lipophilic sedatives that rapidly penetrate the blood:brain barrier to cause unconsciousness and then redistribute to other body tissues like muscle and fat. This terminates the immediate anesthetic effect. These drugs have poor analgesic activity and generally are used with other drugs to create an anesthetic state.

4) Opioids (ie fentanyl, alfentanil, sufentanil, morphine, methadone). Opioids are used extensively in anesthetic practice as a premedication, a supplement to regional or inhalational anesthesia, as the primary anesthetic drug in high doses and as an analgesic for postoperative pain. Only the intraoperative anesthetic use of opioids will be discussed in this chapter.

There are several characteristics of the anesthetic drugs that enhance characterizing pharmacokinetic and pharmacodynamic relationships. These include:

1) Acute intravenous or pulmonary administration.
2) Rapid blood:biophase or site of action equilibration.
3) Rapid dissipation of the degree of drug effect because of redistribution of the drug from the site of action to other body tissues and to a lesser degree elimination from the body.
4) A profound degree of drug effect that allows for quantitation.

The drug effects for the four classes of anesthetic drugs discussed in this chapter represent the spectrum of characteristics that pharmacodynamic measures can have. These include:

1) Continuous vs intermittent drug effect. Continuous measures of drug effect have much greater yield of information for pharmacodynamic modeling compared to intermittent measurement of drug effect.

2) Rapid vs a relatively slow occurrence of the drug effect. Rapidly occurring drug effects (ie 0.5-1 min) will result in a closer relationship between a measured drug blood concentration and the drug effect. If the drug effect is slow in onset (i.e. 3-5 min or longer) special considerations for pharmacodynamic modeling must be considered (effect compartment) or alteratively the drug blood concentrations must be kept relatively constant as the drug effect evolves.

3) Noninvasive vs invasive measurement of drug effect. Less patient or volunteer intervention is desirable, however invasive methodology may yield a higher quality of information.

4) A clinically relevant, interpretable measure vs a surrogate measure of drug effect. Ideally one always will measure the drug effect that is most relevant to the pharmacology of the drug. In many cases, this is not possible. "Surrogate" drug effects are other measurable changes of body physiology or response that are induced by the drug. The clinical meaning or interpretation of the surrogate measure may not be known. On other occasions, the surrogate drug effect will be continuous and information-rich while the ideal drug effect may be intermittent and relatively information-poor. Ideally one desires to characterize how the surrogate measure performs or behaves relative to the desired, ideal drug effect.

In an ideal pharmacodynamic research world, one would desire a continuous noninvasive measure of drug effect that occurs rapidly and is clinically relevant. While some of the anesthetic drugs have this ideal profile, most do not, thus the clinical pharmacologist/anesthesiologist must adapt and be innovative with study methodology. In the following discussion of the four anesthetic drug groups, the characteristics of each measure of drug effect will be indicated along with the use of surrogate drug effects for drugs where the clinical effect is difficult to measure.

MUSCLE PARALYZING DRUGS

Measurement of the degree of neuromuscular junction paralysis involves stimulation of the peripheral nerve innervating the muscle with an electrical current and recording the degree of muscle movement. (Ali and Savarese, 1976). Figure 1 displays the pharmacodynamic data that can be obtained in man. It is possible to obtain the measurement of the degree of paralysis almost continuously (every 10 seconds) with high accuracy. The measurement response is rapid and clinically relevant. The nerve stimulation is modestly invasive, requiring electrodes for stimulation and a force transducer or electromyographic recorder to capture the

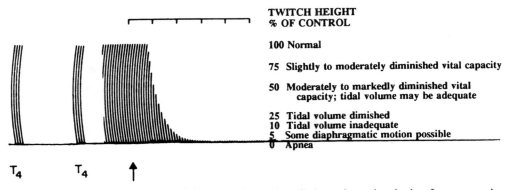

Fig. 1. Correlation of twitch height, clinical relaxation, and ventilation at increasing depths of neuromuscular blockade. A recording of evoked thumb adduction was made in a patient during nitrous oxide-narcotic-barbiturate anesthesia. The single twitch was evoked at 0.15 Hz. At T₄, train-of-four stimulation (2 Hz for 2 seconds) was carried out. Time scale (minutes) at top. At the arrow, pancuronium 0.1 mg/kg, was given intravenously, producing 99 per cent twitch suppression. (Adapted from Ali and Savarese, 1976).

evoked response. Muscle paralysis could be considered a near ideal pharmacodynamic measure.

The degree of muscle paralysis was one of the first drug effect measures to have extensive application of pharmacodynamic modeling concepts. In 1972, Gibaldi, Levy and Hayton used d- tubocurarine data obtained from the literature to explore the relationship of multicompartment pharmacokinetic behavior on drug response. Sheiner and colleagues, (1979) and Hull and colleagues (1978) developed the concept of the "effect compartment" using muscle relaxant pharmacokinetic and pharmacodynamic data. For all nondepolarizing muscle relaxants it is possible to characterize the dose-plasma concentration-degree of paralysis relationship using pharmacodynamic models (Hennis and Stanski, 1985). An excellent example of applying pharmacokinetic and pharmacodynamic models has been provided by Fisher and colleagues (1982). They examined d-tubocurarine dose requirement, pharmacokinetics and pharmacodynamics in neonates (1 day to 2 months of age), infants, (2 months to 1 year), children, (1 years through 12 years) and adults. They found that the volume of distribution at steady-state was greater in neonates than the other groups. The neonates had a neuromuscular junction that was more sensitive to d-tubocurarine, as measured by the serum concentration that resulted in 50% paralysis ($CPSS_{50}$) obtained from pharmacodynamic modeling. The dose that resulted in 50% paralysis, the product of steady-state distribution volume and $CPSS_{50}$ was unaffected by age,predicting no change of d-tubocurarine dose in the neonates. Many other examples of the application of pharmacokinetic and pharmacodynamic concepts to relevant muscle relaxant clinical pharmacology are available in the literature. (Stanski and colleagues, 1979; Martyn and colleagues, 1980; Fisher and colleagues, 1990)

INHALATIONAL ANESTHETICS

For the inhalational anesthetics, pharmacodynamic quantitation is possible using the purposeful movement of a body part in response to noxious perioperative stimulation. Eger, Saidman and Brandstater (1965) defined the minimum alveolar concentration (MAC) of inhalational anesthetics as that end tidal, expired gas concentration required to prevent 50 % of subjects from responding to a painful stimulus with "gross purposeful movement". The MAC concept has three basic components: 1) an all-or-none (quantal) movement response after application of a supramaximal noxious stimulus; 2) quantitation of the biophase concentrations at steady-state via measurement of the end-tidal, expired partial pressures of gas; 3) appropriate mathematical quantitation of the relationship between the end-tidal alveolar concentration of anesthetic and the quantal response.

For determination of MAC in humans, the standard noxious stimulus has been the initial surgical skin incision. In animals the standard stimulus has been application of a surgical clamp to the base of the tail (Quasha, Eger and Tinker, 1980). The MAC concept has been expanded to include other stimuli that are more intense, such as endotracheal intubation and less intense like eye opening (Stoelting, Longnecker and Eger, 1970).

The MAC concept is an example of a pharmacodynamic response that is measured intermittently. It can only be applied on one occasion in a human, the initial skin incision. In animals, multiple stimuli are possible. The response is relatively slow in that the movement response must be observed for at least one minute. Thus, anesthetic gas concentrations must be stable and not changing for meaningful interpretation. It would not be possible to use an effect site concept with changing inhalational anesthetic gas concentrations because the quantal response provides an inadequate amount of information to characterize the biophase response. Thus, a pseudo steady-state of drug concentration in the lungs, blood and biophase must be present to measure MAC. While the movement response is the essence of estimating anesthetic potency this measure is not clinically used in patients. The use of muscle relaxants drugs frequently removes the patient's ability to move as a clinical measure of anesthetic depth. Figure 2 indicates the quantal response/no response data in the estimation of MAC for halothane, halothane with a morphine premedication and halothane with 70% nitrous oxide. This figure demonstrates the marked decrease of halothane MAC with nitrous oxide.

In spite of its simplicity, the MAC concept has proved to be an important experimental tool to understand inhalational anesthetic pharmacology. Table 1 indicates the many clinical situations or anesthetic drug interactions where the potency of the inhalational anesthetic has been increased or decreased. This information has significant relevance in understanding how inhalational anesthetics should be used in patient care.

INTRAVENOUS HYPNOTICS

Pharmacodynamic methodology to quantitate the drug effect of the intravenous hypnotics in man has only recently been proposed. The limited availability of methodology arises

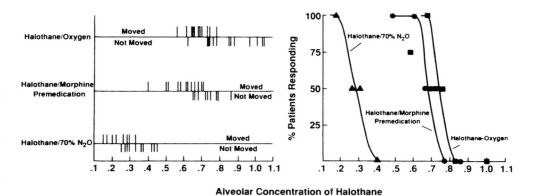

Fig. 2. The minimal alveolar concentration necessary to prevent movement in 50 percent of subjects subjected to a noxious stimulus (MAC) was determined for three combinations of halothane: with oxygen only; with oxygen and a morphine premedication (0.15 mg/kg IM), and with 70 percent nitrous oxide. The anesthetic requirement for halothane is greatly decreased by nitrous oxide, and less so by premedication with morphine. (Reproduced from Miller, R. D. Ed., 1990. Anesthesia, Chap. 30, Fig. 30:8),

TABLE 1. Effect on MAC Factors (study subjects)

Decrease
Hypothermia (animals)
Severe hypotension (animals)
Age (humans)
Narcotics, ketamine (humans, animals)
Benzodiazepines, barbiturates (humans, animals)
Chronic administration of amphetamine (animals)
Reserpine, alpha methyldopa (animals)
Cholinesterase inhibitors (animals)
Intravenous local anesthetics (humans, animals)
Pregnancy (animals)
Hypoxemia (PaO_2(torr) (animals)
Anemia (ml of O_2 per 100 ml blood) (animals)
Alpha-2 agonists (animals)

Increase
Hyperthermia (animals)
Hyperthyroidism (animals)
Alcoholism (humans)
Acute administration of dextroamphetamine (animals)

No effect
Duration of anesthesia (humans, animals)
Sex (humans, animals)
Metabolic acid-base status (animals)
Hypercarbia and Hypocarbia (humans, animals)
Isovolemic anemia (animals)
Hypertension (animals)

MAC - the minimum alveolar concentration of an anesthetic required to abolish movement in 50 percent of patients, in response to a noxious stimulus. (Reproduced from Miller, R. D. Ed., 1990. Anesthesia, Chap. 30, Table 30:1).

from the clinical use of these drugs as a single, intravenous bolus dose to induce the anesthetic state. Plasma concentrations peak within 0.5 minutes and decline rapidly because of drug distribution. The rapidly changing plasma concentrations cause a corresponding fluctuation in the degree of central nervous system (CNS) depression that lags behind the plasma concentration-a rapidly changing, non-steady state clinical situation. The clinical assessment of (CNS) depression is dependant upon application of a relevant noxious stimuli and observation of the clinical response. Clinical end-points that have been used to assess the

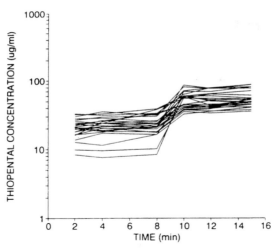

Fig. 3. Measured serum thiopental concentrations vs time for the two target thiopental concentrations in 26 subjects using the computer-controlled infusion pump (Reproduced from Hung and colleagues, 1992).

intravenous hypnotics include: loss of verbal responsiveness, loss of eyelid or corneal reflex or prevention of cardiovascular or movement response to laryngoscopy and tracheal intubation. These are quantal clinical end-points that require a defined period of time (0.5 to 1 minute) to evolve. During this period of time, there are marked changes of both plasma concentration and degree of drug effect when these drugs are given as rapid intravenous bolus doses. The net result is that meaningful pharmacodynamic quantitation cannot be easily performed. Traditional approaches have used dose-response studies to predict the probability of preventing a clinical endpoint in a group of patients. These dose-response studies cannot separate pharmacokinetics and pharmacodynamics.

A new conceptual approach proposed by Hung and colleagues (1992) involves using a computer- controlled infusion pump to rapidly attain, then maintain constant intravenous anesthetic serum concentrations. The computer-controlled infusion pump achieves a constant target serum concentration by using a pharmacokinetic model to choose a loading dose, then constantly changing the maintenance infusion rate every 15 seconds to adjust for drug redistribution and metabolism. Figure 3 displays the thiopental serum concentrations that were obtained in 26 surgical patients. Two different target serum concentrations were achieved in each subject. The computer-controlled infusion pump technology has been reviewed in detail by Shafer and colleagues (1990).

Using the computer-controlled infusion pump to effectively "freeze or clamp" the thiopental serum concentrations, Hung and associates then applied a series of relevant noxious stimuli at one minute intervals: verbal responsiveness, electrical tetanus, trapezius muscle squeeze, direct laryngoscopy and direct laryngoscopy/intubation. These clinical stimuli were applied after the thiopental serum concentration had been maintained for 5 minutes to allow blood:effect site equilibration and achievement of constant drug effect in the biophase or site of action. Thus, when the noxious stimuli are applied, there is no change of plasma or biophase

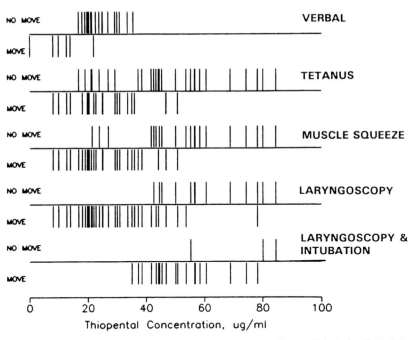

Fig. 4. The move/no move vs serum thiopental concentration for the five different clinical stimuli. Each bar indicates the serum thiopental concentration and response for stimuli applied to an individual patient (Reproduced from Hung and colleagues, 1992).

concentrations between application of the stimuli and observation of the clinical response. Figure 4 displays the thiopental pseudo steady-state serum concentration vs move/no move clinical response relationship obtained in this study. Figure 5 displays this same data converted into the probability of no clinical response vs thiopental serum concentration. This figure demonstrates that the stimuli applied have different degrees of noxiousness and the pharmacodynamic methodology can separate these events. This approach also allows definition of the effective thiopental serum concentrations necessary to prevent clinical responses to relevant stimuli.

OPIOIDS

The opioids have diverse pharmacological effects on the body. These range from analgesia to an anesthetic state in higher doses. There is recently developed methodology for the measurement of pharmacodynamic effects of the anesthetic actions of certain opioids. Alfentail is an opioid that has the rapid rate of blood:brain equilibration ($T_{1/2}$ of 1-2 minutes) (Scott, Ponganis and Stanski, 1985). Ausems and colleagues (1986) have used this characteristic to quantitate alfentanil pharmacodynamics in a clinically relevant environment. Surgical patients received an induction and maintenance anesthetic of alfentanil and 70% nitrous oxide using a bolus induction dose and a variable rate maintenance infusion. The infusion was titrated to the following clinical end-points: 1) an increase in systemic pressure greater than 15 mm Hg above the patient's normal value; 2) heart rate exceeding 90 beats/minute; 3) somatic responses such as body movements, swallowing, coughing, grimacing (minimal muscle paralysis was used); 4) autonomic signs of inadequate anesthesia (lacrimation, flushing, sweating). If any clinical signs occurred, the alfentanil infusion rate was increased, if however, no clinical signs occurred for 15 minutes, the infusion rate was decreased. Arterial alfentanil serum concentrations were measured at times when clinical signs were present and were absent.

Figure 6A displays the alfentanil serum concentration vs clinical response relationship for three single event noxious stimuli: intubation, skin incision and skin closure. Also shown is the logistic regression characterization indicating the probability of no response to each stimulus vs alfentanil serum concentration. Figure 6B displays the probability of no clinical response for 34 patients during the intraoperative surgical procedure where multiple episodes of response and no response were measured in each subject. Figure 6A demonstrates that different surgical stimuli require different alfentanil serum concentrations with much lower opioid concentrations necessary for skin closure relative to skin incision. Figure 6B displays the interpatient pharmacodynamic variability to alfentanil during the interoperative surgical procedure.

Ausems and colleagues (1988) have used the above pharmacodynamic methodology to demonstrate that the method of alfentanil administration (variable rate of infusion vs intermittent bolus) has a clinically significant effect on the quality of the anesthetic. Lemmens and colleagues (1989) have shown that moderate alcohol consumption markedly increases the requirement for alfentanil via a pharmacodynamic mechanism. The methodology indicated above is most applicable to alfentanil that has rapid blood:brain equilibration. For other

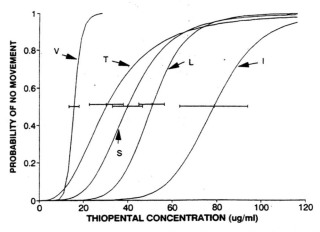

Fig. 5. The predicted probability of no movement vs serum thiopental concentrations function obtained using logistic regression of the data indicated in Fig. 4. The bars indicates the 95% confidence bounds of the Cp$_{50}$ estimate. V=verbal, T=tetanic nerve stimulation, S=trapezius muscle squeeze, L=Laryngoscopy, I=laryngoscopy and intubation. (Reproduced from Hung and colleagues, 1992).

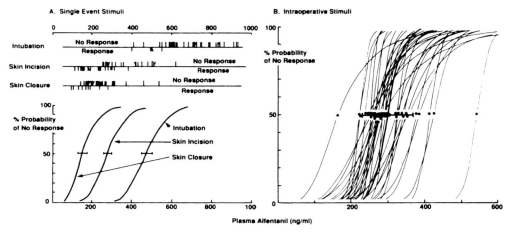

Fig. 6. (A) The relationship between the plasma concentration of alfentanil and response/no response at three specific events of short duration. The quantal data are characterized with logistic regression in the lower panel. Bars indicate the ± SE for the Cp50 (the plasma concentration of alfentanil producing a 50 percent probability of no response). (B) The plasma concentration of alfentanil versus the probability of no response for each of 34 patients during the intra-abdominal phase of lower abdominal surgery. Dots represent the Cp50 values, and the heavy dark line represents the average response of the 34 patients. (Reproduced from Miller, R. D. Ed., 1990. Anesthesia, Chapter 30, Fig. 30:11)

opioids like fentanyl and sufentanil where the blood:brain equilibration is four to five times slower ($T_{1/2}$ of 5 to 7 minutes), it will be more difficult to characterize the same relationship between drug concentrations and clinical responses as has been described with alfentanil because the measured plasma concentration is in a greater disequilibrium with the biophase concentrations.

The two examples of pharmacodynamic analysis for the intravenous anesthetics (thiopental) and opioids (alfentanil) represent new and innovative approaches to capture and characterize anesthetic drug pharmacodynamics using clinical stimuli and responses. In each case, intermittent clinical measures are used. In the final section of this chapter, examples of using surrogate pharmacodynamic measures will be presented.

SURROGATE MEASURES OF OPIOID AND INTRAVENOUS ANESTHETIC DRUG EFFECTS

The electroencephalogram (EEG) has been extensively used in anesthesia as a surrogate pharmacological measure of CNS drug effect. The EEG is a valuable tool because it reflects cerebral physiology, is a continuous and non-invasive measure and changes markedly with the administration of anesthetic drugs. The limitation of the EEG is that it's relationship to traditional measures of CNS depression have not been completely defined. This is especially true when several different drugs are used together to create a defined degree of CNS depression.

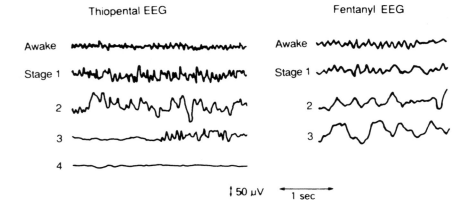

Fig. 7 Increasing plasma concentration of thiopental of fentanyl produce a characteristic progression of changes on the EEG. In stage 1, the frequency and amplitude of waveforms increase (thiopental). In stage 2, both drugs produce a decrease in frequency and an increase in amplitude. In stage 3, thiopental produces a burst-suppression pattern and finally, an isoelectric EEG. Fentanyl has its maximal effect in stage 3 with large, slow delta waves. (Reproduced from Miller, R. D. Ed., 1990. Anesthesia, Chapter 30, Fig. 30:12).

Figure 7 displays the raw EEG changes induced by increasing doses of an intravenous anesthetic (thiopental) or opioid (fentanyl). The EEG patterns differ in that thiopental produces EEG activation at low concentration, then progressive EEG slowing to the point of burst suppression and an isoelectric signal with increased concentration. Fentanyl produces only EEG slowing. To characterize the raw EEG traces, some form of waveform analysis must be utilized. We have found both aperiodic waveform analysis (Gregory and Pettus, 1986) or fast Fourier transformation analysis (Levy and colleagues, 1980) to be useful.

Figure 8 displays the processed EEG for thiopental and fentanyl where the spectral edge (EEG frequency below which 95% of the EEG power exists)is used for fentanyl and the number of waves per second is used for thiopental. Also shown is the arterial serum drug concentration vs time relationship. Pharmacodynamic modeling using the effect compartment concept is necessary to relate the serum concentrations to the continuous EEG drug effect (Sheiner and colleagues, 1979).

Pharmacodynamic analysis of the EEG has generated new and useful clinical pharmacology information. Homer and Stanski (1985) demonstrated that with increasing human age thiopental EEG dose requirement decreases markedly. This decrease in dose requirement resulted from a pharmacokinetic effect: an age-related decline of the rate of thiopental distribution to non-CNS tissues (Stanski and Maitre, 1990). Brain sensitivity, as measured by the EEG was not altered with increasing age as assessed by the thiopental serum concentration needed to achieve half of the maximal EEG slowing. Arden, Holley and Stanski (1986) found similar results with the intravenous anesthetic etomidate. Swerdlow and colleagues (1990) used EEG pharmacodynamic methodology to demonstrate that chronic, heavy alcohol intake did not alter CNS sensitivity to thiopental.

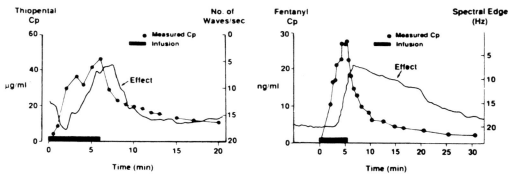

Fig. 8. The relationship between the plasma concentration (Cp) of thiopental or fentanyl and time and the response on the processed electroencephalogram and time. The two drugs were characterized in different ways. Aperiodic waveform analysis provided the number of waves per second produced by thiopental. The fast Fourier transform was used to estimate the spectral edge for fentanyl. Note the biphasic effect of thiopental on the EEG: the number of waves first increases and then decreases as the plasma concentration of thiopental increases. Note also the lag or hysteresis between plasma concentration and EEG effect for each drug. (Reproduced from Miller, R. D. Ed., 1990. Anesthesia. Chapter 30, Fig. 30:13).

    The continuous nature of the EEG signal has been critical in the assessment of the rate of blood:brain equilibration for the three opioids fentanyl, sufentanil and alfentanil (Scott, Ponganis and Stanski, 1985; Scott, Cook and Stanski, 1991). These studies demonstrated the relatively slow blood:brain equilibration of fentanyl and sufentanil ($T_{1/2}$ of 5 to 7 minutes) relative to alfentanil ($T_{1/2}$ of 1-2 minutes). Alfentanil's rapid blood:brain equilibration explains its rapid onset and dissipation of opioid effect and allows the pharmacodynamic modeling of clinical responses as discussed previously.

    There are several important issues that must be addressed when surrogate measures of drug effect, like the EEG, are used in pharmacodynamic analysis. First, there are no standard approaches to deciding which EEG parameter is most representative of the underlying drug effect. To date, empirical approaches have been used to find EEG parameters that have pharmacological relevance. A second important issue is the correlation of the EEG to traditional pharmacological measures of drug effect. To date, limited research has been pursued to understand these relationships. Difficulty in the frequent and accurate measurement of the true, clinically relevant drug effect makes the "calibration" of the surrogate drug effect a challenge. In general, if surrogate drug effects are continuous, relatively noninvasive and occur at serum drug concentrations that are within the "therapeutic window" of clinically relevant drug effects, the surrogate parameters can be extremely helpful in understanding a drug's clinical pharmacology.

    In summary, the drugs used to provide clinical anesthesia have proved to be a fertile therapeutic environment for the development and application of pharmacodynamic research. Because the clinical practice of anesthesia is totally dependant upon potent drugs that cause rapid and profound degrees of drug effect, measurement and quantitation of these drug effects becomes an integrated and relevant component of the practice of medicine. This property, coupled with the conceptual and mathematical advances of pharmacodynamic modeling

(Sheiner and colleagues, 1979), have resulted in pharmacodynamic modeling becoming an integral part of the clinical pharmacology of anesthetic drugs.

ACKNOWLEDGEMENTS

The author acknowledges the support of the National Institute on Aging (R01-AG04595, P01-AG03104), the Veterans Affairs Merit Review grant and the Anesthesiology/Pharmacology Research Foundation.

The editorial assistance of Ms. Georgette Bozovich is also acknowledged.

REFERENCES

Ali, H. H., and J. J. Savarese (1976). Monitoring of neuromuscular function. Anesthesiology, 45, 216-249.

Arden, J. R., F. O. Holley and D. R. Stanski (1986). Increased sensitivity to etomidate in the elderly: Initial distribution vs altered brain response. Anesthesiology, 65, 19-27.

Ausems, M. E., C. C. Hug, Jr., D. R. Stanski and A. G. L. Burm (1986). Plasma concentrations of alfentanil required to supplement nitrous oxide anesthesia for general surgery. Anesthesiology, 65, 362-373.

Ausems, M. E., J. Vuyk, C. C. Hug, Jr. and D. R. Stanski (1988). Comparison of computer-assisted vs intermittent bolus administration of alfentanil as a supplement to nitrous oxide for lower abdominal surgery. Anesthesiology, 68, 851-861.

Eger, E. I., L. J. Saidman and B. Brandstater (1965). Minimum alveolar anesthetic concentration: A standard of anesthetic potency. Anesthesiology, 26, 756-763.

Fisher, D. M., C. O'Keefe, D. R. Stanski, R. Cronnelly, R. D. Miller and G. H. Gregory (1982). Pharmacokinetics and pharmacodynamics of d-tubocurarine in infants, children, and adults. Anesthesiology, 57, 203-208.

Fisher, D. M., P. C. Canfell, M. J. Spellman and R. D. Miller (1990). Pharmacokinetics and pharmacodynamics of atracurium in infants and children. Anesthesiology, 73, 33-37.

Gibaldi, M., G. Levy, and W. Hayton (1972). Kinetics of the elimination and neuromuscular blocking effects of d-tubocurarine in man. Anesthesiology, 36, 213.

Gregory, T. K., and D. C. Pettus (1986). An electroencephalographic processing algorithm specifically intended for analysis of cerebral electrical activity. J. Clin. Mon., 2, 190-197.

Hennis, P. J., and D. R. Stanski (1985). Pharmacokinetic and pharmacodynamic factors that govern the clinical use of muscle relaxants. Seminars in Anesthesia, 4, 21-30.

Homer, T. D. and D. R. Stanski (1985). The effect of increasing age on thiopental disposition and anesthetic requirement. Anesthesiology, 62, 714-724.

Hull, C. J., H. B. Van Beem, K. McLeod, A. Sibbald and M. J. Watson (1978). A pharmacodynamic model for pancuronium. Br. J. Anaesth., 50, 1113-1123.

Hung, O. R., J. R. Varvel, S. L. Shafer and D. R. Stanski (1992). Thiopental pharmacodynamics: II. Quantitation of clinical and EEG depth of anesthesia. Anesthesiology, 77, 237-244.

Lemmens, H. J. M., J. G. Bovill, P. J. Hennis, M. P. R. R. Gladines and A. G. L. Burm (1989). Alcohol consumption alters the pharmacodynamics of alfentanil. Anesthesiology, 71, 669-674.

Levy, W. J., H. M. Shapiro, G. Maruchak and E. Meathe (1980). Automated EEG processing for intraoperative monitoring: A comparison of techniques. Anesthesiology, 53, 223-236.

Martyn, J. A. J., K. Szynfelbein, H. H. Ali, R. S. Matteo and J. J. Savarese (1980). Increased d- tubocurarine requirement following major thermal injury. Anesthesiology, 52, 352-355.

Quasha, A. L., E. I. Eger and J. H. Tinker (1980). Determination and applicaton of MAC. Anesthesiology, 53, 315-334.

Scott, J. C., J. E. Cooke and D. R. Stanski (1991). EEG quantitation of opiate effect:Comparative pharmacodynamics of fentanyl and sufentanil. Anesthesiology, 74, 34-42.

Scott, J. C., K. V. Ponganis and D. R. Stanski (1985). EEG quantitation of narcotic effect:The comparative pharmacodynamics of fentanyl and alfentanil. Anesthesiology, 62, 234-241.

Shafer, S. L., J. R. Varvel, N. Aziz and J. C. Scott (1990). Pharmacokinetics of fentanyl administered by computer-controlled infusion pump. Anesthesiology, 73, 1091-1102.

Sheiner, L. B., D. R. Stanski, S. Vozeh, J. Ham and R. D. Miller (1979). Simultaneous modeling of pharmacokinetics and pharmacodynamics: Application to d-tubocurarine. Clin. Pharmacol. Ther. 25, 358-371.

Stanski, D. R. (1990) In R. D. Miller (Ed.), Anesthesia, 3rd edition, Churchill-Livingston, New York. Chap 30.

Stanski, D. R. and P. O. Maitre (1990). Population pharmacokinetics and pharmacodynamics of thiopental:The effect of age revisited. Anesthesiology, 72, 412-422.

Stanski, D. R., J. Ham, R. D. Miller and L. B. Sheiner (1979). Pharmacokinetics and pharmacodynamics of d-tubocurarine during nitrous oxide-narcotic and halothane anesthesia in man. Anesthesiology, 51, 235-241.

Stoelting, R. K., D. E. Longnecker and E. I. Eger (1970). Minimum alveolar concentrations in man on awakening from methoxyflurane, halothane, ether and fluroxene anesthesia: MAC awake. Anesthesiology, 33, 5-9.

Yakaitis, R. W., C. D. Blitt and J. P. Angiulo (1970). End-tidal halothane concentration for endotracheal intubation. Anesthesiology, 47, 386-388.

PHARMACODYNAMIC/PHARMACOKINETIC RELATIONSHIPS FOR RAPIDLY ACTING DRUGS (NSAIDS) IN RHEUMATOID ARTHRITIS: PROBLEMS AND PRELIMINARY SOLUTIONS

Daniel E. Furst
University of Washington
Seattle, Washington
Virginia Mason Medical Center (VMMC)
1100 Ninth Ave., P.O. Box 900
Seattle, WA 98101

ABSTRACT

The application of pharmacodynamic/pharmacokinetic (PK/PD) principles to anti-inflammatory therapy is hampered by a lack of knowledge about the etiologies of rheumatic diseases and a lack of precise endpoints of response.

For rheumatoid arthritis (RA), for example, the pathogenesis of disease is not well understood, making measurement of surrogate dynamic endpoints difficult. While measurement of T-cell numbers or response is possible, it does not accurately define the best therapeutic intervention.

Likewise, measurement of pharmacodynamic endpoints is inexact. For example, the coefficient of variation of joint tenderness count (a standard measure in RA) is about 25 percent, making measurement of drug effects difficult. And placebo response is also about 20-30 percent, further confounding efficacy.

Even the pharmacokinetics of NSAIDs may be complex and confound the ability to discern PK-PD relationships. Enantiomeric forms of some NSAIDs make previous measurements problematic. Thus, ibuprofen, given as a racemate, is about 60 percent converted in vivo to its active form, while other NSAIDs undergo much less interconversion.

Despite these obstacles, some relationships between response and drug concentrations have been discerned. For example, in two double-blind, cross-over studies, dose-response and serum concentration-response relationships were found for naproxen and carprofen, two NSAIDs. To do this, a nonparametric approach and simple linear relationships were used.

Integration of Pharmacokinetics, Pharmacodynamics, and Toxicokinetics in Rational Drug Development, Edited by A. Yacobi *et al.*, Plenum Press, New York, 1993

Other studies relating to analgesis with NSAIDs have also been examined, as have relationships between salicylate levels and tinnitus.

INTRODUCTION

Documentation of a relationship between pharmacokinetics and pharmacodynamics in rheumatoid arthritis is in its early stages. This review will confine itself to efforts dealing with nonsteroidal anti-inflammatory drugs (NSAIDs) and with rheumatoid arthritis (RA). This is because the relationship between kinetics and dynamics is most easy to document with rapidly acting drugs such as NSAIDs and because rheumatoid arthritis is the prototypic inflammatory disease.

The pharmacokinetic/pharmacodynamic relationship (PK/PD) is difficult to establish in rheumatoid arthritis because:

1. It is hard to relate PK/PD in a disease with a very complex pathogenesis which is not fully understood.
2. The clinical measurements of response in rheumatoid arthritis are inexact, and response is frequently delayed.
3. The pharmacokinetics of NSAIDs may be complex.

Despite these difficulties, some PK/PD relationships have been documented.

PATHOGENESIS OF RHEUMATOID ARTHRITIS

When the pathogenesis of a disease is understood, it is possible to model the relationship between kinetics and the processes leading to the disease. Further, in that circumstance, surrogate measures may be used which correlate with clinical response, making PK/PD modeling even more effective. Unfortunately, this situation is not true for rheumatoid arthritis. There is evidence that there is a genetic background and predisposition in RA (Calin , Elswood and Klorida, 1989). Thus data indicates that HLA-DR4 and HLA-DRl are associated with rheumatoid arthritis and that those with HLA-DR4 have more severe disease (Calin , Elswood and Klorida, 1989).

A complex and interactive immune circuitry exists to start and fuel this disease. The pathogenesis of rheumatoid arthritis involves macrophages, T and B lymphocytes, and polymorphonuclear cells (PMNs). The macrophage, by production of interleukin-l (IL- l) activates B- and T-cells, enhances inflammatory and fibrotic processes through endothelial and fibroblast mediated effects, and diverts hepatic function to acute phase reactive proteins. Interleukin-2 (IL-2) is produced by activated T-cells and amplifies other T-cell responses. Further, this interleukin activates B-cells. The B-cells, in turn, by the production of IL- l, enhance T-cell response. Interferon gamma (IF-gamma) is produced by activated T-cells and amplifies macrophage responses, up-regulates MHC expression, and antagonizes interleukin-4. These and other cytokines result in the expression of receptors on macrophages, T- and B-cells, which facilitate communication between these three groups of cells, further amplifying response (Krane, 1989). Polymorphonuclear cells are also found in great abundance in

Table 1. Variability of Clinical Measures in RA (Furst, 1988)

	C.V. %	"Critical" Change	% Pt. Change*
Morning stiffness	104	100%	17
Onset Fatigue	38	—	—
Joint Tenderness	27	>2 joints	65
Grip Strength	9-25	>11 mmHG	51
ESR	23	>9 mm/hr	17
Walking Time	11	—	—

* Patients changing by critical amount in 7 days

the synovial fluid. These cells appear to be reacting to inflammatory proteins and, in turn, increase inflammatory response through release of collagenase, proteases, and other enzymes (McCarty, 1989). The presence of this inflammatory "soup" means that it will be difficult to find surrogate markers that correlate well with clinical response.

Clinically, the above events result in symmetrical, widespread pain and swelling of the small and large joints of the body. In addition, rheumatoid arthritis is a systemic disease. It affects the eyes, lungs, heart, gastrointestinal tract, kidneys, muscles, bones, nerves, and peripheral vessels (Bacon, 1989). As such, one would hope that clinical measurement of disease would be both accurate and precise. Unfortunately, this is not true. The measures of rheumatoid disease which are clinically in use today include: an addition of the number of tender joints, a summation of the number of swollen joints, the time necessary to walk 50 feet, visual analog scales of disease activity and patient pain, grip strength, erythrocyte sedimentation rate (ESR), and questionnaires measuring the ability to carry on activities of daily living. (Lansbury, Baier and McCracken, 1962; Smythe and Buchanan, 1988). These measures vary spontaneously and are subject to major measurement error, per se (see Table 1) (Furst, 1988). Thus the coefficient of variation (C.V.) of morning stiffness is 100 percent and 17 percent of 499 patients measured one week apart had changes greater than 100 percent in morning stiffness, despite no change in underlying treatment (Furst, 1988). Likewise, as noted in Table 1, the coefficients of variation for other measures vary from as little as 11 percent to as great as 38 percent. An additional complication in the use of these clinical measures is a well-documented circadian rhythmicity in measures of response. Thus grip strength, morning stiffness, and finger joint swelling are all subject to regular and significant circadian rhythms (Kowanko and co-workers, 1982). As swelling is a measure of inflammation, which is usually tender, one would expect very close correlation between joint tenderness and swelling. This is not always so, as documented in a small study of six patients (Spiegel and co-workers, 1987). In this case, it was noted that seven percent of joints were tender without swelling and 16 percent were swollen without tenderness.

Under these circumstances, it is not surprising that it may be difficult to tell active drug from placebo. This is exemplified by a large, well-designed study of sulfasalazine, gold sodium thiomalate, and placebo in rheumatoid arthritis (Williams and co-workers, 1988). This six- month study used placebo as a negative control and gold sodium thiomalate as a positive control. Unfortunately, there was an unusual placebo response making it difficult to tell drug from placebo. Thirty-nine percent of the placebo-treated patients had a 50 percent improvement in joint tenderness, compared to 33 percent of gold sodium thiomalate-treated patients. In this case, there appeared to be no difference between positive and negative controls. Luckily, 57 percent of the sulfasalazine treated patients had a 50 percent improvement in joint tenderness, which was significantly better than placebo. Changes in other measures were of borderline significance. Thus, despite a well-designed trial, and because the measurements of disease have inherent variability, it may be difficult to tell whether a drug is effective in rheumatoid arthritis. Fortunately, most trials are more like that comparing methotrexate to placebo. In that parallel, six-month study, there are clear differences between drug and placebo (Williams and co-workers, 1985). Eleven percent of placebo-treated patients had a 50 percent improvement in joint tenderness count while 32 percent of patients on methotrexate had this degree of response. Joint swelling response also separated drug from placebo. On the other hand, patient assessment of disease severity did not separate drug from placebo. This result is not atypical of trials in rheumatoid arthritis, where some measures of response separate drug from control, whereas others do not. It is for this reason that rheumatologists frequently measure the nine response measures mentioned previously, in the hopes that a majority of them will "point" to drug efficacy (or lack thereof).

Are there objective measures which may be useful? One objective measure is the erythrocyte sedimentation rate (ESR). As noted in Table 1 above, this measure has a coefficient of variation which is not very different from other clinical measures. Further, it responds to treatment more slowly than clinical measures, thus making it a less than ideal measure.

A commendable goal in RA treatment would be to decrease the rate of bony destruction associated with the disease. Standardized measures of bony erosion have been developed and tested (Sharp and co-workers, 1985). One study examined variability by using three blinded observers and hand x-rays of 52 patients. The x-rays were read blindly six weeks apart. Interobserver coefficients of variation (CV) were between 19 and 35 percent, and intraobserver CV was 27 percent (Sharp and co-workers, 1985). Once again, this measurement is not easy to use, and once again, carefully designed trials, plus long duration of follow-up, have enabled standardized x-ray comparisons to separate drug from placebo (Larsen, Horton and Osborne, 1983). A one-year study demonstrated that gold sodium thiomalate prevented the appearance of new erosions to a larger degree than did placebo or oral gold (28 percent versus 64 percent and 42 percent, respectively).

PHARMACOKINETIC COMPLICATIONS

While there are newly discovered complications in the appropriate measurement of rapidly acting drugs in rheumatoid arthritis, this area of measurement is relatively easy to solve. Recent evidence has documented that most NSAIDs, which are given as racemic mixtures, consist of an active and inactive (or less active) enantiomer (Knihinickik, Williams and Day, 1989). For ibuprofen, there is reversible, in vivo conversion of the (R) enantiomer (inactive) to the (S) isomer, (which is active). This interconversion means that measurement of total ibuprofen concentrations will be an inaccurate reflection of active drug. In essence, the R ibuprofen is a reversible prodrug for the active form. Other NSAIDs which are given as enantiomers are not converted but are excreted differentially (Jamali and co-workers, 1988). Thus it is important to understand the underlying composition of the drug which is given and to measure it appropriately.

Further, a biologic effect of the drug may outlast its serum concentrations. Dromgoole et al. (1982) demonstrated this for tolmetin. Although tolmetin concentrations in the synovial fluid were below measurement sensitivity, prostaglandin concentrations remained low for many hours. If one believes that prostaglandin concentrations in synovial fluid reflect a biological response, this prolonged effect might complicate the kinetic/dynamic relationship. In fact, an 18-patient, double-blind, cross-over, two-week clinical study, comparing ibuprofen (with a serum half life of one to two hours) given twice daily versus four times a day, showed no differences (Jalali and co-workers, 1986).

ATTEMPTS AND EARLY SUCCESSES AT DOCUMENTING PHARMACOKINETIC/PHARMACODYNAMIC RELATIONSHIPS

Early attempts at measuring dose-response relationships were occasionally successful. Thus differences were found between 2.4 and 5.4 g/day aspirin, between 50 and 300 mg/day phenylbutazone, and between 1200 and 2400 mg/day ibuprofen.[17] On the other hand, no dose-response relationships were found for meclofenamate, tolmetin, flurbiprofen, or piroxicam (Day and co-workers, 1982). An attempt by Grennan et al. (1983) to correlate ibuprofen AUC with response was only marginally successful. Similar attempts by Baber et al. (1979) and Ekstrand et al. (1980) for indomethacin were unsuccessful.

Day and colleagues (1982) approached the problem using 24 patients in a double-blind, Latin-square comparison of 250, 750, and 1500 mg/day naproxen. The usual standard

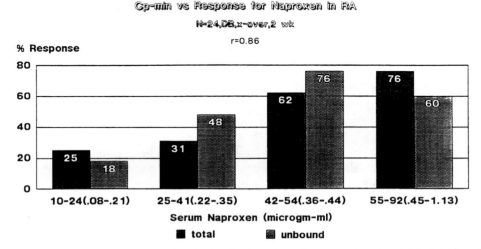

Figure 1. Minimum plasma concentration (total and unbound) vs. % response in a double blind, Latin-square comparison of three naproxen doses in 24 RA patients (Day and co-workers, 1982).

measures of efficacy were tested and showed a statistical, but not convincing, dose- response relationship. For example, the joint tenderness count went from 71 (at prestudy flare) to 53 on 250 mg/day naproxen, 45 on 750 mg/day naproxen, and 46 on 1500 mg/day naproxen. In an attempt to improve results, a non-parametric approach was used for statistical analysis. Patients were defined as responders or nonresponders using a defined, summed efficacy score, with the result seen in Figure 1. The percentage responding patients increased from 25 percent to 31 percent, to 59 percent, to 75 percent as total naproxen concentration increased by quartile. Interestingly, unbound naproxen concentrations gave no better results than total concentration. This encouraging result was confirmed in a serum concentration and dose-response study of carprofen (Furst et al., 1988). Again, a multiple cross-over, randomized, block design comparison study was carried out of 100, 300, 600 and 800 mg/day carprofen. Similar response relationships were found for six of the nine efficacy measures. When using the non parametric analysis, the percent responders rose from 38.1 percent to 50 percent to 59.1 percent, when patients were divided into three equal groups. While no dose or serum concentration to toxicity relationship was found in the naproxen study, a hint of such a realtionship was found for carprofen (Day et al., 1982; Furst et al., 1988). While 27 percent of patients on placebo had an adverse experience, a rough dose-adverse experience relationship for carprofen was found during the active treatment. Thus 10 percent of patients had an adverse experience on 100 mg/day carprofen, 22 percent on 300 mg/day carprofen, 33 percent on 600 mg/day carprofen, and 26 percent on 800 mg/day carprofen.

CONCLUSIONS

There are a number of significant problems when describing the pharmacokinetic/pharmacodynamic relationship for NSAIDs in rheumatoid arthritis. While formidable, these problems have already, to some extent, been overcome. The methodologies already described in previous chapters of this book should make it possible to successfully model this relationship for rapidly acting drugs such as NSAIDs in rheumatoid arthritis. Once this challenge has been met, it will be time to examine the relationships among disease-modifying anti-rheumatic drugs, whose onset of response is often delayed by three to six months.

REFERENCES

Baber, N., L. Halliday, and W. J. A. Van den Heuvel (1979). Indomethacin in rheumatoid arthritis: Clinical effects, pharmacokinetics and platelet studies in responders and non-responders. Ann. Rheum. Dis., 38, 128-137.

Bacon, P. A. (1989). Extra articular rheumatoid arthritis. In D. J. McCarth (Ed.), Rheumatoid Arthritis and Allied Conditions, 11th ed. Lea & Febiger, Philadelphia, pp. 1967-1988.

Calin, A., J. Elswood, and P. T. Klorida (1989). Destructive arthritis, rheumatoid factor and HLA-DR4. Arth. Rheum., 32, 1221-1225.

Day, R. O., D. E. Furst, S. H. Dromgoole, B. Kamm, R. Roe, and H. E. Paulus (1982). Relationship of serum naproxen concentration to efficacy in rheumatoid arthritis. Clin. Pharmacol. Ther., 31, 733-740.

Day, R. O., G. G. Graham, D. Bieri, M. Brown, D. Cairns, G. Harris, J. Hounsell, S. Platt-Hepworth, R. Reeve, P. N. Sambrook, and J. Smith (1989). Concentration-response relationships for salicylate induced ototoxicity in normal volunteers. Br. J. Clin. Pharmacol., 28, 695-702.

Dromgoole, S. H., D. E. Furst, R. K. Desiraju, R. K. Nayak, M. A. Kirschenbaum, and H. E. Paulus (1982). Tolmetin kinetics and synovial fluid prostaglandin E levels in rheumatoid arthritis. Clin. Pharmacol. Ther., 32, 371-377.

Ekstrand, R., G. Alvan, M. L'Orme, R. Lewander, L. Palmer, and B. Sorby (1980). Double-blind dose response study of indomethacin in rheumatoid arthritis. Eur. J. Clin. Pharmacol., 17, 437-442.

Furst, D. E (1988). Clinical evaluation of drugs in rheumatoid arthritis. Adv. Inflamm. Res., 12, 227-238.

Furst, D. E., J. R. Caldwell, M. P. Klugman, D. Enthoven, K. Rittweger, R. Scheer, E. Sarkissian, and S. Dromgoole (1988). Serum concentration and dose-response relationships for carprofen in rheumatoid arthritis. Clin. Pharmacol. Ther., 44, 186-194.

Grennan, D. M., L. Aarons, M. Siddigui, M. Richards, R. Thompson, and C. Hingham (1983). Dose-response study with ibuprofen in rheumatoid arthritis: Clinical and pharmacokinetics. Br. J. Clin. Pharmacol., 15, 311-316.

Jalali, S., J. G. MacFarlane, E. M. Grace, and Y. B. Kassam (1986). Frequency of administration of short half-life nonsteroidal antiinflammatory analgesics (NSAIDs): Studies with ibuprofen. Clin. Exp. Rheum., 4, 91-93.

Jamali, F., B. W. Berry, M. R. Tehrani, and A. S. Russell (1988). Stereoselective pharmacokinetics of flurbiprofen in humans and rats. J. Pharm. Sci., 77, 666-669,

Knihinickik, R. D., K. M. Williams, and R. O. Day (1989). Chiral inversion of 2- arylproprionic acid non-steroidal anti-inflammatory drugs - 1. Biochem. Pharmacol., 38, 4389-4395.

Kowanko, I. C., M. S. Knapp, R. Pownall, and A. J. Swanell (1982). Domiciliary self-measurement in rheumatoid arthritis and the demonstration of circadian rhythmicity. Ann. Rheum. Dis., 41, 453-455.

Krane, S. M. (1989). Mechanisms of tissue destruction. In D. J. McCarth (Ed.), Rheumatoid Arthritis and Allied Conditions, 11th ed. Lea & Febiger, Philadelphia, pp. 698-714.

Lansbury, J., H. N. Baier, and S. McCracken (1962). Statistical study of variation in systemic and articular indexes. Arth. Rheum., 5, 445-456.

Larsen, A., J. Horton, and C. Osborne (1983). Auranofin compared with intramuscular gold in the long-term treatment of rheumatoid arthritis: an x-ray analysis. In H. A. Capell, D. S. Cole, K. K. Manghani, and R. W. Morris (Eds.), Auranofin. Excerpta Medica. Amsterdam. pp. 264-277.

McCarty, D. J. (1989). Clinical picture of rheumatoid arthritis. In D. J. McCarth (Ed.), Rheumatoid Arthritis and Allied Conditions, 11th ed. Lea & Febiger, Philadelphia, pp. 715-743.

Sharp, J. T., G. B. Bluhm, A. Brook, A. C. Brower, M. Corbett, J. L. Decker, H. K. Genant, J. P. Gofton, N. Goodman, A. Larsen, M. D. Lidsky, P. Pussila, A. S. Weinstein, B. N.

Weissman, and D. Y. Young (1985). Reproducibility of multiple-observer scoring of radiologic abnormalities in the hands and wrists of patients with RA. Arth. Rheum., 28, 16-25.

Smythe, H. A., and W. W. Buchanan (1988). An experiment in reducing interobserver variability of the examination for joint tenderness. J. Rheum., 15, 492-494.

Spiegel, T. M., W. King, S. R. Weiner, and H. E. Paulus (1987). Measuring disease activity: comparison of joint tenderness, swelling and ultrasonography in rheumatoid arthritis. Arth. Rheum., 30, 1283-1288.

Williams, H. J., J. R. Ward, S. L. Dahl, D. O. Clegg, R. F. Willkens, T. Oglesby, M. H. Weisman, S. Schlegel, R. M. Michaels, J. C. Luggen, M. J. Egger (1988). A controlled trial comparing sulfasalazine, gold sodium thiomalate and placebo in RA. Arth. Rheum., 31, 702-713.

Williams, H. J., R. F. Willkens, C. O. Samuelson, G. S. Alarcon, M. Guttadauria, C. Yarboro, R. P. Polisson, S. R. Weiner, M. E. Luggen, L. M. Billingsley, D. L. Dahl, M. J. Egger, J. C. Redding, and J. R. Ward (1985). Comparison of low-dose oral pulse methotrexate and placebo in the treatment of rheumatoid arthritis: a controlled clinical trial. Arth. Rheum., 28, 721- 730.

THE VALUE OF PLASMA-WARFARIN MEASUREMENT

Robert A. O'Reilly
Departments of Medicine, Santa Clara Valley Medical Center,
San Jose, and the Stanford University Medical Center, Stanford, and the
California Institute for Medical Research, San Jose, CA 95128

INTRODUCTION

For the last 30 years I have measured the plasma concentration of warfarin in man and animal and correlated it with the pharmacologic effect (O'Reilly, 1986). This effect of oral anticoagulants like warfarin is measured by the one-stage prothrombin time in plasma, which is easily quantitated. In the therapeutic monitoring of oral anticoagulants, the prothrombin time must be utilized and not the blood concentrations of the drug. Both the therapeutic efficacy and the clinical safety of these drugs in patients is achieved only by the careful control of the prothrombin time within narrow limits. The correlation of the plasma concentration of warfarin and the prothrombin-time response has yielded insights on the clinical use of racemic warfarin. For each of the entities described herein, the tables of data and the illustrations may be found in the original publications cited in the references.

LINK'S RABBITS

Link (1943) isolated the hemorrhagic agent dicumarol from spoiled sweet-clover hay by using the one-stage prothrombin time in "reactor" rabbits as a bioassay. Link fed normal rabbits single test doses of spoiled hay extracts. Only the rabbits with marked "reactor responses" of the prothrombin times were used in his subsequent experiments. To determine if the difference in prothrombin-time response in reactor and nonreactor rabbits was related to the rate of metabolic disposition of dicumarol, we measured the plasma concentrations of dicumarol in 20 normal rabbits after large single oral doses.

The prothrombin-time responses showed a wide range, of which the reactor and nonreactor designations were the extreme ends. The reactor rabbits had high plasma concen-

Integration of Pharmacokinetics, Pharmacodynamics, and Toxicokinetics in Rational Drug Development, Edited by A. Yacobi et al., Plenum Press, New York, 1993

trations of dicumarol and slow clearance of the drug, whereas the nonreactor rabbits had lower concentrations of dicumarol and more rapid clearance of drug (O'Reilly, Pool and Aggeler, 1968). Thus, the marked variation of the pharmacologic responses in Link's rabbits resulted from a pharmacokinetic basis in the metabolic disposition of dicumarol.

CLINICAL PHARMACOLOGY OF WARFARIN

By 1961, the oral anticoagulant most commonly used in the U.S.A. was racemic warfarin. Despite its clinical popularity, there was no published method for its measurement. We successfully modified the method for dicumarol for the measurement of warfarin in human plasma (O'Reilly and co-workers, 1962). The error introduced by the nonspecificity of these spectrophotometric methods was lessened by the experimental use of single doses of the drugs. Accordingly, we gave single doses of racemic warfarin orally and intravenously to many normal human subjects. The nearly identical results obtained from both routes of administration indicated essentially 100% bioavailability and complete gastrointestinal absorption (O'Reilly, Aggeler and Leong, 1963). The biologic half-life of warfarin in plasma was directly correlated with the prothrombin response in the normal subjects. Those subjects with a longer half-life of warfarin had a greater area under the curve for the prothrombin response and those with the more rapid half-life had a smaller response of the one-stage prothrombin time.

The mean biologic half-life of warfarin in blood for normal human subjects was 36 hours. This finding was independent of the route of administration, size of the dose, or the pharmacokinetic model used (O'Reilly, Welling and Wagner, 1971). Additionally, we found a high degree of binding of racemic warfarin to plasma albumin, over 99% (O'Reilly, 1967). Thus, the low intrinsic clearance of racemic warfarin and its affinity for plasma albumin could explain the prolonged biologic effect and half-life of drug in plasma, the small volume of distribution of the drug (12% of body weight or the albumin space), and the absence of unchanged warfarin in red blood cells, cerebrospinal fluid, and urine (O'Reilly, 1986).

LOW-DOSE METHOD OF INITIATION OF LONG-TERM THERAPY

The long half-life of warfarin, 36 hours, makes it one of the few drugs administered at time intervals shorter than its half-life. Thus, I reasoned that the administration of small daily doses of warfarin could lead to its accumulation in the body and to a progressive rise in its blood concentrations and in its pharmacologic effect. In separate experiments daily doses of 15 mg and 10 mg of racemic warfarin were administered to 15 normal subjects. The mean time to achieve a therapeutic prolongation of the prothrombin times was 3 days with the 15-mg dose and 5 days with the 10-mg dose, compared to 1 day with a very large loading dose (O'Reilly and Aggeler, 1968a). These data clearly showed that therapeutic anticoagulation could be achieved without using large and dangerous loading doses, because plasma concentrations of warfarin accumulated with small, daily doses of the drug. A pharmacokinetic model was developed that showed a linear relationship of the logarithm of the drug concentration in plasma and the degree of inhibition of the rate of synthesis of the prothrombin complex (Nagashima, O'Reilly and Levy, 1969).

WARFARIN RESISTANCE IN MAN AND RAT

I took care of a patient who required the largest dose of warfarin ever recorded: 145 mg per day for eight years. This remarkable dose size caused no side effects in the patient. His blood concentrations of warfarin were within the range expected for this dose size (O'Reilly and co-workers, 1964). His dose- response curve was parallel to that of normal subjects but displaced, as is seen in altered affinity of a drug for its receptor site. I also studied another patient who required 80 mg per day of warfarin to achieve therapeutic anticoagulation, also a remarkable dose and again without any side effects (O'Reilly, 1970).

All the known relatives of both patients were studied with a single large dose of racemic warfarin. They all had 48-hour plasma concentrations of warfarin within the range for normal subjects. The response of the one-stage prothrombin activity for 34 of the family members was within the range of normal subjects, $82\pm4\%$ (mean $\pm$ SEM) reduction in 48 hours, whereas 26 of the family members had the same degree of resistance as the propositi, only 10% reduction at 48 hours. This marked bimodal distribution of the 48-hour prothrombin activity allowed an unambiguous genetic assessment of these data (O'Reilly, 1974). The pedigree of the second kindred showed four generations with nearly a 50% frequency of transmission of the resistant response and male-to-male transmission in two instances. These data are consistent with an autosomal dominant transmission of a simple mendelian gene (O'Reilly, 1976).

I bred wild rats from Scotland, who had resistance to warfarin as a rodenticide, with normal Sprague-Dawley rats for 5 generations of back crosses. The fifth generation was docile and albino, had "normal" blood levels of warfarin, autosomal dominant transmission of the resistance, and an altered receptor site for warfarin (Pool and co-workers, 1968). The warfarin receptor site is the pathway for the reactivation of vitamin K, the enzyme vitamin K epoxide reductase. In all experiments performed the results in man and rat have been identical. Hence, an excellent animal model exists for the study of warfarin resistance.

STEREOSELECTIVE DRUG INTERACTIONS WITH RACEMIC WARFARIN

Warfarin is a racemic mixture composed equally of two enantiomorphs. For over 20 years I have studied the interaction of phenylbutazone with racemic warfarin in man. The original studies showed marked augmentation of the prothrombin time in the presence of decreased plasma levels of racemic warfarin during phenylbutazone administration (O'Reilly and Aggeler, 1968b). These data were interpreted as displacement of the highly protein-bound warfarin by the second drug that was even more highly protein-bound, phenylbutazone. The next study with the separated enantiomorphs of warfarin in normal human subjects showed marked augmentation of the prothrombin time and a marked increase of the blood levels of S- warfarin. With R-warfarin and phenylbutazone there was no alteration of the prothrombin time and decreased concentrations of R-warfarin. These data suggested inhibition of the metabolic disposition of S-warfarin and induction of the metabolic disposition of R-warfarin (O'Reilly and co-workers, 1980). The next study measured the unbound clearance of R- and S-warfarin. The peak unbound concentrations of both R- and S-warfarin were higher during phenylbutazone administration, as a result of non-stereoselective displacement from plasma albumin. The unbound clearance of the more potent S-warfarin was decreased fourfold during phenylbutazone administration, due to inhibition of the metabolic pathways of S warfarin to its 6- and 7-hydroxywarfarin metabolic products (Banfield and co-workers, 1983). The unbound clearance of R-warfarin was essentially unchanged during phenylbutazone administration, due to the marginal effect of phenylbutazone on its metabolic disposition. These effects of phenylbutazone on racemic warfarin were due to a combination of displacement of protein-bound warfarin and inhibition of metabolic disposition. Phenylbutazone displaced R-warfarin from its plasma binding sites which left more unbound R-warfarin available for hepatic elimination (Tucker and Lennard, 1990). The clearance of the more active S-warfarin was markedly reduced by phenylbutazone, due to the highly stereoselective inhibition of the metabolism of S-warfarin. The details of this complicated interaction of phenylbutazone and racemic warfarin in man required the successive measurement of plasma warfarin concentrations for the total drug, for the separated R and S- warfarin enantiomorphs, and for unbound R- and S-warfarin clearance.

SUMMARY

The measurement of racemic warfarin in the plasma of man for the last 30 years has been useful in understanding its clinical pharmacology. This understanding was established by correlating the blood concentrations of unchanged warfarin with its pharmacologic effect, the inhibition of the one-stage prothrombin time. These data allowed us to initiate therapy with small daily doses of warfarin, to establish the absence of a pharmacokinetic basis for warfarin resistance in man and rat, and to evaluate stereoselective drug interactions with racemic warfarin. We commend the study of racemic warfarin to all students of pharmacology and all practitioners of therapeutics. This drug is a model system in man and animal for probing the mechanisms of pharmacologic problems, because of the ready quantitation of the pharmacologic effect and of the drug itself (O'Reilly and Aggeler, 1970).

ACKNOWLEDGEMENTS

Supported in part by U.S.P.H.S Grant GM 32165-08.

REFERENCES

Banfield, C., R. A. O'Reilly, E. Chan, and M. Rowland (1983). Phenylbutazone-warfarin interaction in man: further stereochemical and metabolic considerations. Br. J. Clin. Pharmacol., 16, 669.

Link, K. P. (1943). Anticoagulant from spoiled sweet clover hay. Harvey Lect., 39, 162.

Nagashima, R., R. A. O'Reilly, and G. Levy (1969). Kinetics of pharmacologic effects in man: the anticoagulant action of warfarin. Clin. Pharmacol. Ther., 10, 22.

O'Reilly, R. A. (1967). Studies on the coumarin anticoagulant drugs; interaction of human plasma albumin and warfarin sodium. J. Clin. Invest., 46, 329.

O'Reilly, R. A. (1970). The second reported kindred of hereditary resistance to oral anticoagulant drugs. N. Engl. J. Med., 282, 1448.

O'Reilly, R. A. (1974). Drug interactions involving oral anticoagulants. Cardiovasc. Cl., 6, 23.

O'Reilly, R. A. (1976). Vitamin K and the oral anticoagulant drugs. Annu. Rev. Med., 27, 245.

O'Reilly, R. A. (1986). Drug induced vitamin K deficiency, resistance, and drug interactions. In W. H. Seegers and D. A. Walz (Eds.), Prothrombin and Other Vitamin K Proteins, Vol. 11, CRC Press, Boca Raton, pp. 37-46.

O'Reilly, R. A., and P. M. Aggeler (1968a). Studies on coumarin anticoagulant drugs: initiation of warfarin therapy without a loading dose. Circulation, 38, 269.

O'Reilly, R. A., and P. M. Aggeler (1968b). Phenylbutazone potentiation of anticoagulant effect: fluorometric assay of warfarin. Proc. Soc. Exp. Biol. Med., 128, 1080.

O'Reilly, R. A., and P. M. Aggeler (1970). Determinants of the response to oral anticoagulant drugs in man. Pharmacol. Rev., 22, 35.

O'Reilly, R. A., P. M. Aggeler, and L. S. Leong (1963). Studies on the coumarin anticoagulant drugs: pharmacodynamics of warfarin in man. J. Clin. Invest., 42, 1542.

O'Reilly, R. A., J. G. Pool, and P. M. Aggeler (1968). Hereditary resistance to coumarin anticoagulant drugs in man and rat. Ann. NY Acad. Sci., 151, 913.

O'Reilly, R. A., P. G. Welling, and J. G. Wagner (1971). Pharmacokinetics of warfarin following intravenous administration to man. Thromb. Diath. Haemorrh., 25, 178.

O'Reilly, R. A., P. M. Aggeler, M. S. Hoag, and L. Leong (1962). Studies on the coumarin anticoagulant drugs; the assay of warfarin and its biologic application. Thromb. Diath. Haemorrh., 8, 82.

O'Reilly, R. A., P. M. Aggeler, M. S. Hoag, L. S. Leong, and M. L. Kropatkin (1964). Hereditary transmission of exceptional resistance to coumarin anticoagulant drugs:first reported kindred. N. Engl. J. Med., 271, 809.

O'Reilly, R. A., W. F. Trager, C. H. Motley, and W. Howald (1980). Stereoselective interaction of phenylbutazone with C12-/C13-warfarin pseudoracemates in man. J. Clin. Invest., 65, 746.

Pool, J. G., R. A. O'Reilly, L. J. Schneiderman, and M. Alexander (1968). Warfarin resistance in the rat. Am. J. Physiol., 215, 627.

Tucker, G. T., and M. S. Lennard (1990). Enantiomer specific pharmacokinetics. Pharmacol. Ther., 45, 309.

CLINICAL PHARMACODYNAMICS OF CARDIOVASCULAR AGENTS: FOCUS ON SUDDEN CARDIAC DEATH

Dan M. Roden
Departments of Medicine and Pharmacology
Vanderbilt University
School of Medicine
Nashville, TN 37232

ABSTRACT

Sudden death due to ventricular tachyarrhythmias is common in patients with advanced coronary artery disease. Three strategies might be useful: slowing progression of coronary atherosclerosis (e.g. antihypertensive or lipid-lowering agents); antiarrhythmic therapy; or elimination of transient factors which trigger fatal arrhythmias (e.g. antiplatelet drugs or ß-blockers). For each of these classes of compounds, an easily measured response variable, such as heart rate, blood pressure, ECG interval, frequency of ambient arrhythmia, or bleeding time, is available and the links between drug concentrations and response are readily determined. However, the common extrapolation that these responses are necessarily accompanied by a decrease in sudden death is unfounded. In addition, patients who are at risk for sudden death have an underlying cardiac substrate which can fluctuate over seconds to years, resulting in both loss of drug efficacy and increased drug toxicity. Thus evaluation of interventions designed to reduce sudden death must be performed in patients at risk, using death as the study end-point. This approach also permits assessment of compounds whose only therapeutic action might be to reduce sudden death.

INTRODUCTION

Like many other forms of therapy discussed in this book, agents used to treat cardiovascular disease are often directed at a readily identifiable symptom, such as angina, pulmonary congestion, or palpitations. Patients can gauge the severity of symptoms and their response to a variety of interventions. In addition, objective measures, such as myocardial

Integration of Pharmacokinetics, Pharmacodynamics, and Toxicokinetics in Rational Drug Development, Edited by A. Yacobi et al., Plenum Press, New York, 1993

207

ischemia during a standardized exercise test, left ventricular filling pressure, or arrhythmia frequency or rate recorded during long term ambulatory electrocardiographic monitoring, can also be used as response variables in the development of cardiovascular therapies directed at the symptoms.

However, unlike many areas of therapeutics discussed here, cardiovascular drugs may also be directed at asymptomatic abnormalities whose treatment is thought to reduce cardiovascular morbidity. Frequently, the assumption is made that treatment of a well-recognized cardiovascular risk factor, such as hypertension or hypercholesterolemia, necessarily reduces cardiovascular risk. Although this may seem rational, trials to test that such a therapeutic strategy does indeed produce long term benefit are necessary. For example, as discussed below, although ventricular ectopic beats are a recognized risk factor for cardiovascular mortality in patients convalescing from myocardial infarction, a test of the hypothesis that arrhythmia suppression would reduce risk has generated new information on the dangers of antiarrhythmic therapy. The remainder of this review will focus on the way in which critical evaluation of the relationship between plasma drug concentrations of antiarrhythmic drugs and their effects can be exploited to develop new information on drug action.

Response Variables in Antiarrhythmic Therapy

Available antiarrhythmic drugs act by blocking one or more ion channels in cardiac cell membranes. These blocking actions at the cellular level then result in typical changes on the surface electrocardiogram, which can be used to monitor drug therapy. Sodium channel blockers slow cardiac propagation and widen the QRS. This action is often exaggerated at fast rates (Hondeghem, 1987). Potassium channel block results in delayed repolarization and prolongation of the QT interval. Again, these effects are frequency-dependent but in this case are exaggerated at slower rates (Hondeghem and Snyders, 1989). Beta blockers slow heart rate, particularly with exercise, and calcium channel blockers such as verapamil slow conduction in the atrioventricular node, resulting in prolongation of the PR interval. These electrocardiographic changes are global indices of drug effect. Measures of drug action at a local level can be obtained either through specialized intracardiac recordings, most often performed in an electrophysiology laboratory, or through the use of the technique of signal-averaged electrocardiography, which is a noninvasive method of detecting slow conduction which may promote reentrant arrhythmias in the ventricle. These more specialized indices of drug action may in the future serve as more sensitive indicators of drug action at diseased (target) tissue. Invasive electrophysiologic studies can also be used to assess drug actions on electrically inducible arrhythmias, while ambulatory electrocardiography can be used to determine drug actions on spontaneously occurring arrhythmias. The latter approach may be confounded by highly variable arrhythmia frequency. Moreover, ascertainment bias (patients tend to seek treatment at a time of maximal symptoms), and regression to the mean can result in overestimation of the effects of interventions. Finally, if an aim of antiarrhythmic therapy is reduction of mortality due to arrhythmias, then trials using death as an endpoint must be conducted. These can be performed in large numbers of patients at low risk of death using an intervention without any major risk of serious toxicity. Alternatively, smaller numbers of patients at high risk of cardiac death can be studied. One technological advance which may permit such trials to proceed is the increasing availability of automatic implantable cardiovertor defibrillators (ICDs). Widespread use of ICDs in high risk patients may eventually allow placebo controlled trials of drug efficacy, using ICD discharge as a surrogate for prevention of serious arrhythmia or death.

Failure of Drug Action to Correlate with Effect: Chirality

As with other forms of pharmacodynamic modelling, interesting information can be derived when plasma concentrations of drugs do not correlate well with effect. One example is the relationship between plasma concentrations of verapamil and PR interval prolongation. Here, the concentration-response curve for intravenous drug is consistently an order of magnitude or so to the left of that for oral drug (Echizen, Vogelgesang and Eichelbaum, 1985). These route-dependent pharmacodynamics are determined by the differences in electrophysiologic potency and in disposition of *l*- and *d*-verapamil (Eichelbaum, Mikus and Vogelgesang, 1984). The *l*-isomer is more potent a calcium channel blocker than the *d*-isomer, but undergoes more extensive first pass hepatic metabolism. Thus, shortly after an intravenous bolus of verapamil measured plasma concentration is 50% *d*-verapamil and 50% *l*-verapamil. However, during oral treatment, measured plasma verapamil is actually proportionally more of the less potent *d*-isomer. These studies illustrate that isomers can differ both in their pharmacologic effects and in their disposition. If isomers do not differ in their pharmacologic effects, then differences in their disposition become less important as determinants of net drug effect. For cardiovascular agents, alpha blockers, beta blockers, calcium channel blockers, and blockers of certain potassium channels display marked stereoselectivity, with ratios of activity between isomers (eudismic ratios) of 50-100 (Turgeon, Thompson, and Roden, 1990). On the other hand, for antiarrhythmics which have sodium channels as their primary electrophysiologic target, eudismic ratios are usually <5, arguing against a prominent role for chirality during treatment with these commonly-used antiarrhythmics. However, an individual isomer may still be responsible for some non-cardiovascular form of drug toxicity. Hence, since racemic compounds may carry a risk of unusual or unanticipated pharmacodynamics, with either cardiovascular or noncardiovascular endpoints, they should therefore in general be avoided.

Failure of Drug Action to Correlate with Effect: Active Metabolites

In early clinical trials, plasma concentrations of the potent sodium channel blocking antiarrhythmic encainide and resultant QRS prolongation showed excellent correlation (Roden and others, 1980). However, occasional outlier patients whose plasma concentrations were strikingly elevated, but whose electrocardiograms were unaffected were identified. This failure of plasma drug concentration to correlate well with effects in all patients was one of the first clues which led to identification of polymorphic metabolism of this compound (Roden and others, 1986). In over 90% of patients, encainide is rapidly biotransformed to two active metabolites, O-desmethyl encainide (ODE) and 3-methoxy-O-desmethyl encainide (MODE). ODE and MODE are more potent sodium channel blockers than encainide in vitro, and their plasma concentrations are higher than those of parent drug, so they likely mediate the effects of encainide therapy in these extensive metabolizer (EM) patients. In less than 10% of patients, the enzyme responsible for encainide O-demethylation is absent on a genetic basis. In these poor metabolizers (PM) subjects, encainide clearance is reduced, plasma encainide accumulates to high concentrations, and arrhythmias are suppressed. The clinical consequences of the P4502D6 polymorphism, inhibition of P4502D6 by other drugs (such as ultra low dose quinidine), and the molecular genetics of this defect have been the subject of intense study in a number of laboratories (Eichelbaum and Gross, 1990; Roden, 1988) and only a few examples will be described here.

The clinical consequences of the P4502D6 polymorphism will depend on whether alternate forms of drug elimination are available and whether substrate biotransformation by P4502D6 results in metabolites which are less potent than, equally potent to, or more potent than the parent drug. For example, flecainide is a P4502D6 substrate and its metabolites are inactive. However, the major route of flecainide elimination is renal. Thus, flecainide accumulation, with attendant cardiovascular toxicity, might be expected almost exclusively in patients with advanced renal failure in whom P4502D6 activity is also absent, either because of the PM phenotype (Mikus and others, 1989) or because of concomitant drug therapy (Birgersdotter and others, 1990).

When the relationship between plasma concentration of propafenone and QRS prolongation was examined, no correlation was found (Siddoway and others, 1987). However, when patients then underwent P4502D6 phenotyping, two separate correlations were found. In subjects with the EM phenotype, the slope of the concentration- ΔQRS plots was steeper than that in the subjects with the PM phenotype; at any given concentration, QRS was greater in EMs than in PMs. These data provided evidence that active metabolites generated by P4502D6 contribute to the pharmacologic effects of propafenone therapy. Subsequent studies have confirmed that propafenone 5-hydroxylation is P4502D6-mediated (Funck-Brentano and others, 1989) and that 5-hydroxy propafenone is as potent a sodium channel blocker as the parent drug (Thompson and others, 1988). The polymorphism has a different impact on propafenone pharmacodynamics when a different response variable, exercise heart rate reduction due to ß-blockade, is used. Here, the parent drug is much more potent a ß-blocker in vitro and the extent of ß-blockade in man was well-correlated with plasma concentrations of the parent drug. In PM subjects, in whom plasma concentrations of propafenone are higher than in EM subjects, the extent of beta blockade was greater (Lee and others, 1990). Since PM subjects also demonstrate statistically significantly more side effects during chronic propafenone therapy, this phenotypic different in ß-blockade may be clinically important. As well, the ß-blocking properties of propafenone reside almost exclusively in the S-(+)-isomer, while the two isomers are equipotent as sodium channel blockers (Kroemer and others, 1989). A more detailed discussion of genetic metabolic polymorphism as related to propafenone can be found in a subsequent chapter, pages 231-233.

Inferences on the role of active metabolites during drug therapy can be drawn from studies such as those outlined above. However, the best way to determine the clinical effects of metabolites is to administer them to patients. When single intravenous doses of ODE were administered to patients, its subsequent clearance to MODE was found to be P4502D6-dependent (Barbey and others, 1988). Since ODE is much more potent a sodium channel blocker than MODE, chronic therapy in PM subjects would be associated with marked drug accumulation and toxicity. On the other hand, MODE disposition was not found to depend on the P4502D6 polymorphism. MODE also produced electrocardiographic changes (prolongation of repolarization) dissimilar to those produced by ODE and in dogs MODE facilitates cardiac defibrillation while ODE impairs it (Fain and others, 1986). These animal and clinical data, then, suggested that MODE might be a suitable candidate for further drug development, while ODE certainly was not. A further detailed discussion of encainide and its metabolites can be found on pages 229-231.

Although it is increasingly recognized that active drug metabolites may contribute to the chronic effects of drug therapy, it should be appreciated that these interactions are not necessarily additive. For example, the lidocaine metabolite glycinexylidide (GX) can, under appropriate in vitro conditions, actually reverse sodium channel block produced by lidocaine (Bennett, Woosley and Hondeghem, 1988). This interaction not only provides evidence for a common receptor site for such agents on sodium channels, but it also raises the possibility that even inactive metabolites might compete with parent drug to modulate drug actions at the receptor level. It is also well-recognized that lidocaine clearance is reduced during long infusions, and competition between metabolites and parent drugs for access to hepatic metabolizing enzyme systems has been proposed (LeLorier and others, 1977). Another example of an interaction between parent drug and metabolites is the decrease in procainamide renal clearance and prolongation of procainamide elimination half-life by concomitant administration of N-acetyl procainamide (Funck-Brentano and others, 1989). Thus, intensive evaluation of the relationship between plasma concentration and effect can be exploited not only to optimize drug delivery methods as described in other chapters and to study drug delivery to receptor sites, but also to detect interesting anomalies which can then provide major clues to mechanisms which modulate drug action.

Failure of Drug Action to Correlate with Effect: End-Organ Variability

Another source of variability in plasma concentration-effect relations is variability in end organ responsiveness. For example, an important area in contemporary antiarrhythmic therapeutics is the relationship between drug concentration and change in the QT interval, since one major thrust in drug development is toward potassium channel blockers, whose major electrocardiographic effect is QT prolongation. These drugs are particularly attractive because they produce a range of desirable pharmacologic effects, such as suppression of ischemic-mediated arrhythmias and facilitated defibrillation; however, as a class, they appear to have the potential liability of markedly prolonging the QT interval and thereby resulting in development of polymorphic ventricular tachycardia, the "Torsades de Pointes" syndrome (Roden, 1990). When Holford and colleagues (1981) compared the time course of changes in repolarization following oral and intravenous quinidine, they inferred that intravenous drug was delivered from a central site to an effector site rapidly, within minutes. Since the slopes of the IV and oral concentration-response curves were different, a role for active metabolites in mediating the repolarization changes produced by quinidine was suggested. Four active metabolites have been identified and their effects characterized in animal models (Drayer and others, 1978) and in vitro (Thompson and others, 1987). However, none exerts more potent electrophysiologic effects than the parent drug, and importantly, no differences in the free plasma concentrations of parent drug or metabolites are found in patients who develop

Torsades de Pointes during quinidine therapy compared to patients who tolerate quinidine therapy without marked QT interval prolongation (Thompson and others, 1988b). Thus, in this case, it is unlikely that variability in drug effect (in this case, delayed repolarization) can be attributed to pharmacokinetic phenomena. Rather, variability in the end organ response to a given concentration of drug appears responsible. Further evidence for such variability has been developed during a trial of a newer potassium channel blocker, sematilide, in patients with ventricular arrhythmias (Wong and others, 1989). Here again, the relationship between plasma drug concentration and QT prolongation was variable, with some patients showing exaggerated responses and arrhythmias at "usual" plasma concentrations. Since sematilide is largely excreted unchanged and does not have a chiral center, end organ variability in response to the QT-prolonging actions of this compound appears to be an important factor in modulating its pharmacologic actions in man.

Unanticipated Responses During Long-Term Treatment: The Problem of the Moving Target

Potent sodium channel blockers such as encainide and flecainide are highly effective suppressors of nonsustained ventricular ectopic activity (Anderson and others, 1981; Roden and others, 1980). The presence of these arrhythmias in a patient convalescing from myocardial infarction is a marker for an increased risk of sudden (presumably arrhythmia- mediated) cardiac death (Bigger and others, 1984; Ruberman and others, 1977). Therefore, the Cardiac Arrhythmia Suppression Trial (CAST) tested the hypothesis that suppression of these arrhythmias would result in decreased sudden death. In CAST, a drug regimen which suppressed ventricular ectopic activity in patients convalescing from a myocardial infarction was first identified in an open-label study phase. Then, patients were randomly assigned in a double-blind fashion to continue that drug regimen or a corresponding placebo. In spring 1989, the encainide and flecainide arms were discontinued because they were found to increase mortality 2-3 fold compared to placebo (CAST investigators, 1989). A third drug, moricizine, continues to be tested in a modified trial design.

Continued analysis of the CAST database has yielded a number of tantalizing suggestions to explain the mortality increment produced by these drugs. First, the survival curves for the drug- and placebo-treated patients divert continually over the year of treatment. This, in turn, suggests that some as yet unidentified intercurrent factor triggers fatal arrhythmias more often in the presence of drug treatment than in the presence of placebo. Two recent reports from CAST investigators support the notion that intercurrent myocardial ischemia is a likely candidate for such a trigger. Echt and colleagues (1991) found that the sum of deaths plus nonfatal myocardial infarctions plus angina was equivalent in the drug and the placebo treated groups, suggesting that myocardial ischemia was more likely to result in death in the drug-treated group while it was more likely to result in angina or a nonfatal myocardial infarction in the placebo treated group. Similarly, Platia and coworkers (1991) identified a non-Q wave infarction as a very potent risk factor for increased mortality during active drug treatment. Since a non-Q wave infarct is thought to be more likely to be associated with continued myocardial ischemic events, this analysis also suggests a role for myocardial ischemia. Other factors which could trigger fatal arrhythmias more often in patients treated with encainide or flecainide compared to those treated with placebo include adrenergic surges, post-myocardial infarction healing, or myocardial stretch. Obviously, further studies both in the experimental laboratory and in man to further elucidate the mechanisms underlying the mechanism of the adverse drug effect in CAST will provide information important for the further development of antiarrhythmic drugs.

Intensive study of the relationship between plasma concentration of cardiovascular agents and resultant pharmacologic effects can explain some of the variability in response to these agents. Some of this variability lies at a pharmacokinetic level; that is, it is attributable to generation of drug metabolites, to the use of racemic compounds, or to delayed drug delivery to a non- central effector site. On the other hand, other variability appears more related to variability in the end organ. The pharmacodynamic response variables we use are frequently surrogates for the true effect we seek, reduction in cardiovascular mortality. As CAST has highlighted, end organ response to therapy may change in a time frame of seconds to years. Thus, studies of the pharmacokinetics and pharmacodynamics of cardiovascular therapy have pointed out the need for compounds with wide margins between efficacy and toxicity, under a range of experimental and clinical conditions, which can then be used to reduce cardiovascular morbidity and mortality in large numbers of patients.

REFERENCES

Anderson, J. L., J. R. Stewart, B. A. Perry, D. D. Van Hamersveld, T. A. Johnson, G. J. Conard, S. F. Chang, D. C. Kvam, and B. Pitt (1981). Oral flecainide acetate for the treatment of ventricular arrhythmias. N. Engl. J. Med., 305, 473-477.

Barbey, J. T., K. A. Thompson, D. S. Echt, R. L. Woosley, and D. M. Roden (1988). Antiarrhythmic activity, electrocardiographic effects and pharmacokinetics of the encainide metabolites O-desmethyl encainide and 3- methoxy-O-desmethyl encainide in man. Circulation, 77, 380-391.

Bennett, P. B., R. L. Woosley, and L. M. Hondeghem (1988). Competitive interactions of lidocaine (L) and one of its metabolites, glycine xylidide (GX), with cardiac sodium channels. Circulation, 78, 692-700.

Bigger J. T., Jr., J. L. Fleiss, R. Kleiger, J. P. Miller, L. M. Rolintzky, and Multicenter Post-Infarction Research Group (1984). The relationship among ventricular arrhythmias, left ventricular dysfunction, and mortality in the 2 years after myocardial infarction. Circulation, 69, 250-258.

Birgersdotter, U. M., J. Turgeon, W. Wong, and D. M. Roden (1990). Stereoselective genetically-determined interaction of flecainide and quinidine. Clin. Res., 38, 339A.

Drayer, D. E., D. T. Lowenthal, K. M. Restivo, A. Schwartz, and M. M. Reidenberg (1978). Steady state serum levels of quinidine and active metabolites in cardiac patients with varying degrees of renal function. Clin. Pharmacol. Ther., 24, 31-39.

Echizen, H., B. Vogelgesang, and M. Eichelbaum (1985). Effects of d,l- verapamil on atrioventricular conduction in relation to its stereoselective first-pass metabolism. Clin. Pharmacol. Ther., 38, 71-76.

Echt, D. S., P. R. Liebson, B. Mitchell, R. W. Peters, D. Obias-Manno, A. H. Barker, A. Arensberg, A. Baker, L. Friedman, H. L. Greene, M. L. Huther, D. W. Richardson, and the CAST Investigators (1991). Mortality and morbidity in patients receiving encainide, flecainide, or placebo: The Cardiac Arrhythmia Suppression Trial. N. Engl. J. Med., 324, 781-788.

Eichelbaum, M., and A. S. Gross (1990). The genetic polymorphism of debrisoquine/sparteine metabolism—clinical aspects. Pharmacol. Ther., 46, 377-394.

Eichelbaum, M., G. Mikus, and B. Vogelgesang (1984). Pharmacokinetics of (+)-,(-)- and (±)-verapamil after intravenous administration. Br. J. Clin. Pharmacol., 17, 453-458.

Fain, E. S., P. Dorian, J-M. Davy, R. E. Kates, and R. A. Winkle (1986). Effects of encainide and its metabolites on energy requirements for defibrillation. Circulation, 73, 1334-1341.

Funck-Brentano, C., H. K. Kroemer, R. L. Woosley, and D. M. Roden (1989). Genetically-determined interaction between propafenone and low dose quinidine: role of active metabolites in modulating net drug effect. Br. J. Clin. Pharmacol., 27, 435-444.

Holford, N. H. G., P. E. Coates, T. W. Guentert, S. Riegelman, and L. B. Sheiner (1981). The effect of quinidine and its metabolites on the electrocardiogram and systolic time intervals: concentration—effect relationships. Br. J. Clin. Pharmacol., 11, 187-195.

Hondeghem, L. M. (1987). Antiarrhythmic agents: modulated receptor applications. Circulation, 75, 514-520.

Hondeghem, L. M., and D. J. Snyders (1990). Class III antiarrhythmic agents have a lot of potential, but a long way to go: reduced effectiveness and dangers of reverse use-dependence. Circulation, 81, 686-690.

Kroemer, H. K., C. Funck-Brentano, D. J. Silberstein, A. J. J. Wood, M. Eichelbaum, R. L. Woosley, and D. M. Roden (1989). Stereoselective disposition and pharmacological activity of propafenone enantiomers. Circulation, 79, 1068-1076.

Lee, J. T., H. T. Kroemer, D. Silberstein, C. Funck-Brentano, M. D. Lineberry, A. J. J. Wood, D. M. Roden, and R. L. Woosley (1990). Genetically determined polymorphism of propafenone metabolism accounts for variable beta-blockade in man. N. Engl. J. Med., 322, 1764-1768.

LeLorier, J., D. Grenon, Y. Latour, G. Caillé, G. Dumont, A. Brosseau, and A. Solignac (1977). Pharmacokinetics of lidocaine after prolonged intravenous infusions in uncomplicated myocardial infarction. Ann. Int. Med., 87, 700-702.

Mikus, G., A. S. Gross, J. Beckmann, R. Hertrampf, U. Gundert-Remy, and M. Eichelbaum (1989). The influence of the sparteine/debrisoquin phenotype on the disposition of flecainide. Clin. Pharmacol. Ther., 45, 562-567.

Platia, E. V., R. W. Henthorn, Y. Pawitan, T. A. Buckingham, M. D. Carlson, J. L. Anderson, P. E. Carson, and CAST Investigators (1991). Cardiac Arrhythmia Suppression Trial (CAST): Baseline predictors of highest mortality. JACC, 17, 230A.

Roden, D. M. (1988). Encainide and related antiarrhythmic drugs. ISI Atlas of Science, 374-380.

Roden, D. M. (1990). Clinical features of arrhythmia aggravation by antiarrhythmic drugs and their implications for basic mechanisms. Drug Dev. Res., 19, 153-172.

Roden, D. M., A. J. J. Wood, G. R. Wilkinson, and R. L. Woosley (1986). Disposition kinetics of encainide and metabolites. Am. J. Cardiol., 58, 4C- 9C.

Roden, D. M., S. B. Reele, S. B. Higgins, R. Mayol, R. Gammans, J. A. Oates, and R. L. Woosley (1980). Total suppression of ventricular arrhythmias by encainide. N. Engl. J. Med., 302, 877-882.

Ruberman, W., E. Weinblatt, J. D. Goldberg, C. W. Frank and S. Shapiro (1977). Ventricular premature beats and mortality after myocardial infarction. N. Engl. J. Med., 297, 750-757.

Schulze, R. A., J. O. Humphries, L. S. C. Griffith, and others (1977). Left ventricular and coronary angiographic anatomy. Relationship to ventricular irritability in the late hospital phase of acute myocardial infarction. Circulation, 55, 839-843.

Siddoway, L. A., K. A. Thompson, C. B. McAllister, T. Wang, G. R. Wilkinson, D. M. Roden, and R. L. Woosley (1987). Polymorphism of propafenone metabolism and disposition in man: clinical and pharmacokinetic consequences. Circulation, 75, 785-791.

The Cardiac Arrhythmia Suppression Trial (CAST) Investigators (1989). Preliminary report: Effect of encainide and flecainide on mortality in a randomized trial of arrhythmia suppression after myocardial infarction. N. Engl. J. Med., 321, 406-412.

Thompson, K. A., I. A. Blair, R. L. Woosley, and D. M. Roden (1987). Comparative electrophysiologic effects of quinidine, its major metabolites and dihydroquinidine in canine cardiac Purkinje fibers. J. Pharmacol. Exp. Ther., 241, 84-90.

Thompson, K. A., D. H. S. Iansmith, L. A. Siddoway, R. L. Woosley, and D. M. Roden (1988a). Potent electrophysiologic effects of the major metabolites of propafenone in canine Purkinje fibers. J. Pharmacol. Exp. Ther., 244, 950- 955.

Thompson, K. A., J. J. Murray, I. A. Blair, R. L. Woosley, and D. M. Roden (1988b). Plasma concentrations of quinidine, major metabolites, and dihydroquinidine in patients with Torsades de Pointes. Clin. Pharmacol. Ther., 43, 636-642.

Turgeon, J., K. T. Murray, and D. M. Roden (1990). Effects of drug metabolism, metabolites and stereoselectivity on antiarrhythmic drug action. J. Cardiovasc. Electrophysiol., 1, 238-260.

Wong, W., H. N. Pavlou, and D. M. Roden (1989). Pharmacology of sematilide, a class III procainamide analog, in man. 62nd Annual Scientific Sessions, American Heart Association. Circulation, 80, SII-326.

THE BENZODIAZEPINES: KINETIC-DYNAMIC RELATIONSHIPS

David J. Greenblatt
Division of Clinical Pharmacology
Department of Pharmacology and Experimental Therapeutics
Tufts University School of Medicine
and New England Medical Center Hospital
Boston, MA 02111

ABSTRACT

The primary pharmacologic actions of the benzodiazepine derivatives include: reduction of anxiety, induction of sleep, and anti-seizure effects. Establishing kinetic-dynamic relationships for this class of drugs is a particular challenge, since reliable quantitation of these primary pharmacologic actions is difficult to achieve. This chapter reviews methodologic issues in studying the pharmacokinetic profile and the pharmacodynamic properties of benzodiazepine derivatives, and methods for quantitative linkage of plasma concentrations with clinical effects.

INTRODUCTION

Benzodiazepine derivatives have been available and in clinical use since 1960. Thirteen different derivatives are used in the United States (Table 1) and many others are available in other nations. (Greenblatt and others, 1983)

The primary pharmacologic actions of the benzodiazepine derivatives include: anti-anxiety effects, induction of sleep, and anti-seizure effects. Whether these actions constitute desired therapeutic effects as opposed to undesired side effects depends on the clinical situation. For example, sedation and sleep are therapeutically desired when a benzodiazepine is taken to induce sleep in a patient with insomnia. On the other hand, the same pharmacologic actions constitute unwanted side effects if they produce daytime drowsiness, sedation, difficulty concentrating, or impaired psychomotor performance. Likewise, memory impairment maybe a desired effect of a benzodiazepine if given as a premedication or induction

Integration of Pharmacokinetics, Pharmacodynamics, and Toxicokinetics in Rational Drug Development, Edited by A. Yacobi *et al.*, Plenum Press, New York, 1993

217

TABLE 1. Benzodiazepines Available in the U.S.

chlordiazepoxide
diazepam
oxazepam
flurazepam
clonazepam
lorazepam
prazepam
halazepam
temazepam
alprazolam
triazolam
quazepam
estazolam

agent prior to a surgical or endoscopic procedure, or prior to cardioversion; amnesia is an unwanted side effect in an ambulatory, working individual who wishes to have unimpaired mentation.

In any case, reliable, replicable, and precise quantitation of the clinical actions of benzodiazepines is notoriously difficult. A number of methods have been used to translate the effects of benzodiazepines into quantitative measures that can be used for clinical or research purposes (Greenblatt and others, 1991a). Each method has significant limitations and drawbacks, but many have been utilized, either alone or in combination, to enhance understanding of the relation of the pharmacokinetic properties of benzodiazepine derivatives to their pharmacodynamic actions.

QUANTITATION OF PHARMACODYNAMIC RESPONSE

Methodologic options for quantitation of the pharmacodynamic response to benzodiazepine derivatives can be divided into the subjective, the semi-objective, and the objective.

Subjective measures

Subjective measures of response depend on the subject's or the patient's own perception of drug effects, or the effect perceived by an observer. Self ratings may focus on a patient's global assessment of the degree of clinical improvement produced by a benzodiazepine in the treatment of anxiety or panic disorder (Ballenger and others, 1988). Ratings may also focus on very specific descriptors of drug effect, including those related to therapeutic actions (such as anxiety or tension), as well as those which may be interpreted as side effects (sedation, fatigue, difficulty concentrating, etc.). Methods are available to translate the perceptions into numbers, including discrete numerical ratings provided by a patient or observer, or by continuous ratings based on instruments such as visual analogue scales (Lapierre and others, 1990). Whatever particular method is chosen, subjective response ratings have the benefit of focusing on the most important primary pharmacologic actions of the drug, such as reduced anxiety or tension, or increased sedation or difficulty concentrating. An important drawback of these approaches is that absolute scores have relatively little meaning, and only with great difficulty can they be compared between patients or between studies. Subjective ratings in general are only meaningful when expressed as change scores relative to some well-established pre-drug baseline score. Interpretation of changes attributable to active drug therapy also requires careful evaluation of the placebo response, which must be documented under double-blind conditions. Other problems may arise in comparisons of different populations, such as young versus elderly individuals, or healthy normal controls versus those with psychopathology. Differences between groups in the interpretation of rating scale items may complicate interpretation of drug effects.

Semi-objective measures

A variety of psychomotor testing procedures, measurements of visual and auditory fusion frequency, and assessment of information acquisition and recall (i.e. memory) comprise a large group of semi-objective methods to quantitate response to benzodiazepines (Johnson and Chernik, 1982; Koelega, 1989; Ghoneim and Mewaldt, 1990). Using these procedures, absolute scores in themselves may have meaning, making it possible to compare different study populations, as well as results from different laboratories. However, the semi-objective approaches also have drawbacks. Practice or adaptation effects are of considerable importance, particularly in the context of psychomotor testing procedures such as: the digit symbol substitution test, tests of reaction time, tracking tasks, computation tests, or more complicated assessments of performance such as simulated driving. Repeated exposure to these testing procedures in general leads to improvement in performance over time in the absence of drug treatment. These practice effects must be accounted for in any study design, usually by allowing subjects to practice and adapt to the task before entering a double-blind trial. Assessment of drug-induced changes require reliable assessment of drug-free or pre-drug baseline performance. Additional methodologic problems are encountered when study populations differ in their intrinsic baseline performance capacity in the absence of drug treatment. It is not established how drug-related changes should be appropriately interpreted and compared between populations whose baseline performance differs. Finally, drug-related alterations in performance on laboratory testing procedures do not necessarily apply to tasks encountered in real life. For example, drug-induced impairment of performance on a driving simulator does not automatically imply that an individual's performance will be equally impaired while actually operating an automobile. As opposed to the laboratory situation, a significant error during real-life automobile operation can have fatal consequences. Awareness of these hazards, and the resulting vigilance that they provoke, may counteract impairment due to a benzodiazepine medication. The reverse may also be true. A very subtle degree of drug-induced impairment that is undetectable by a laboratory test, or does not reach statistical significance, may actually be highly important and dangerous in the context of actual automobile operation.

Objective measures

Measurement methods that are largely or completely objective are being increasingly utilized in studies of the pharmacodynamics of benzodiazepines. These methods include: quantitative analysis of the electroencephalogram (EEG), measurement of saccadic eye movement velocity, postural sway, and plasma concentrations of various endogenous hormones (Greenblatt and others, 1989a; Hommer and others, 1986; Roy–Byrne and others, 1990). These approaches have the benefit of being essentially uninfluenced by adaptation or practice effects, and having little or no response to placebo. Under usual circumstances, the methods provide very reliable quantitative response ratings. There is still a need to establish measures within a given individual in the pre-dose baseline state. Furthermore, these objective measures may be criticized in that they are not necessarily related to primary sedative or anxiolytic actions of the benzodiazepines. Nonetheless, these objective measurement techniques are highly promising in the research context, particularly in light of recent studies suggesting that some objective outcome measures may be directly intercorrelated with the primary actions of the drug class.

QUANTITATION OF PLASMA CONCENTRATIONS AND PHARMACOKINETICS

The pharmacokinetic properties of the various benzodiazepines, both after single doses and at steady state during multiple dosage, have been the subject of extensive research in many parts of the world (Greenblatt and others, 1983; Greenblatt and Shader, 1987). The ease and accuracy of these studies has improved over the years in parallel with technologic improvements in analytical chemistry. The earliest cornerstone of analytical methodology in this context was gas chromatography with electron caption detection, and this continues to be one of the most important analytical tools for pharmacokinetic studies for benzodiazepines. The availability of capillary column technology has allowed enhancement of accuracy and sensitivity in some laboratories. High pressure liquid chromatography has also become an important analytic option. Nonspecific assay techniques, such as radioreceptor assays, have also received some attention, but the potential nonspecificity of receptor or immunoassays always raises doubts as to how quantitative plasma concentrations should be interpreted.

The analytic needs in the context of pharmacokinetic studies of benzodiazepines depend on the particular drug under consideration, and whether the study is a single or multiple dose study. It is essential that any clinically important pharmacologically active metabolites be measured along with the parent drug. As an example, a single- dose study of 5 mg of diazepam in a human will require analytical sensitivity in the range of 1-200 ng/ml for the parent drug, and 1-30 ng/ml for the major metabolite desmethyldiazepam. During multiple dosage, there is accumulation of both diazepam and desmethyldiazepam. Steady state concentrations of both of these compounds typically range from 200 to 1000 ng/ml with chronic treatment using usual therapeutic doses. At the other extreme is a benzodiazepine such as triazolam, for which single therapeutic doses require analytic sensitivity in the range of 0.2-10 ng/ml. Since the

Table 2. Plasma Concentration Ranges for Representative Benzodiazepines

Drug	Plasma level range (ng/ml)	
	Single-dose	Multiple-dose
diazepam	1-200	200-1000
desmethyldiazepam*	1-30	200-1000
lorazepam	1-30	5-80
alprazolam	1-30	5-120
triazolam	0.2-10	0.2-10

*Major metabolite of diazepam

drug is non-accumulating, the required analytic range is the same when the drug is taken repeatedly. Table 2 shows typical concentration ranges encountered following single and multiple doses of several representative benzodiazepines.

KINETIC-DYNAMIC RELATIONSHIPS

The medical literature contains many studies simultaneously evaluating the kinetic and dynamic properties of benzodiazepines. Outcome measures include the subjective, the semi-objective, and the objective approaches described above; in many studies, more than one approach is used simultaneously. We will not attempt a complete review of the literature, but rather point out some important methodologic issues.

Of the many mathematical approaches available to link a drug's plasma concentration to the time-course of its clinical effects, no one method is clearly the most appropriately applied to studies of benzodiazepines. The applicability of a particular model is entirely dependent on the design of the study, the drug under study, the dose, the route of administration, the timing and duration of plasma sampling, the range of plasma concentrations encountered, and the type of pharmacodynamic outcome measure that is utilized. Models used in the medical literature range from straightforward linear models to relatively complex mathematical relationships (Greenblatt and others, 1989a, 1991b). In some studies, inappropriately complex mathematical models have been forced on sets of data that do not warrant such models. This may lead to misleading conclusions about kinetic-dynamic relationships. We suggest that the choice of the appropriate mathematical model should be based on initial visual inspection of the data, and should be the simplest model that provides an adequate explanation of the apparent relationship. It is possible that even within a given study, different models, with different mathematical parameters, may be required for different outcome measures.

The relation of plasma benzodiazepine concentrations to concentration at the target organ, and subsequently to the degree of benzodiazepine receptor occupancy, may be of concern in the context of kinetic-dynamic studies. Experimental data repeatedly indicates that, after the attainment of distribution equilibrium, plasma concentrations of benzodiazepines are directly proportional to concentrations in brain (Barnhill and others, 1990). Brain concentrations, in turn, directly reflect the degree of benzodiazepine receptor occupancy (Miller and others, 1987). However, following single doses of some benzodiazepines, there may be a significant delay in attainment of distribution equilibrium. That is, even after a rapid intravenous bolus dose, a delay may be encountered in the time necessary for the drug to fully equilibrate between plasma and brain (Greenblatt and Sethy, 1990). This is reflected in a delay in the onset of maximal clinical activity. For certain highly lipid- soluble benzodiazepines, such as diazepam, this time delay is negligible; however, for less lipid-soluble drugs, such as lorazepam, the delay in attainment of maximal pharmacologic activity may be delayed up to 30 min following a single intravenous dose (Greenblatt and others, 1989b). In kinetic-dynamic studies that focus on the initial time period after intravenous drug administration, mathematical models must be modified to compensate for the time delay for drug to equilibrate between plasma and the "effect compartment".

Finally, most kinetic-dynamic studies of benzodiazepines focus upon acute single doses. The phenomenon of acute tolerance may disrupt plasma level-effect relationships even after single doses (Smith and others, 1984). The problem is much greater during chronic dosage of benzodiazepines, during which the development of tolerance to pharmacologic effects—particularly nonspecific sedative effects—can cause a shift in the concentration-response relationship simply as the consequence of chronic exposure (Smith and Kroboth, 1987). The molecular mechanisms of tolerance have been described previously, and are explained by receptor downregulation as opposed to pharmacokinetic changes (Miller and others, 1988). In any case, this phenomenon greatly complicates kinetic-dynamic studies during chronic dosage of benzodiazepines.

ACKNOWLEDGEMENTS

This work was supported in part by grants MH-34223 and DA-05258 from the United States Department of Health and Human Services. The author is grateful for the continuing collaboration of Richard I. Shader, Jerold S. Harmatz, and Lawrence G. Miller.

REFERENCES

Ballenger, J. C., G. D. Burrows, R. L. DuPont, I. M. Lesser, R. Noyes, Jr., J. C. Pecknold, A. Rifkin, and R. P. Swinson (1988). Alprazolam in panic disorder and agoraphobia: results from a multicenter trial. I. Efficacy in short-term treatment. Arch. Gen. Psychiatry, 45, 413-422.

Barnhill, J. G., D. J. Greenblatt, L. G. Miller, A. Gaver, J. S. Harmatz and R. I. Shader (1990). Kinetic and dynamic components of increased benzodiazepine sensitivity in aging animals. J. Pharmacol. Exp. Ther., 253, 1153-1161.

Ghoneim, M. M., and S. P. Mewaldt (1990). Benzodiazepines and human memory: a review. Anesthesiology, 72, 926-938.

Greenblatt, D. J., and V. H. Sethy (1990). Benzodiazepine concentrations in brain directly reflect receptor occupancy: studies of diazepam, lorazepam, and oxazepam. Psychopharmacology, 102, 373-378.

Greenblatt, D. J., and R. I. Shader (1987). Pharmacokinetics of antianxiety agents. In H. Y. Meltzer (Ed.), Psychopharmacology: The Third Generation of Progress. Raven Press, New York. pp. 1377-1386.

Greenblatt, D. J., R. I. Shader, and D. R. Abernethy (1983). Current status of benzodiazepines. N. Engl. J. Med., 309, 354-358, 410-416.

Greenblatt, D. J., B. L. Ehrenberg, J. Gunderman, A. Locniskar, J. M. Scavone, J. S. Harmatz, and R. I. Shader (1989a). Pharmacokinetic and electroencephalographic study of intravenous diazepam, midazolam, and placebo. Clin. Pharmacol. Ther., 45, 356-365.

Greenblatt, D. J., B. L. Ehrenberg, J. Gunderman, J. M. Scavone, N. T. Tai, J. S. Harmatz, and R. I. Shader (1989b). Kinetic and dynamic study of intravenous lorazepam: comparison with intravenous diazepam. J. Pharmacol. Exp. Ther., 250, 134-140.

Greenblatt, D. J., J. S. Harmatz, and R. I. Shader (1991a). Clinical pharmacokinetics of anxiolytics and hypnotics in the elderly. Therapeutic considerations (Parts I and II). Clin. Pharmacokinet., 21, 165-177, 262-273.

Greenblatt, D.J., J. S. Harmatz, L. Shapiro, N. Engelhardt, T. A. Gouthro and R. I. Shader (1991b). Sensitivity to triazolam in the elderly. N. Engl. J. Med., 324, 1691-1698.

Hommer, D. W., V. Matsuo, O. Wolkowitz, G. Chrousos, D. J. Greenblatt, H. Weingartner, and S. M. Paul (1986). Benzodiazepine sensitivity in normal human subjects. Arch. Gen. Psych., 43, 542-551.

Johnson, L. C., and D. A. Chernik (1982). Sedative-hypnotics and human performance. Psychopharmacology, 76, 101-113.

Koelega, H. S. (1989). Benzodiazepines and vigilance performance: a review. Psychopharmacology, 98, 145-156.

Lapierre, K. A., D. J. Greenblatt, J. E. Goddard, J. S. Harmatz, and R. I. Shader (1990). The neuropsychiatric effects of asparatame in normal volunteers. J. Clin. Pharmacol., 30, 454-460.

Miller, L. G., D. J. Greenblatt, J. G. Barnhill, and R. I. Shader (1988). Chronic benzodiazepine administration. I. Tolerance is associated with benzodiazepine receptor downregulation and decreased gamma-aminobutyric acid$_A$ receptor function. J. Pharmacol. Exp. Ther., 246, 170-176.

Miller, L. G., D. J. Greenblatt, S. M. Paul, and R. I. Shader (1987). Benzodiazepine receptor occupancy in vivo: correlation with brain concentrations and pharmacodynamic actions. J. Pharmacol. Exp. Ther., 240, 516-522.

Roy-Byrne, P. P., D. S. Cowley, D. J. Greenblatt, and R. I. Shader (1990). Reduced benzodiazepine sensitivity in panic disorder. Arch. Gen. Psychiatry, 47, 534-540.

Smith, R. B., and P. D. Kroboth (1987). Influence of dosing regimen on alprazolam and metabolite serum concentrations and tolerance to sedative and psychomotor effects. Psychopharmacology, 93, 105-112.

Smith, R. B., P. D. Kroboth, J. T. Vanderlugt, J. P. Phillips, and R. P. Juhl (1984). Pharmacokinetics and pharmacodynamics of alprazolam after oral and IV administration. Psychopharmacology, 48, 452-456.

THE INTEGRATION OF PHARMACODYNAMICS AND PHARMACOKINETICS IN RATIONAL DRUG DEVELOPMENT

Sally Usdin Yasuda
Sorell L. Schwartz
Anton Wellstein
Raymond L. Woosley

The Department of Pharmacology
Georgetown University Medical Center
Washington, D.C. 20007

INTRODUCTION

Pharmacokinetic and pharmacodynamic analyses have been found to be valuable components of new drug development programs. This chapter will describe developments in pharmacokinetic and pharmacodynamic studies that have taken place in recent years. An understanding of the relationship between pharmacokinetics and pharmacodynamics and the integration of each type of study will allow even greater contributions to drug development and pharmacological research.

PHARMACOKINETIC MODELING

The most commonly used methods to describe the pharmacokinetic characteristics of drugs are the empirical model and the compartmental model. Another, the physiologically-based model, has been used in toxicology but has not been applied extensively in clinical pharmacologic research.

The compartmental approach to pharmacokinetics is a familiar model of drug disposition. One- and two-compartment models are applicable for most drugs that are used clinically. The two-compartment model utilizes a "theoretical" central compartment, perhaps representing the blood and highly perfused organs such as the heart, lungs, liver and kidneys, and

Integration of Pharmacokinetics, Pharmacodynamics, and Toxicokinetics in Rational Drug Development, Edited by A. Yacobi *et al.*, Plenum Press, New York, 1993

a peripheral compartment, which consists of less rapidly perfused tissues such as fat, muscle and skin (Jusko, 1986). The modeling of drug concentrations in the various compartments has been a very useful tool for derivation of numerical values to describe pharmacokinetic characteristics of drugs, based on plasma concentrations of the drugs. These values include clearance (a direct indication of elimination rate) and volume of distribution (a direct assessment of equilibrium distribution of the drug). The compartmental approach to modeling allows the derivation of numerical values that are potentially applicable to clinical decision making and dosage estimation.

Application of pharmacokinetics has been very useful in the clinical setting. First approximations can be made of what is likely to happen when a drug is given in different dosing regimens or to different types of patients. When plasma concentrations are monitored, the dose can be adjusted based on specific patient pharmacokinetic parameters. These data are also useful in predicting the plasma concentrations that are likely to occur in disease states. For example, by accounting for expected changes in clearance, estimates of the pharmacokinetics of a renally eliminated drug can be made for dosage prediction in patients with renal disease. By accounting for expected alterations in liver blood flow and intrinsic clearance of drugs in patients with liver disease, the dosing of hepatically eliminated drugs can be predicted. Similar projections can be made for patients with congestive heart failure with secondary effects on renal function and/or hepatic function.

The use of phamacokinetic data has clearly played a role in these instances. Such data has also been applied clinically to rapidly and safely achieve and maintain effective drug concentrations. Based on the recognition that lidocaine displays two-compartment kinetics, pharmacokinetic principles were used to propose and test a rational loading regimen for lidocaine (Benowitz, 1974; Stargel and co-workers, 1981). The plasma concentration curve follows a two-compartment model after rapid intravenous administration of lidocaine. Initial high plasma concentrations fall rapidly as the drug distributes into peripheral compartments and then more slowly as it is eliminated by the liver. Early clinical experience with lidocaine given as a rapid intravenous single large dose frequently resulted in toxicity. Pharmacokinetic principles suggest that a sustained effect could be achieved if both the central and peripheral compartments were loaded sequentially. This was tested in a clinical study in which, by administering a series of loading injections and a maintenance infusion, the total volume of distribution was filled, and a relatively constant level of lidocaine was maintained during the 12 hours of this study (Stargel and co-workers, 1981). Early studies such as this have been verified by many larger studies to show that compartmental pharmacokinetics can be used to improve the clinical utility of a drug (Wyman and co-workers, 1983).

Those same approaches have been used in the design of dosing regimens during drug development. Pharmacokinetic modeling of data from single doses has been used to project the accumulation to steady state with infusions or multiple doses. In this way, one can estimate the dose and dosing frequency required to reach a target concentration range in plasma.

Physiologically-based pharmacokinetic (PBPK) modeling represents a new approach to pharmacokinetic analysis. In this method a computer model takes into account disposition of the drug in arterial and venous blood, as well as the kidneys, adipose tissue, muscle, liver, target tissue and all other organs and tissues to which the drug is known to distribute. For drugs administered through the gastrointestinal tract, an absorption component is included.

Using traditional pharmacokinetic approaches, pharmacokinetic values may be mathematically derived. In contrast, the PBPK model uses actual data including the size of an organ or a tissue, clearance data from animal or clinical studies, and distribution data, usually from animal studies, to determine the expected plasma to tissue (site of action of the drug) ratio. Utilization of all available pharmacokinetic data from a variety of both animal and clinical studies should result in the generation of more specific and accurate predictions than are available from traditional single or multiple-dose pharmacokinetic studies. The PBPK model appears to be of greatest value in describing the pharmacokinetic behavior of very complex drugs.

Physiologically-based pharmacokinetic modeling has been used extensively in toxicology. More recently, this approach has been used to study the pharmacokinetics of the antiarrhythmic agent, amiodarone (Hou and co-workers, 1990). Amiodarone is one of the most effective antiarrhythmic agents but one of the most complex drugs available in terms of its pharmacokinetics, pharmacodynamics, and antiarrhythmic effects (Barbey and Woosley, 1986; Mason, 1987). Traditionally its pharmacokinetics have been considered to follow a three-compartment model, distributing slowly to poorly perfused tissue such as adipose tissue. It has extremely variable pharmacokinetic behavior. The oral bioavailability varies from 20 to 70 percent, and the elimination half-life ranges from 8 to 107 days. Efficacy after oral dosing is delayed in onset and requires several days to become apparent. The reasons are unproven but may be due in part to poor bioavailability, the time required for distribution to the heart, and accumulation of desethylamiodarone, an active metabolite. Therefore, onset of clinical effect is difficult to predict. Current practice utilizes a series of decremental loading doses to achieve an early therapeutic effect (Siddoway and co-workers, 1983). Because of the complex pharmacokinetics of amiodarone, dosing is a challenge when traditional methods of dosage adjustment and monitoring of plasma concentrations are attempted. However, these complex pharmacokinetic factors have been incorporated into the PBPK model and applied clinically (Hou and co-workers, 1990).

The time course of plasma concentrations of desethylamiodarone predicted by the PBPK model for an intravenous amiodarone dose of 400 mg is in good agreement with data observed when patients had been given this dose (Hou and co-workers, 1990). Figure 1 shows that the computer-simulated concentrations of desethylamiodarone in blood or various tissues are in good agreement with the concentrations that are observed (Hou and co-workers, 1990). This agreement is closer than that achievable using two- or three-compartment mathematical modeling and could lead to better understanding of the concentration-effect relationships observed with amiodarone.

The pharmacokinetic modeling of amiodarone is one of the most complex that could be analyzed using PBPK modeling. This model has been utilized to predict appropriate clinical dosing in a small number of patients with atrial fibrillation or atrial flutter (Hou and co-workers, 1991). Certainly, less complex pharmacokinetic problems could easily be studied using physiologically-based pharmacokinetic modeling.

In PBPK modeling it is imperative to use pharmacokinetic data from as many sources as possible. A future goal for this type of analysis would be to include drug action, or pharmacodynamic modeling, into the pharmacokinetic model. Computer analysis of this combination of data would yield projections of the pharmacokinetic/pharmacodynamic

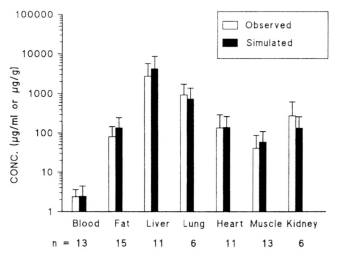

Fig. 1. Blood and tissue concentrations of desethylamiodarone in 15 patients receiving long-term oral amiodarone compared to data simulated by a PB-PK model (Modified from Hou and and co-workers, 1990).

profiles of drugs and make possible the design of clinical efficacy studies and predictions of drug effects in various clinical settings.

RELATIONSHIPS BETWEEN PLASMA CONCENTRATION, DOSE, AND EFFICACY

The application of pharmacokinetics in drug development or in the clinical setting requires the demonstration of a reliable concentration-response relationship for the particular drug. Therefore, it is important to understand the methods for examining relationships between plasma concentration, efficacy and dosage, and how these relationships can be utilized to identify confounding factors in a clinical database. An examination of these relationships can also aid in identifying confounding factors in drug development, such as the role of active metabolites, chirally specific actions or stereospecific clearances of drugs, and nonlinearity of pharmacokinetics and/or pharmacodynamics. These factors can often explain discrepancies in concentration-response relationships. Polymorphic metabolism of drugs is now recognized as a contributor to such discrepancies, and it can have clinically relevant consequences. Because a therapeutic end point is often not available to measure drug efficacy, surrogate markers for drug action are often used. Electrocardiographic intervals are surrogates for the actions of many drugs that affect ion channels, including antiarrhythmic drugs, as well as some antihistaminic drugs. In many cases the electrocardiogram can be used as a surrogate for drug efficacy or drug toxicity.

During depolarization of the cardiac cells, there is an inward movement of sodium, which causes the upstroke or phase zero of the action potential. This corresponds to the QRS interval on the surface electrocardiogram. In the absence of structural heart block, the duration of the QRS interval is generally a measure of sodium channel activity. Excessive dosages of drugs that block sodium channels widen the QRS duration. Some drugs such as encainide or flecainide widen QRS even at usually effective dosages. The PR interval is also an end point that can be examined as a surrogate marker for drug action; it is prolonged by calcium channel blockade and/or beta-adrenergic blockade. However, the use of this marker is complex because the PR interval is also influenced by changes in autonomic tone. The duration of the QT interval is roughly equivalent to the duration of cardiac repolarization. Repolarization occurs due to the movement of several ions, especially potassium. The activity of drugs that alter repolarization, either by lengthening or shortening it, can be detected by looking at the surface electrocardiogram for effects on the QT interval. Prolongation of electrocardiographic intervals on the surface electrocardiogram generally correlates with drug actions that have been observed *in vitro* and are consistent with clinical effects. In such cases they are useful surrogate markers for efficacy and safety.

Encainide is an antiarrhythmic drug for which the QRS interval is a reasonably reliable surrogate marker for drug action. The pharmacokinetics of this drug are quite complex and its action is markedly influenced by its metabolism. As previously discussed by Roden (pages 209 and 210), encainide is metabolized by O-demethylation and by N-demethylation. O-demethylation to O-des-methylencainide (ODE) is the major pathway for metabolism in 93 percent of the population (McAllister et al., 1986; Woosley et al., 1986; Cary et al., 1984). The cytochrome P450 isozyme responsible for the O-demethylation of encainide is known as P4502D6 and is responsible for the metabolism of other antiarrhythmic agents, as well as some beta-adrenergic receptor antagonists (beta-blockers) and many tricyclic antidepressants (Gonzalez and Meyer, 1991; Kalow, 1987). The oxidative metabolism of the antihypertensive agent debrisoquine has been used as a marker for P4502D6. Therefore this metabolic pathway is known as the debrisoquine oxidative pathway of drug metabolism. This pathway is genetically determined and functionally absent in 7 percent of the Caucasian population classified as poor metabolizers (PMs). In PMs, N-demethylation of encainide predominates, resulting in the production of small amounts of N-desmethylencainide, which is most likely an inactive metabolite (McAllister and co-workers, 1986). However, in this group, encainide also accumulates, resulting in sodium channel blockade. In patients who can form ODE, it is subsequently converted to 3-methoxy-O-desmethylencainide (MODE) by the same pathway responsible for the formation of ODE (McAllister and co-workers, 1986; Cary and co-workers, 1984). For encainide, both ODE and MODE are pharmacologically active and have different electrophysiologic effects compared to the parent compound (Cary and co-workers, 1984).

The presence of active metabolites following administration of encainide was suggested by analysis of pharmacokinetic/pharmacodynamic relationships obtained during the infusion of encainide in patients with stable ventricular ectopic depolarizations (VEDs) (Cary and co-workers, 1984). In this study, VED frequency was compared to simultaneously determined plasma concentrations of encainide, ODE, and MODE. A counterclockwise hysteresis loop was observed for encainide (Figure 2), such that even though the encainide concentrations early after infusion were quite high, there was very little suppression of VED, but later, when the plasma levels of encainide were decreasing, an antiarrhythmic effect and QRS prolonga-

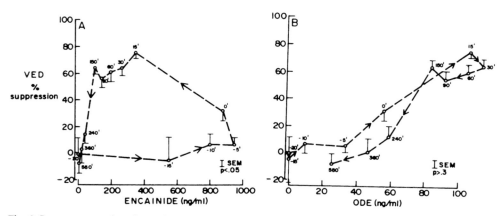

Fig. 2. Percent suppression of VED in relation to plasma concentrations of (A) encainide and (B) ODE after infusion of encainide in extensive metabolizers. The points are connected in the order of time at which they were obtained. (Reprinted from Cary et al., 1984)

tion were observed. When ODE levels were examined in the same patients given encainide, development of the antiarrhythmic effect was observed as the ODE levels increased, and the antiarrhythmic effect declined as the ODE levels declined. Therefore, there was a much better correlation between the clinical response and ODE concentrations than between response and plasma concentrations of the parent compound, leading to the hypothesis that ODE is the active agent in this clinical setting. This was later confirmed when ODE was given intravenously to similar patients (Barbey and co-workers, 1988). In this way, surrogate markers of efficacy can be used in combination with pharmacokinetic measures to identify potentially active metabolites and the presence of a pro-drug.

Encainide, ODE, and MODE are all sodium channel blockers, of which ODE is the most potent (Woosley and co-workers, 1988). In addition to sodium channel blockade, MODE alters refractoriness and prolongs the QT interval on the surface electrocardiogram. Because this pharmacologic profile appeared desirable, studies were conducted to evaluate the clinical antiarrhythmic actions of MODE. Previous clinical studies evaluated the pharmacokinetic characteristics of MODE following single intravenous doses of MODE administered to patients with stable high frequency VEDs (Barbey and co-workers, 1988). The pharmacokinetics after single doses were analyzed and modeled. Those data were then used to design loading and maintenance infusions that should reach target blood levels for patients with ventricular arrhythmias (Roden and co-workers, 1989). These doses were increased until side effects occurred or arrhythmia suppression was achieved. Electrophysiologic data were obtained during pseudo-steady-state conditions as evidence of pharmacologic activity during each maintenance infusion. The infusion regimens, based on pharmacokinetic data and a targeted concentration of MODE, were able to predict the observed plasma concentrations of MODE attained during the efficacy study (Figure 3).

This protocol for drug administration rapidly produced blood levels in the desired range, resulting in the desired pharmacologic effects. A fairly constant plasma concentration and drug effect were produced and maintained throughout the infusion. This administration

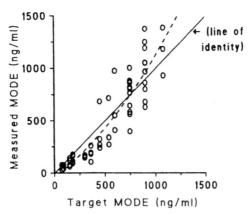

Fig. 3. Relationship between predicted and observed plasma MODE concentrations. (Reprinted from Roden and co-workers, 1989).

regimen was also used to examine the pharmacologic effects of MODE on arrhythmias such as ventricular ectopic depolarizations, and to determine the relationship between that action and other surrogate markers of drug action, such as QRS prolongation. In this model the plasma concentration-effect relationship can also be examined. The relationship between pharmacokinetics and pharmacodynamics can be used to predict dosing requirements.

The previous studies exemplified how pharmacokinetic data can be used to help design dosing regimens for subsequent efficacy studies in patients with severe arrhythmias. However, pharmacokinetic data may have transiently misled drug development in the case of the antiarrhythmic agent, propafenone, as was briefly discussed by Roden (see page 210).

In an early study assessing the clinical pharmacokinetics of propafenone, patients with ventricular arrhythmias received 3 to 7 days of each dose of propafenone in progressively increasing daily oral doses of 300 mg, 450 mg, 600 mg, and 900 mg (Connolly and co-workers, 1983). A nonlinear relationship was observed between propafenone dose and steady state plasma concentrations. In addition, intrasubject variability was observed in steady state plasma concentrations, therapeutic concentrations, and half-life of elimination. As a result, caution in making dosage adjustments was advised, with the observation that a doubling of the dose would more than double the plasma concentration of propafenone. These observations generated concern among investigators that slow titration with small dose increments would be necessary.

A great deal of evidence suggests that propafenone is metabolized by P4502D6 (Funck-Brentano and co-workers, 1990). A comparison of dosage and trough plasma concentrations of propafenone in relationship to debrisoquine metabolic phenotype indicated a linear relationship in the poor metabolizers (Siddoway and co-workers, 1987). However, a disproportionate (nonlinear) doubling of plasma concentration was observed after a 50 percent increase in dose for the extensive metabolizers, suggesting that although active metabolites are formed, P4502D6 is saturated at higher propafenone dosages. However, in a parallel dosage comparison, a linear relationship between propafenone dosage and clinical effect

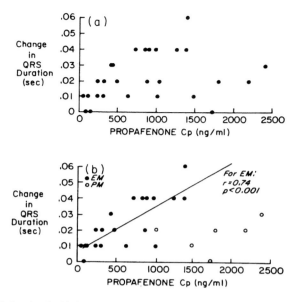

Fig. 4. Change in QRS duration in relation to plasma propafenone concentration (Cp). *a*, Data for all patients; *b*, data for extensive metabolizers of P4502D6 (open circles) and poor metabolizers (closed circles), with linear regression fit for extensive metabolizers. (Reprinted from Siddoway and co-workers, 1987).

(suppression of ventricular ectopic depolarizations) was observed (Salerno and co-workers, 1984). This demonstrates that the interpretation of nonlinearity of pharmacokinetics must be carefully and clinically assessed. The discrepancy was based on the fact that the metabolite was active but proportionally less was present at high doses of propafenone.

Siddoway et al. (1987) also assessed the effect of debrisoquine metabolic phenotype on clinical response to propafenone. Their early clinical experience had detected an unusually long half-life of propafenone in a patient who was a known poor metabolizer of debrisoquine. In a group of patients with ventricular arrhythmias treated with propafenone, no correlation was observed between propafenone plasma concentration and change in QRS interval, the surrogate end point (Figure 4). However, if this analysis is corrected for metabolic phenotype, by separately analyzing data for the patients who are poor or extensive metabolizers of propafenone, a very good correlation exists between plasma propafenone concentration and QRS widening for the extensive metabolizers. A similarly good but very different relationship was found in the poor metabolizers. Because the concentrations required for QRS widening in the poor metabolizers are much higher than those in the extensive metabolizers, the presence of active metabolites contributing to the clinical effect in extensive metabolizers is suggested. Since 5-hydroxy-propafenone (5HP) was only seen in the plasma of extensive metabolizers and not PMs, and 5HP is active in animal models, these results support the hypothesis that the metabolite contributes to the clinical actions of propafenone. Because the poor metabolizers are missing the enzyme required for formation of 5HP, a higher plasma concentration of the parent is required in this population to achieve a clinical effect.

These studies demonstrate that the initially misleading results of pharmacokinetic studies were clarified by subsequent pharmacodynamic studies. Later in the drug's development, the relationship between pharmacologic effects and pharmacokinetic characteristics was very helpful in understanding the clinical pharmacology of propafenone.

A closer examination of the clinical pharmacology of propafenone led to yet another interesting observation. Although propafenone is a structural analog of beta-blockers, the early clinical data using single doses indicated that it had 1/40 the potency of propranolol (McLeod, Stiles and Shand, 1984). This was consistent with *in vitro* studies which concluded that propafenone had very weak beta-blocking activity (McLeod, Stiles and Shand, 1984) However, an interesting phenomenon was observed in a careful study of the beta-blocking actions of propafenone. Beta-blockade was determined by maximum exercise heart rate and by isoproterenol sensitivity, the dose ratio (DR) of isoproterenol required to raise the heart rate 25 beats per minute during drug administration (propafenone) compared to during control (placebo) administration over a range of propafenone plasma concentrations and dosages (Lee and co-workers, 1988 and 1990). Schild analysis was then used to determine potency of beta-blockade. As determined by a right shift in the isoproterenol dose response curve (an increase in the DR), and by a reduction in maximum exercise heart rate, both poor and extensive metabolizers of propafenone had measurable dose-related beta-blockade. The extent of beta-blockade was much greater in poor metabolizers, who had significantly higher plasma levels of propafenone than the extensive metabolizers. In fact, *in vitro* receptor binding studies show that the active metabolite 5-hydroxypropafenone, which is present in the extensive metabolizers but not in the poor metabolizers, is much less potent as a beta-blocker than the parent compound. Results from phase I and phase II studies did not indicate that beta-blockade had occurred because the data from poor and extensive metabolizers were averaged. Because this effect occurs in only 7 percent of the population, it is easily overlooked when the data are averaged. The beta-blocking action was identified only when the poor metabolizer phenotype was studied in greater detail. Thus for drugs undergoing oxidative metabolism, determination of metabolic phenotype is important in the interpretation of pharmacokinetic data and in the application of such data to clinical trials or drug therapy.

RECEPTOR OCCUPANCY AS A MARKER FOR *IN VIVO* ACTIVITY

Consideration of pharmacodynamic end points requires an assessment of drug effect at its site of action. Although clinical efficacy is the ideal end point, it is not always readily observed during clinical trials and surrogate markers for efficacy are often used. For example, blood pressure reduction may be monitored as a surrogate end point for reduction of longterm sequelae of hypertension. Also, reduction of plasma lipid levels for the management of hypercholesterolemia is a surrogate end point for prevention of related morbidity.

The radioreceptor assay of antagonist activity present in patients' plasma during drug therapy can be used as a pharmacodynamic/pharmacokinetic model (Wellstein and co-workers, 1985a). This is a three-dimensional model that takes into account plasma concentration of a drug, characteristics of the binding of that drug at a specific receptor, and the clinically measured effect of the drug. Radioreceptor assays can be surrogates for drug action and alternatives to chemical methods of detection of plasma concentrations of drugs, and may be useful in early stages of drug development. Such studies are useful when the interaction of drugs with receptors is equally quantified by a variety of measurements, from *in vitro* receptor binding assays to effect measurements in man (Wellstein and co-workers, 1985b). For example, for beta-blockers, the Ki values detected from radioreceptor assay are in agreement with those obtained from Schild analysis of isoproterenol sensitivity testing (Wellstein, Belz and Palm, 1988). In these studies, the *in vitro* pharmacodynamics of antagonist present in plasma is linked to the time course of drug effect in man, and this model can be used to predict the time course of the clinical effects, thereby helping in the design of clinical trials. Radioreceptor assays have been used in this way to quantify drug effects at beta-1 and beta-2 adrenergic receptors and muscarinic cholinergic receptors (M1, M2, and M3) in man (Pitschner and co-workers, 1988, 1989a and 1989b; Wellstein and co-workers, 1984).

The radioreceptor assay relies on the competition between antagonist in the plasma and a radioligand specific for the receptor of interest (Wellstein and co-workers, 1984). Rather than describing this competition in terms of inhibition, the results are expressed as occupancy of the receptor *in vitro* by antagonist present. This gives a determination of the potential pharmacologic activity present in the plasma that is assumed to be in equilibrium with the effect compartment.

Many pharmacokinetic studies examine plasma concentration kinetics of a drug, i.e., a measure of drug concentration in the plasma compartment. This is often compared to the time course of effect (the change in response in the effect compartment) which may not be parallel with the plasma concentration time course. In contrast, the time course of receptor occupancy is a direct measure of the time course of agonist or antagonist activity in the plasma and in the effect compartment.

For most drugs, it is possible to assay the presence of parent compound in the plasma. If the parent compound is the only one that is measured in the assay, and if the parent compound is the only active agent, excellent correlations are usually seen between plasma concentration and drug effects. However, many drugs have active metabolites or act selectively at different receptor subtypes to produce a clinical effect, resulting in poor concentration-response relationships. If the chemical detection method measures both enantiomers of a racemic mixture, only one of which is active, a discrepancy between plasma levels and clinical response will be observed (Wellstein and co-workers, 1984). Similarly, the method of chemical detection may not be sensitive enough to detect very low concentrations of a drug. In such cases the time course of the clinical effect may not agree with that of the plasma concentration. Because receptor occupancy measures only non- protein bound active drug that has high affinity for the receptor of interest, occupancy is determined by the presence of any active compound, including both the parent compound and active metabolites. Therefore, in such cases, receptor occupancy would account for many of the observed differences between the time course of clinical effects and the plasma concentration kinetics.

Propranolol is a classical drug for which a discrepancy is observed between the time course of plasma concentration (t = 4 hours) and the time course of clinical effects (t = 10.5

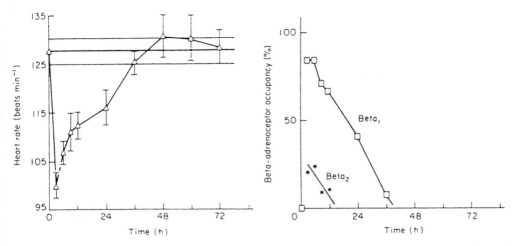

Fig. 5. Reduction of exercise tachycardia (left panel) and relative *in vitro* beta-adrenoceptor occupancy (right panel) after a single 200 mg oral dose of atenolol. (Reprinted from Wellstein and co-workers, 1987).

hours) (Wellstein and co-workers, 1985a). However, the radioreceptor assay can be used to explain this discrepancy. For example, following a single oral dose of propranolol, a decrease in maximum exercise-induced heart rate occurred within 1 to 5 hours and then fell off slowly over the next 36 hours (Wellstein and co-workers, 1987). Plasma samples collected at each exercise time point were analyzed in an *in vitro* radioreceptor assay. In this *in vitro* assay, radioligand is displaced from beta-adrenergic receptors by active antagonist present in the plasma collected from the subjects who had received propranolol. A determination of occupancy of the beta-adrenergic receptors by the antagonist present showed that the time course for occupancy paralleled the time course of effects of propranolol on heart rate. The duration of the effect depends on the degree of initial receptor occupancy, and therefore depends on the dose of drug used (Wellstein and co-workers, 1985b). A perfect concordance was found between occupancy measured *in vitro* at beta-1 (rat parotid gland) or at beta-2 (rat reticulocytes) adrenergic receptors, in agreement with the lack of selectivity of propranolol at beta-adrenergic receptors (Wellstein and co-workers, 1985b).

Atenolol given to normal volunteers shows similar effects on heart rate (Wellstein and co-workers, 1987). However, the beta-adrenergic radioreceptor assay can be used in this case to determine subtype selectivity of this drug. Figure 5 shows marked differences in the selectivity of atenolol for beta-1 and beta-2 adrenergic receptors. *In vitro* receptor occupancy at the beta-1 adrenergic receptor by antagonist from plasma of volunteers having taken atenolol correlates best with its effects on heart rate. This is in agreement with other *in vitro* and clinical measurements of the selective effect of atenolol on heart rate. However, as shown in this figure, subtype selectivity is not complete; occupancy at beta-2 adrenergic receptors is evident and may be clinically relevant at high concentrations of atenolol. Thus, the radioreceptor assay can be used to demonstrate relative subtype selectivity of clinically relevant doses of drugs.

CONCLUSION

From the integration of pharmacokinetic and pharmacodynamic analyses, i.e. inter-relating concentration, drug action, and *in vitro* receptor binding, hypotheses can be tested in the evaluation of the clinical pharmacology of drugs. Furthermore, computer modeling such as physiologically-based pharmacokinetic modeling, and basic pharmacologic methods, like radio receptor binding and Schild plot analysis, can be used to observe and quantify drug action in man, making drug development more efficient and productive and safer.

REFERENCES

Barbey, J. T., and R. L. Woosley (1986). Pharmacokinetic approach to amiodarone dosage selection. Clin. Prog. Electrophysiol. Pacing, 4, 310-317.

Barbey, J. T., K. A. Thompson, D. S. Echt, R. L. Woosley, and D. M. Roden (1988). Antiarrhythmic activity, electrocardiographic effects and pharmacokinetics of the encainide metabolites O-desmethyl encainide and 3- methoxy-O-desmethyl encainide in man. Circulation, 77, 380-391.

Benowitz, N. L. (1974). Clinical applications of the pharmacokinetics of lidocaine. In K. L. Melmon (Ed.) Cardiovascular Drug Therapy (Cardiovascular Clinics). Vol. 6. F. A. Davis, Philadelphia.

Carey, E. L., H. J. Duff, D. M. Roden, R. K. Primm, G. R. Wilkinson, T. Wang, J. A. Oates, and R. L. Woosley (1984). Encainide and its metabolites. Comparative effects in man on ventricular arrhythmia and electrocardiographic intervals. J. Clin. Invest., 73, 539-547.

Connolly, S. J., R. E. Kates, C. S. Lebsack, D. C. Harrison, and R. A. Winkle (1983). Clinical pharmacology of propafenone. Circulation, 68, 589- 596.

Funck-Brentano, C., H. K. Kroemer, J. T. Lee, and D. M. Roden (1990). Propafenone. N. Engl. J. Med., 322, 518-525.

Gonzalez, F. J., and U. A. Meyer (1991). Molecular genetics of the debrisoquin-sparteine polymorphism. Clin. Pharmacol. Ther., 50, 233-237.

Hou, Z. Y., N. J. Balter, R. L. Woosley, and S. L. Schwartz (1990). A Physiologically-Based Pharmacokinetic (PB-PK) Model for Desethylamiodarone. Circulation, 82 (Suppl III), 196 (Abstract).

Hou, Z. Y., S. J. Huang, S. A. Chen, C. W. Chiou, S. L. Lin, M. Lin, M. S. Chang, S. L. Schwartz, R.. L. Woosely, and C. Y. Chen (1991). Application of a simulated myocardial concentration-based amiodarone regimen in atrial fibrillation/flutter. Circulation, 84(Suppl II), II-714.

Jusko, W. J. (1986). Guidelines for collection and analysis of pharmacokinetic data. In W. E. Evans, J. J. Schentag, and W. J. Jusko (Eds.), Applied Pharmacokinetics. Applied Therapeutics, Inc., Spokane, Washington, pp. 9-54.

Kalow, W. (1987). Genetic variation in the human hepatic cytochrome P450 system. Eur. J. Clin. Pharmacol., 31, 633-641.

Lee, J. T., H. K. Kroemer, D. J. Silberstein, C. Funck-Brentano, M. D. Lineberry, A. J. J. Wood, D. M. Roden, and R. L. Woosley (1990). The role of genetically determined polymorphic drug metabolism in the beta-blockade produced by propafenone. N. Engl. J. Med., 322, 1164-1168.

Lee, J. T., M. D. Lineberry, C. Funck-Brentano, P. L. Chaffin, D. M. Roden, and R. L. Woosley (1988). Propafenone-induced ß-blockade in extensive and poor metabolizer subjects. Circulation, 78(Suppl II), II-499.(Abstract)

Mason, J. W. (1987). Amiodarone. N. Engl. J. Med., 316, 455-466.

McAllister, C. B., H. T. Wolfenden, W. S. Aslanian, R. L. Woosley, and G. R. Wilkinson (1986). Oxidative metabolism of encainide: Polymorphism, pharmacokinetics and clinical considerations. Xenobiotica, 16, 483-490.

McLeod, A. A., G. L. Stiles, and D. G. Shand (1984). Demonstration of beta adrenoceptor blockade by propafenone hydrochloride: clinical pharmacologic, radioligand binding, and adenylate cyclase activation studies. J. Pharmacol. Exp. Ther., 228, 461-466.

Pitschner, H. F., and A. Wellstein (1988). Dose response curves of pirenzipine in man in relation to M1- and M2-cholinoceptor occupancy. Naunyn Schmiedebergs Arch. Pharmacol., 338, 207-210.

Pitschner, H. F., B. Schulte, M. Schlepper, D. Palm, and A. Wellstein (1989a). AF-DX 116 discriminates heart from gland M2-cholinoceptors in man. Life Sci., 45, 493-498.

Pitschner, H. F., M. Schlepper, B. Schulte, C. Volz, D. Palm, and A. Wellstein (1989b). Selective antagonists reveal different functions of M cholinoceptor subtypes in humans. Trends Pharmacol. Sci., (Suppl), 92-96.

Roden, D. M., J. T. Lee, R. L. Woosley, and D. S. Echt (1989). Antiarrhythmic efficacy, clinical electrophysiology, and pharmacokinetics of 3-methoxy-O-desmethyl encainide (MODE) in patients with recurrent sustained ventricular tachycardia or fibrillation. Circulation, 80, 1247-1258.

Salerno, D. M., G. Granrud, P. Sharkey, R. Asinger, and M. Hodges (1984). Controlled trial of propafenone for treatment of frequent and repetitive ventricular premature complexes. Am. J. Cardiol., 53, 77-83.

Siddoway, L. A., C. B. McAllister, G. R. Wilkinson, D. M. Roden, and R. L. Woosley (1983). Amiodarone dosing: a proposal based on its pharmacokinetics. Am. Heart J., 106, 951-956.

Siddoway, L. A., K. A. Thompson, C. B. McAllister, T. Wang, G. R. Wilkinson, D. M. Roden, and R. L. Woosley (1987). Polymorphism of propafenone metabolism and disposition in man: clinical and pharmacokinetic consequences. Circulation, 75, 785-791.

Stargel, W. W., D. G. Shand, P. A. Routledge, A. Barchowsky, and G. S. Wagner (1981). Clinical comparison of rapid infusion and multiple injection methods for lidocaine loading. Am. Heart J., 102, 872-876.

Wellstein, A., D. Palm, G. Weimer, M. Schafer-Korting, and E. Mutschler (1984). Simple and reliable radioreceptor assay for beta-adrenoceptor antagonists and active metabolites in native human plasma. Eur. J. Clin. Pharmacol., 27, 545-553.

Wellstein, A., D. Palm, G. G. Belz, and H. F. Pitschner (1985a). Receptor binding characteristics and pharmacokinetic properties as a tool for the prediction of clinical effects of ß-blockers. Arzneimittelforschung, 35, 2-6.

Wellstein, A., D. Palm, H. F. Pitschner, and G. G. Belz (1985b). Receptor binding of propranolol is the missing link between plasma concentration kinetics and effect-time course in man. Eur. J. Clin. Pharmacol., 29, 131-147.

Wellstein, A., D. Palm, G. G. Belz, R. Butzer, R. Polsak, and B. Pett (1987). Reduction of exercise tachycardia in man after propranolol, atenolol and bisoprolol in comparison to beta-adrenoceptor occupancy. Eur. Heart J., 8(Suppl M), 3-8.

Wellstein, A., G. G. Belz, and D. Palm (1988). Beta adrenoceptor subtype binding activity in plasma and beta blockade by propranolol and beta-1 selective bisoprolol in humans. Evaluation with Schild-Plots. J. Pharmacol. Exp. Ther., 246, 328-337.

Woosley, R. L., D. M. Roden, G. H. Dai, T. Wang, D. C. Altenbern, J. Oates, and G. R. Wilkinson (1986). Co-inheritance of the polymorphic metabolism of encainide and debrisoquin. Clin. Pharmacol. Ther., 39, 282-287.

Woosley, R. L., A. J. J. Wood, and D. M. Roden (1988). Encainide. N. Engl. J. Med., 318, 1107-1115.

Wyman, M. G., R. L. Slaughter, D. A. Farolino, S. Gore, D. S. Cannom, B. N. Goldreyer, and D. Lalka (1983). Multiple bolus technique for lidocaine administration in acute ischemic heart disease. II. Treatment of refractory ventricular arrhythmias and the pharmacokinetic significance of severe left ventricular failure. J. Am. Coll. Cardiol., 2, 764-769.

CONCENTRATION-CONTROLLED TRIALS: BASIC CONCEPTS, DESIGN, AND IMPLEMENTATION

Lilly P. Sanathanan *
Carl C. Peck
Food and Drug Administration
Rockville, MD 20857

ABSTRACT

A Concentration-Controlled Trial (CCT) is one where subjects are assigned to prede-termined levels of average plasma drug concentration. These target concentrations are achieved (within reasonable ranges) by an individualized pharmacokinetically (PK) control-led dosing scheme. In a recent paper (Sanathanan and Peck, 1991), we have investigated the sample size efficiency of the Randomized CCT (RCCT) design in comparison to the traditional Randomized Dose-Controlled Trial (RDCT). We have pointed out that in addition to safety concerns which strongly suggest the use of CCTs for drugs with narrow therapeutic windows, sample size considerations favor the choice of CCTs in many situations. In particular, substantially smaller sample sizes are possible with CCTs which are designed to minimize the interindividual PK variability within comparison groups and consequently decrease the variability in clinical response within these groups. In a subsequent paper (Sanathanan and co-workers, 1991), we proposed a Phase II randomized concentration-con-trolled titration design with the objective of streamlining the drug development process. In this chapter we present a brief overview of the basic concepts underlying the design and implementation of CCTs.

---

* This work was performed while the author was employed by the Food and Drug Administration. Dr. Sanathanan is presently affiliated with IBRD (Institute for Biological Research and Development, Inc.) Blue Bell, PA.

Integration of Pharmacokinetics, Pharmacodynamics, and Toxicokinetics in Rational Drug Development, Edited by A. Yacobi *et al.*, Plenum Press, New York, 1993

239

INTRODUCTION

The traditional approach to drug development has been to evaluate the effectiveness of a new drug using the randomized dose-controlled trial (RDCT) design, involving comparison of a single dose group with placebo, or comparison of multiple dose groups. The RDCT design often leads to large variability in response within comparison groups, a substantial part of which can be due to inter-individual pharmacokinetic (PK) variability. An alternative to this situation is offered by the Randomized Concentration-Controlled Trial (RCCT), proposed by Peck (1990). In this design, subjects are randomly assigned to predetermined levels of average plasma drug concentration including or excluding the zero concentration or placebo group. These target concentrations are achieved (within reasonable ranges) by an individualized pharmacokinetically (PK) controlled dosing scheme. If plasma concentrations are more strongly related to drug response than are doses, as is often the case, it is clear that the RCCT design has an advantage over the RDCT design in that it is able to decrease the variability in response within comparison groups by minimizing the variability in plasma concentrations within these groups.

EFFICIENCY OF RCCT

The efficiency of RCCT vs. RDCT in terms of sample size requirements for detecting a possible concentration-related effect was derived by Sanathanan and Peck (1991) using the pharmacodynamic model for theophylline (Figure 1) as an example. Specifically, let N_C and N_D be sample sizes required for RCCT and RDCT respectively, to achieve the same power with an α-level significance test of the hypothesis that $\beta=0$, where β is the slope of the linear portion of the relationship between concentration and effect. The ratio N_D/N_C is defined as the efficiency, Eff, of RCCT vs. RDCT. Thus, Eff >1 implies that the sample size required for RDCT is larger compared to RCCT or that RCCT is more efficient than RDCT.

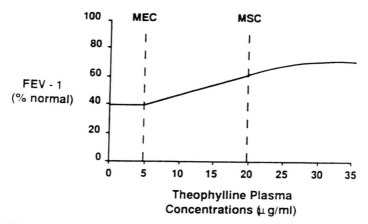

Fig. 1. Theophylline pharmacodynamic model relating FEV-1 measurements, as a percent of normal, to plasma concentrations, where MEC and MSC are minimum effective and safe concentrations, respectively.

Let C_i be the steady state concentration value to which the ith individual is randomized. For example, in a theophylline study, one might consider randomizing individuals to one of four target concentrations: 5,10,15, and 20 µg/ml. In order to make a fair comparison of the RCCT and RDCT designs, the dose levels D_i for the RDCT design are chosen to yield average concentrations equal to C_i in the RCCT design. The steady state concentration C of a drug obeying linear kinetics is given by

$$C = \frac{D}{CL} \qquad (1)$$

where D is the infusion rate for IV infusion and CL is clearance which can be regarded as a random variable varying over individuals given the same dose. It follows from (1) that $E(C) = DE\,(1/CL)$ where E denotes expected value or mean. Thus, D_i should be chosen such that $D_i = C_i/E\,(1/CL)$.

The linear part of the RCCT model is given by

$$R = Baseline + \beta\,(C\text{-}MEC) + e \qquad (2)$$

where R denotes response to the drug at steady state concentration C, MEC denotes "Minimum Effective Concentration", ß is the slope of the linear relationship, and e is error distributed with mean 0 and variance σ_e^2 representing intra-subject variability in response plus measurement error.

The linear part of the RDCT model is given by

$$R = Baseline - \beta\,(D/CL\text{-}MEC) + e \qquad (D\ fixed,\ CL\ random) \qquad (3)$$

The main distinction between the RCCT and RDCT designs is that the RDCT design leads to a larger variance [Var (R)] for the response variable due to inter-subject variability in clearance. Specifically, from equations (2) and (3) it follows that

$$for\ RDCT,\ \ Var(R) = \sigma_e^2 + \beta^2\,Var(1/CL)D^2 \qquad (4)$$

and

$$for\ RCCT,\ \ Var(R) = \sigma_e^2 \qquad (5)$$

Equations (4) and (5), in turn, lead to the following expression for efficiency of RCCT vs RDCT

$$Eff = 1 + \frac{\beta^2\ CV_{CL}^2\ \sum C_i^2(C_i - C_{av})^2}{\sigma_e^2\ \sum(C_i - C_{av})^2} \qquad (6)$$

where C_i values are the concentrations chosen for the RCCT trial, C_{av} is the average concentration, CV_{CL} is the coefficient of variation for clearance, ß is the slope of the linear PK model, and σ_e^2 is the intra-subject variance (including variability due to measurement error) in PD response, and CL is assumed to have a log normal distribution.

241

It is evident from equation (6) that RCCT is always more efficient than RDCT. The extent of improvement due to RCCT is determined by the second term in equation (6). Greater efficiency for RCCT results from (a) a larger PK variability as reflected by the presence of CV_{CL}^2 in the numerator and (b) a stronger PD relationship as manifested by a steeper slope and a lower intra-subject variance.

The quantities appearing in equation (6) are unit dependent, and some form of normalization is necessary to achieve an equivalent form of equation (6) that is independent of units. Let W denote the width of the therapeutic range given by MSC (Maximum Safe Concentration) - MEC. The maximum PD effect equals ßW and one can relate σ_e to this maximum PD effect by defining CV_e as $\sigma_e/\beta W$. CV_e can be viewed as a measure of the strength of the PD relationship, capturing both the magnitude and variability of PD response. Further, let $S_i = C_i/W$, and let S_{av} be the average of the S_i values. Then equation (6) reduces to

$$Eff = 1 + \frac{CV_{CL}^2 \; \Sigma \; S_i^2(S_i - S_{av})^2}{CV_e^2 \; \Sigma \; (S_i - S_{av})^2} \qquad (7)$$

and the quantities appearing in equation (7) are all unit-free. From equation (7) it is clear that the wider the range of concentrations used, or the higher the concentrations (compared to the width of the therapeutic range) explored, the greater is the efficiency of RCCT. Higher concentrations may be required for demonstration of the efficacy of a drug. However, this can pose a safety problem for a drug with a narrow therapeutic window. In such situations, the RCCT design offers a distinct advantage in that higher concentrations can be achieved with RCCT more precisely, and hence safely, or alternatively, the RDCT design would be necessarily limited by low concentrations to allow an adequate safety margin. This type of gain in efficiency is a bonus and is not reflected in our computations, which are dependent on the assumption that in the RDCT design doses equivalent to concentrations in the RCCT design can be administered safely.

EFFICIENCY RESULTS

Plausible values for efficiency based on the theophylline data provided in Peck et al. (1989) ($\beta = 1.43\%$ *FEV-1 per* µg/ml; MEC = 5µg/ml; MSC = 20µg/ml; Intercept = 40% normal FEV-1; σ_e = 8% FEV-1 units) are shown in Table 1 for varying values of CV_{CL}. For the theophylline example, $\Sigma S_i^2 (S_i - S_{av})^2 / \Sigma (S_i - S_{av})^2$ equals 0.92 which is close to 1. This is probably typical (unless the therapeutic range is narrow compared to MEC) in which case Eff is approximately $1 + CV_{CL}^2/CV_e^2$. For theophylline, CV_{CL} is approximately 0.50 and CV_e is approximately 0.40, and thus, Eff is roughly equal to 2.6. Table 1 also contains efficiency values in the presence of inter-subject PD variability (incorporated into the PD model by allowing the slope ß to be a random variable varying over the different individuals in the trial. Figure 2 contains a graphic representation of the effect of PK/PD variability on the efficiency of RCCT vs RDCT. The efficiency of RCCT vs. RDCT is less sensitive to increases in PD

242

TABLE 1. Effects of PK/PD Variability on Efficiency of RCCT vs RDCT

PK Variability $CV_{cl}{}^{*}$	PD Variability $CV_{s}{}^{*}$	Theoretical -Linear Model
20%	Zero	1.27
20%	20%	1.24
20%	50%	1.18
50%	Zero	2.66
50%	20%	2.52
50%	50%	2.11
50%	70%	1.92
70%	Zero	4.25
70%	20%	3.97
70%	50%	3.18
70%	70%	2.80

* CV_{cl} and CV_{s} are expressed as percentages here, although they appear as proportion in the analytical expressions given in the text.

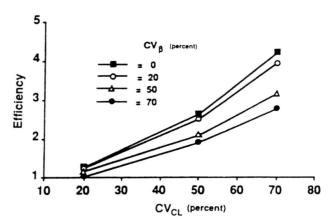

Fig. 2. Effects of PK/PD variability on efficiency of RCCT vs RDCT

variability, as shown in Table 1 and Figure 2. Specifically, it is seen from Table 1 that the efficiency value of 2.7 resulting from 50% CV_{CL} and zero PD variability is reduced to only 2.1 and 1.9 with the addition of 50% and 70% PD variability respectively. This is in contrast to the sharp increase in efficiency from 1.2 to 3.2 corresponding to an increase from 20% PK variability to 70% PK variability in the presence of 50% PD variability. The results in Table 1 are based on the strictly linear PD model. Simulations were done on the basis of the threshold model with the plateau constraint (as shown in Figure 1). These results were very close to the analytical results and are therefore not presented here.

The expression for the efficiency of RCCT vs RDCT given by equation (6) is based on the IV route of administration, and reflects the inter-subject variability in clearance only. This expression can be generalized to the oral route by taking into account the inter-subject variability in extent of absorption in addition to clearance. In the presence of either PK variability alone or PK plus PD variability, the efficiency EFF$_{PO}$ of RCCT vs RDCT for the oral route is related to the efficiency, Eff$_{IV}$ for the IV route, as follows:

$$Eff_{PO} = 1 + \frac{(Eff_{IV}-1)((CV_F^2+1)(CV_{CL}^2+1)-1)}{CV_{CL}^2} \qquad (8)$$

where CV_F is the coefficient of variation for the extent of systemic bioavailability F. F and CL are assumed to have log normal distributions. For a numerical illustration, consider the case of 50% PK and 50% PD variability. From Table 1, Eff$_{iv}$ equals 2.11. Additionally, for the oral route, suppose there is a 50% coefficient of variation in bioavailability (some of this variability could arise from noncompliance). Then, Eff$_{PO}$ = 3.49. In other words, with 50% variability in clearance, 50% variability in bioavailability, and 50% PD variability, one would need roughly 3.5 times as many patients for the RDCT design, compared to the RCCT design. Thus, there is a substantial gain in efficiency from using RCCT in such situations. Moreover, for a drug with a narrow therapeutic window, requiring high concentrations for demonstration of efficacy, RCCT may be a preferable design from the ethical (safety) as well as practical standpoint.

DESIGN CONSIDERATIONS

The RCCT and RDCT designs discussed thus far are parallel group designs. Design issues such as the choice of specific concentrations/doses and in particular, the inclusion/exclusion of the placebo group are common to RCCT and RDCT. The issue of optimal design in the absence of specific information regarding the threshold and plateau regions is not straightforward. However, we note that it is a good idea to include the placebo arm in the first efficacy trial, if feasible, to get around the uncertainty regarding the linear range. By the same token, it would also be desirable to include a concentration near MSC in the first efficacy trial. For the first efficacy trial, we would also recommend two additional concentrations between the zero concentration and MSC, to gain information on the shape of the concentration - response curve. Reasonable choices of concentrations would be MSC, MSC/2, MSC/4, and

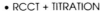

- RCCT + TITRATION

- EXIT RULE FOR NONREPONDERS AND TOXIC CASES

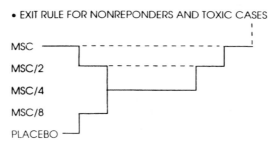

Fig. 3. Randomized concentration—controlled titration design (RCCTD) for Phase II.

MSC/8 or placebo (if feasible). This type of geometric spacing has some justification on the basis of an Emax model.

Sanathanan and co-workers (1991) discuss an efficient variant of the strictly parallel RCCT design, referred to as the randomized concentration-controlled titration design (RCCTD). This design is appropriate for Phase II of drug development and is basically an RCCT design with two parallel arms, one arm that is assigned to the maximum safe concentration (MSC) and a placebo arm. The proposed modification of this simple RCCT is to include an exit rule (for ethical reasons) that allows for dose reduction on the MSC arm and dose escalation on the placebo arm (Figure 3). It is further proposed that a titration design be incorporated within the exit rule, to provide information on the concentration-response relationship. Specifically, subjects failing on placebo (within a certain period of time) can be titrated through increasing concentrations until MSC (or even greater than MSC, if tolerated) is reached, if the subject fails at all intermediate concentrations. The number of intermediate concentrations to be included in the titration design can be flexible. Typically, up to three geometrically spaced intermediate concentrations (MSC/8, MSC/4, MSC/2) should suffice. One can also limit the number of intermediate concentrations to one or two per individual in order to shorten the trial duration. This can be done by assigning a given individual (failing on placebo) to one or two of the pre-specified intermediate concentrations at random, before eventually titrating this individual to the highest concentration, if necessary.

The RCCTD essentially consists of two parts. The first part is represented by a simple RCCT (proper blinding is assumed) with a fixed duration at the end of which the end points for placebo and MSC, including time to failure, can be determined. As soon as this part is completed, the blind can be broken, and an assessment can be made about the efficacy of the drug. Thus, this design can help determine if a drug is therapeutically useful, early in drug development. The second part is designed to give information on concentration response for a rational choice of dose or concentration in Phase III. Details regarding the analysis of data generated by a Phase II RCCTD trial and translating the optimal concentration based on such a trial to an optimal dose for a Phase III trial are discussed by Sanathanan and co-workers (1991).

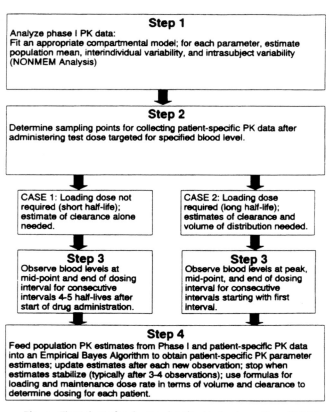

Step 1

Analyze phase I PK data:
Fit an appropriate compartmental model; for each parameter, estimate population mean, interindividual variability, and intrasubject variability (NONMEM Analysis)

Step 2

Determine sampling points for collecting patient-specific PK data after administering test dose targeted for specified blood level.

CASE 1: Loading dose not required (short half-life); estimate of clearance alone needed.

CASE 2: Loading dose required (long half-life); estimates of clearance and volume of distribution needed.

Step 3
Observe blood levels at mid-point and end of dosing interval for consecutive intervals 4–5 half-lives after start of drug administration.

Step 3
Observe blood levels at peak, mid-point, and end of dosing interval for consecutive intervals starting with first interval.

Step 4
Feed population PK estimates from Phase I and patient-specific PK data into an Empirical Bayes Algorithm to obtain patient-specific PK parameter estimates; update estimates after each new observation; stop when estimates stabilize (typically after 3–4 observations); use formulas for loading and maintenance dose rate in terms of volume and clearance to determine dosing for each patient.

Fig. 4. Flow chart of main steps involved in implementing a RCCT.

In general, RCCTD is appropriate for Phase II, while the parallel RCCT design may be an attractive option for Phase III. The CCT approach may also be utilized in Phase I for drugs with narrow therapeutic windows.

IMPLEMENTATION OF CCTS

The target concentration value for each individual in a CCT can be achieved via an appropriate adaptive dosage control scheme, such as the empirical Bayes algorithm explained by Peck and others (1991). The empirical Bayes procedure takes into account a limited number of measured drug concentrations at informative times after initiation of therapy, along with population kinetic parameters adjusted for patient characteristics derived from a similar patient population. Computer routines for implementing this algorithm are available and references to these have been provided by Peck (1986). With reasonably good information on population kinetics from Phase I trials, it is possible to achieve the targeted concentrations within 15% - 25% CV, using a small number of informative blood level observations from each individual (Peck and others, 1991). Estimates of inter-individual and intra-individual variability are automatically incorporated into the Bayesian algorithm for adaptive dosing. If these estimates are not available, one can use default values (e.g. 50% coefficient of variation for inter-individual variability and 20% coefficient of variation for intra-individual variability). In most situations, the steady state average concentration (given by dose rate/clearance) is the appropriate target value. To achieve this target, it is sufficient to obtain an estimate of clearance for each individual (unless a loading dose is required because of a long half-life, in which case an estimate of the volume of distribution would also be needed). The flow chart depicted in Figure 4 outlines the main steps involved in implementing a CCT.

DISCUSSION

CCTs are recommended primarily for shortening the drug development time. The randomized concentration controlled titration design (RCCTD) is seen to be an appealing design for Phase II. It combines the desirable features of a dose titration design with those of a basic RCCT design. The adaptive control scheme once put in place, may become so routine that it may not add to the complexity of the design. Data analysis and dose selection based on CCTs can also be handled with existing methodology. However, until a system is put in place for routine use, the CCT approach may be underutilized.

REFERENCES

Peck, C. C. (1986). Bayesian pharmacokinetics. Evolution and start of the art. In Young, Ingalls, and Hawkins (Eds.), Simulation at the Frontiers of Science. Eastern Simulation Conference, Norfolk, Virginia. Soc. Comp. Sim., San Diego. pp. 17-20.

Peck, C. C. (1990). The randomized concentration-controlled clinical trial: an information-rich alternative to the randomized placebo-controlled clinical trial. Clin. Pharmacol. Ther., 47, 126.

Peck, C. C., D. Z. D'Argenio, and J. Rodman (1991). Analysis of pharmacokinetic data for individualizing drug dosage regimens. In W. E. Evans, J. J. Schentag and W. J. Jusko (Eds.), Applied Pharmacokinetics, 3rd ed. Applied Therapeutics, Inc. Vancouver, Washington. Chapter 3.

Peck, C. C., D. P. Conner, and M. G. Murphy (1989). Bedside Clinical Pharmacokinetics: Simple Techniques for Individualizing Therapy. Applied Therapeutics, Inc. Vancouver, Washington.

Sanathanan, L. P., and C. C. Peck (1991). The randomized concentration- controlled trial: an evaluation of its sample size efficiency. Controlled Clinical Trials, 12, 780-794.

Sanathanan, L. P., C. C. Peck, R. Temple, R. Lieberman, and G. Pledger (1991). Randomization, PK-controlled dosing, and titration: an integrated approach for designing clinical trials. Drug Information Journal, 25, 425- 431.

OPPORTUNITIES FOR INTEGRATION OF PHARMACOKINETICS, PHARMACODYNAMICS AND TOXICOKINETICS IN RATIONAL DRUG DEVELOPMENT

Carl C. Peck[1], William H. Barr[2] Leslie Z. Benet[3],
Jerry Collins[1], Robert E. Desjardins[4], Daniel E. Furst[5],
John G. Harter[1], Gerhard Levy[6], Thomas Ludden[1],
John H. Rodman[7], Lilly Sanathanan[1,8], Jerome J. Schentag[9],
Vinod P. Shah[1], Lewis B. Sheiner[10], Jerome P. Skelly[1],
Donald R. Stanski[11], Robert J. Temple[1], C.T. Viswanathan[1],
Judi Weissinger[1], Avraham Yacobi[4]

[1] Center for Drug Evaluation and Research, FDA, Rockville, MD 20857
[2] School of Pharmacy, Virginia Commonwealth University, Richmond, VA 23298
[3] School of Pharmacy, University of California, San Francisco, CA 94143
[4] American Cyanamid Co., Pearl River, NY 10965
[5] Ciba-Geigy Pharmaceuticals, Summit, NJ 0790
[6] State University of New York at Buffalo, Amherst, NY 14260
[7] St. Jude Children's Research Hospital, Memphis, TN 38105
[8] Present address: IBRD, Irvine, CA 92715
[9] SUNY Clinical Pharmacokinetics Lab. at Millard Fillmore Hospital, Buffalo, NY 14209
[10] University of California Medical Center, San Francisco, CA 94143
[11] Department of Anesthesia, VA Hospital, Palo Alto, CA 94304

This report derives from the conference on "The Integration of Pharmacokinetic, Pharmacodynamic and Toxicokinetic Principles in Rational Drug Development," held on April 24-26, 1991 in Arlington, VA. The conference was sponsored by the American Association of Pharmaceutical Scientists, U.S. Food and Drug Administration and the American Society for Clinical Pharmacology and Therapeutics.

Integration of Pharmacokinetics, Pharmacodynamics, and Toxicokinetics in Rational Drug Development, Edited by A. Yacobi et al., Plenum Press, New York, 1993

249

THE OBJECTIVES OF THE CONFERENCE WERE:

- To identify the roles and the interrelationships between pharmacokinetics (PK), pharmacodynamics (PD) and toxicokinetics (TK) in the drug development process.

- To evolve strategies for the effective application of the principles of pharmacokinetics, pharmacodynamics and toxicokinetics in drug development, including early clinical trials.

- To prepare a report on the use of pharmacokinetics and pharmacodynamics in rational drug development as a basis for the development of future regulatory guidelines.

The new drug development process involves a series of developmental and evaluative steps carried out (in the United States) under an Investigational New Drug application (IND) and leading to submission of a New Drug application (NDA). The steps involved in this process and FDA evaluation are illustrated in Figure 1 and are summarized below. The process includes preclinical research and development, and clinical trials commonly divided into Phases 1, 2, and 3, and NDA review by FDA. For drugs that are shown to be effective and that can be administered with acceptable toxicity, the process results in NDA approval and marketing of the drug.

    A. Preclinical studies: The purposes of these studies in experimental animals are to demonstrate, directly or indirectly, the biological activity against the targeted disease; to provide data for toxicity and safety evaluation; and to provide PK and PD data which may be helpful in human dosing regimen development and dose escalation strategies.

    B. Clinical studies, Phase 1: These studies in healthy volunteers or patients are intended to define the initial parameters of toxicity, the tolerated dose range and general PK and PD characteristics of the drug. The studies also provide information on relevant PK and PD in special populations and on candidate drug delivery systems.

    C. Clinical studies, Phase 2: These studies in patients are to assess the drug's therapeutic effectiveness and to develop a rational dosing strategy for Phase 3 studies, by providing information on dose-concentration-response relationships suitable for designing dosage optimization/individualization strategies applicable in Phase 3.

    D. Clinical studies, Phase 3: These studies in patients are designed to document the clinical safety and efficacy, further refine the dose-concentration-response relationships and allow qualitative and quantitative assessment of adverse drug reaction rates.

    E. Drug labeling/individualization of dosing: On the basis of data obtained in clinical studies, product information for labeling is generated to provide individualized dosing strategies for optimal use of the new drug.

250

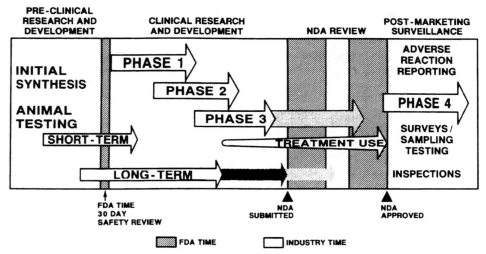

PRE-CLINICAL
RESEARCH AND
DEVELOPMENT
CLINICAL RESEARCH
AND DEVELOPMENT
NDA REVIEW
POST-MARKETING
SURVEILLANCE

INITIAL
SYNTHESIS

ANIMAL
TESTING

PHASE 1

PHASE 2

PHASE 3

SHORT-TERM

TREATMENT USE

LONG-TERM

ADVERSE
REACTION
REPORTING

PHASE 4

SURVEYS/
SAMPLING
TESTING

INSPECTIONS

FDA TIME
30 DAY
SAFETY REVIEW

NDA
SUBMITTED

NDA
APPROVED

FDA TIME   INDUSTRY TIME

Fig. 1. A schematic depiction of the new drug development process.

We believe that the application of PK, PD and TK principles and procedures to the development of a new drug is essential. Incorporation of PK and PD studies along with TK studies in each of these phases, coupled with appropriate and timely evaluation so as to influence subsequent drug development procedures, may lead to earlier identification of optimal dosing regimens, and may contribute to shortening the overall time of drug development. Of equal importance, the increased understanding of drug action derived from PK/PD based drug development leads to a more informative drug development program, especially as regards identification of drug dosage regimens that result in optimal therapeutic outcome through strategies for individualization of dosage. The establishment of this PK/PD information base during premarketing drug development provides an essential framework for continued refinement and improvement during post marketing drug use.

Figure 2 outlines opportunities for incorporation of these PK, PD and TK assessments in different stages of premarketing drug development. This report summarizes the rationale for incorporating PK, PD and TK in each phase of the drug development process and identifies specific kinds of studies that can/should be carried out.

I. PRECLINICAL PHARMACOKINETIC AND PHARMACODYNAMIC STUDIES

The objectives of preclinical pharmacokinetic and metabolism studies are to obtain information which is useful for: a) toxicity and safety evaluation studies in animals, by supporting study design, dosing regimen development and interpretation of toxicity data; and b) initial safety and tolerance studies in man, by providing pharmacokinetic and pharmacodynamic data that may be helpful in dosing regimen development and dose escalation in normal

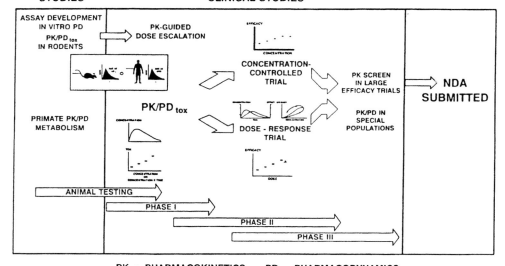

PK = PHARMACOKINETICS   PD = PHARMACODYNAMICS

Fig. 2. Schematic depicting opportunities for incorporation of PK, PD and TK assessments in drug development.

subjects and patients. Informative preclinical information can be helpful in expediting the drug development process.

The following specific kinds of studies will often be of value.

A. **Development of methodologies for quantitation of drug and metabolite concentrations in biologic fluids.**

The availability of specific and sensitive analytical procedures is essential to start any pharmacokinetic or pharmacodynamic research and development program for a new drug. When a major metabolite(s) is (are) known, particularly if pharmacologically active, an appropriate method should be developed for its (their) identification and quantitation in biologic fluids. If the drug and/or its metabolite(s) exhibit chirality, the assay should be stereospecific.

Note: Throughout this report, systemic drug concentrations may be used interchangeably with blood, plasma or serum measurements, depending upon which fluid of measurement is most convenient or useful for the drug under study. When analytical methods are developed in plasma or serum, it is useful to know the partition parameter into red blood cells so that drug clearances from blood by organs of elimination may be evaluated relative to organ blood flows.

B. **Mass balance-metabolism profile and metabolite pharmacology: determination of metabolic pathways and qualitative and/or quantitative measurement of major metabolites in blood, plasma or serum, urine, and other relevant fluids or tissues.**

252

In order to fully understand and interpret toxicology studies, it is essential to determine the fate (absorption, distribution, metabolism and elimination) of the drug in the species used in toxicology testing; it is especially important to discover interspecies differences, including differences from humans. Identification and pharmacologic characterization of individual metabolites is key in comparing results of preclinical studies with those of human studies.

C. **Pharmacokinetics and biological fluid concentration monitoring.**

Development of a pharmacokinetic data base, which characterizes the time-course of drug and metabolite(s) following multiple doses, supports the dosing regimens chosen and is needed to substantiate the extent and duration of exposure in animal toxicology species. Such a data base may also allow results using one dosage form to be extrapolated to another, or may facilitate extrapolation from different animal species to man.

D. **Relation of systemic drug concentrations to pharmacodynamic endpoints.**

Determination of systemic drug concentration ranges that are associated with pharmacological action and toxicological effects of a drug [or its metabolite(s)] may aid in development of human dosing regimens and may indicate the likely steepness of the dose response curve in man. For planning dose escalation in Phase 1 studies in normal subjects and patients, for example, the AUC of LD_{10} in mice of certain oncologic drugs has been shown to correlate with the AUC of the maximum tolerated dose of those drugs in patients.

E. **Systemic drug concentration monitoring in long-term toxicology studies.**

Concentration monitoring is used to determine extent of exposure during safety evaluation studies. This information will allow better interspecies comparisons than simple dose/body-weight comparisons. Knowledge of the intensity and duration of drug exposure is essential for substantiating safety assessments and will assist in interpretation of unanticipated toxicity.

F. **Protein binding.**

In vitro studies are undertaken to determine the extent of binding to proteins and unbound plasma concentration ranges associated with pharmacological action or toxicity of the drug. The quantitated free fraction values and their concentration dependence can be used to estimate the plasma concentrations of the free drug, which are associated with pharmacological action or toxicity.

G. **Tissue distribution.**

This study is usually conducted with a radiolabeled drug to determine the time course, persistence and potential accumulation of the drug and/or its metabolite(s) in various parts of the animal body. The disposition information can support a metabolism study in man using radiolabeled compound by providing dosimetry data.

H. **Placental transfer kinetic studies may complement reproduction studies.**

II. PHASE 1 STUDIES

The objective of Phase 1 clinical development is to define the initial parameters of toxicity, tolerance and their relation to dosage and the relevant pharmacokinetics of the drug.

These studies are usually carried out in healthy volunteers but in the development of drugs to treat AIDS and cancer, where the drugs under study are often highly toxic, Phase 1 investigations are undertaken in patients. It is important to realize that "Phase 1" refers both to a stage of development (earliest human exposure) and a kind of study (loosely, any clinical pharmacology), that may occur throughout the clinical development of the drug. The initial (early Phase 1) rising dose-tolerance and pharmacokinetic studies are utilized to establish the appropriate dosing program to be incorporated in Phase 2 studies. Further Phase 1 studies in volunteers and patients, usually carried out during and even after the Phase 2 and 3 clinical studies, are intended to characterize the drug's PK and PD in special populations, to optimize the drug delivery system, and to probe potential drug-drug and drug-disease interactions that might be expected to perturb the PK/PD relationship of the drug.

The sequence and timing of Phase 1 studies relative to other phases will depend upon the Clinical Development Plan, which will differ depending upon pharmacologic class and pharmacokinetic characteristics of the drug. It is important to incorporate PK/PD studies in the very first dose-tolerance studies in humans since this offers a unique (possibly one-time only) opportunity to evaluate drug concentration-acute toxic effect relationships of poorly tolerated doses which will be avoided in subsequent studies.

The following description of Phase 1 studies does not necessarily reflect the order in which they will be done. The major aims in Phase 1 studies include the following:

- To determine the tolerability and acute toxicity of the drug in normal subjects as a function of dose, duration of dosing, and, where possible, as a function of plasma concentration, prior to initiating Phase 2 studies in patients.

- To characterize the pharmacokinetics of the drug after a single dose as a function of dose size and, where appropriate after multiple doses.

- To characterize the acute pharmacologic effects, and their dose- and plasma concentration-relationships to both the desired clinical outcome and adverse effects.

- To assess the suitability (probable predictive value for humans) of the animal models used in toxicology studies with respect to comparability of exposure to the drug and its metabolites.

- To evaluate the bioavailability of dosage forms and drug delivery system(s) to be used in clinical studies, including assessment of the effects of food and other clinical variables on the rate and extent of absorption.

- To identify special populations or clinical conditions that result in altered pharmacokinetics/pharmacodynamics, requiring dose adjustment during clinical use.

- To initiate development of a PK/PD knowledge base for development of algorithms for initiation and adjustment of dosing in individual patients.

The following is a list of the types of studies that relate to these aims.

A. **Dose-escalation tolerance studies using a variety of designs to expose patients to increasing single, and subsequently multiple doses of drug. Often the same patient may receive several doses of the drug.**

These studies can yield at least three kinds of information:

1. Dose- and concentration-toxicity relationships:

Tolerance studies in humans reveal the first and often the only systematic information in humans at doses near or above maximum tolerated doses, making it possible to correlate acute toxicity with dose and, even better, plasma concentrations of the drug. In addition to systematic blood sampling for PK analysis, whenever possible, in these studies, a blood sample should be taken at each time that an adverse effect is observed. It may also be useful to measure active metabolite(s) at the time of an adverse effect.

2. Dose- and concentration-effect (or surrogate for effect) relationship:

If a clinically relevant pharmacologic effect can be measured in healthy volunteers and examining it will not compromise the safety outcomes of the study, an initial PK/PD model can be developed. A placebo group (zero dose) may contribute to the validity of such an effort. Where clinically relevant effects are not readily measured, it may be possible in preclinical animal studies to develop surrogate measures which can be used to relate PK parameters to pharmacologic effects. For many drugs, it will not be possible to develop PK/PD models of therapeutic efficacy in Phase 1, but a unique opportunity is lost if PK/PD models of acute or subacute toxicity and of some efficacy-related target organ effect(s) are not forthcoming from Phase 1 investigations.

3. Describing the dose-concentration relationship:

Single dose ranging oral studies can yield estimates of PK parameters such as CL/F, V/F, apparent half-lives, and CLr, as well as the variability and linearity with respect to dose of these parameters in a limited population. The relatively high doses usually employed in dose tolerance tests provide a unique opportunity to study the linearity of pharmacokinetics at concentrations that might occur clinically only through overdosing. Adequate systemic drug concentrations should be obtained following high doses for a sufficiently long period of time so that extrapolated areas will represent only a small fraction of the total area and so that multiple half-lives of disposition may be accurately estimated. The latter is important for determining the relevance of particular half-lives with respect to clearance. If this study is large enough, it may adequately characterize dose proportionality of the drug, but even a small study should detect significant non-linearity. Parallel measurements of acute drug effects, if possible, will provide data for PD modeling.

B. **Pharmacokinetic studies to characterize dose and time dependencies or non-linearities in the same individual after increasing single doses and multiple doses.**

In these studies it is important to cover the full range of doses likely to be used clinically. These studies can yield at least 2 kinds of information:

1. Dose-linearity over the therapeutic range after single doses. Crossover single dose studies in healthy volunteers encompassing the dose range anticipated to be studied in Phases 2 and 3 provide information on linearity of PK systems and intra-and intersubject variability. If low intersubject variability is encountered in the initial dose-escalation tolerance study such that linearity can be reliably demonstrated, or if PK screening data show clear linearity, these additional crossover single dose studies may not be necessary. This may be especially true if the initial tolerance studies can be designed to allow more than one dose per individual.

2. Dose linearity/dose-concentration relationship following multiple dosing. At a dose in the upper end of the anticipated clinical dose range, PK linearity can be evaluated by comparing the PK following a single dose to that during a dosing interval (relevant to the anticipated clinical studies) at steady state in the same volunteers. Multiple dose oral studies yield measures of CL/F and apparent half-life. Linearity of CL/F with increasing concentrations, stability with time of PK parameters or their time dependency (metabolic inhibition, induction) can be determined.

C. **Intravenous single dose study (with comparison to oral dosing) to rigorously characterize PK.**

This study can establish the absolute bioavailability of the drug and a precise model for the disposition characteristics of the drug. When an I.V. solution can be devised, a crossover study of an intravenous dose with an oral dose in healthy volunteers will provide unambiguous measures of F, CL, V and allows characterization of the absorption time-course profile of the oral dose. Metabolite profiles following oral and I.V. drug administration may provide information on the nature and site of biotransformation. These studies are critical to complete characterization of the PK and are also important in dosage form development.

To facilitate this goal the regulatory agencies should review and attempt to minimize any barriers to I.V. studies in humans for scientific purposes.

D. **Radioactive tracer studies to assess mass balance and further characterize metabolism and routes of elimination.**

Determination of mass balance and the time course of elimination of drugs and major metabolites is highly desirable. If most of the drug and its metabolites can be accounted for in blood and urine (with guidance provided by animal studies), it may not be necessary to utilize tracer studies. They will be helpful, however, where there is insufficient information on the routes and metabolic pathways of elimination from non-labeled studies.

It may be useful in some cases to combine administration of an oral radiolabeled dosage form with an I.V. dosage form, particularly when there is significant first-pass metabolism, but adequate chemical methods for the identification and quantification of metabolites are not available. Comparison of metabolite ratios following I.V. and oral dosing is important in evaluating first pass metabolism. If the drug is optically active, chiral assays may be employed to investigate stereospecific differences in biotransformation.

E. Evaluation of the suitability of preclinical animal models to predict pharmacologic effects in humans.

Data from studies described in paragraphs A-D, that characterize the pharmacokinetics of the drug, can be used to evaluate the suitability of preclinical animal species used in toxicity studies.

Differences in pharmacokinetics between the small number of animals available for toxicity testing and man may lead to toxicity data that are of limited relevance to clinical use. An adequate preclinical animal model is one that can be dosed such that it will attain blood or tissue levels of drug and active metabolites at least equal to, and preferably higher, than those attained in humans during therapeutic usage. While this issue is often most critical with respect to the interpretation of carcinogenicity and reproduction studies, it is pertinent also to the earliest human studies. If humans form a major metabolite not seen in animals it may be necessary to study the metabolite in animals by direct administration. However, this would not account for possible reactive intermediate metabolites.

Measures such as AUC, C_{max}, C_{min}, average steady state concentrations and degree of fluctuation may be used to compare systemic exposure in toxicology species and humans. Plasma protein binding and the plasma: red blood cell concentration ratio may be factors that influence the concentration of the drug in a target site. The frequency of dosing in the animal model compared to dosage regimens used clinically may be critical in terms of effective exposure because of differences in half-lives and therefore, in degrees of concentration fluctuation at fixed dosage intervals.

The qualitative and quantitative comparisons of active and potentially active metabolites with those found in early studies in humans are necessary to validate the animal model. Consideration should be given to chirality of active metabolites.

A complete understanding of the pharmacokinetics of the drug in both preclinical animals models and humans, including delineation of the relative drug distribution to the organs and routes of elimination, is important to all subsequent development, particularly in anticipating drug and disease state perturbations of PK/PD relationships that should be evaluated in late Phase l studies.

F. Evaluation of the drug formulations and delivery systems.

The importance of the dosage form is often unappreciated, leading to premature commitment to suboptimal formulations. It is unwise to prematurely commit to a particular dosage form prior to full characterization of PK/PD relationships, particularly GI absorption and first-pass elimination characteristics. It is advisable to initiate clinical studies in man using an experimental dosage form that is likely to have good systemic availability based on in vitro stability and dissolution data, and that is flexible in dosage. This is often a solution, suspension or "neat" capsule. Even these dosage forms must be considered with caution until absolute bioavailability and its variability are documented. Drugs delivered as solutions may have limited bioavailability due to instability in the gastric or intestinal environment. Some suspensions have poor dissolution and absorption due to the suspending agent or decreased effective surface area.

To maximize flexibility and ability to act on information attainable in early studies, the final dosage form can be chosen just prior to the conduct of clinical trials in Phase 3, even though candidate formulations may have to be developed earlier for stability studies. The final dosage form should be based on PK/PD relationships established in Phase 1/2. Significant differences in rate and extent of absorption between the formulation used in clinical studies and the formulation to be marketed should be avoided, because they may complicate interpretation of the trials. Because it is not always feasible to develop the final dosage form prior to Phase 3 clinical studies, it is critical to establish the bioavailability relationships of the to-be-marketed form to the dosage forms used in trials and to evaluate the clinical importance of differences.

The effect of food on the availability of the clinical dosage form should, if at all possible, be known before the pivotal clinical trials are carried out. The effects of food on the systemic availability of a drug may be quite complex. The sponsor should consider the physical-chemical properties of the drug, the performance characteristics of the dosage form and the degree of first pass metabolism in selecting an appropriate test meal(s) for a new drug product. A high fat meal may not be appropriate in all circumstances. Details on the types of food studies that should be done on the marketed dosage form have been listed in the AAPS/FDA Workshops on "In Vitro and In Vivo Testing and Correlation for Oral Controlled/Modified-Release Dosage Forms" (Skelly et al., 1990).

G. **Studies in special populations to identify patient characteristics that influence pharmacokinetics and/or pharmacodynamics and therefore require altered dosing or special monitoring.**

Depending on the pharmacologic class and the pharmacokinetic and metabolic characteristics of the drug, studies should be carried out in those types of individuals likely to exhibit clinically significant deviations from usual PK/PD behavior. These include patients with dysfunction of the drug elimination systems (e.g., hepatic and renal) that are relevant to the drug; patients with disease states that alter distribution (e.g., obesity or congestive heart failure), patients with genetically determined drug metabolism rates or patients who are likely to be taking concomitant medication that may interact with the drug. The development plan should also address, using specific studies, or population approaches (see Phases 2,3 below), methods that allow effects of age, race, body weight and gender to be evaluated. Studies in pediatric and elderly patients are essential when drug use is likely in these age ranges, the therapeutic index is narrow and/or pharmacokinetic variability is high.

Study of these patient and clinical variables is intended to provide information for the package insert to assist the clinician in tailoring drug dosage to optimize therapeutic outcome in individual patients. Therefore, the determinants of drug dosing rate should use those patient variables that would normally be conveniently available to or measurable by the practitioner (for example, age, body weight, creatinine clearance, etc.).

III. PHASE 2 AND 3 STUDIES

With the exception of drugs for a few diseases such as AIDS or cancer, Phase 2 studies are the first controlled trials in individuals with the disease or condition intended to be treated by the drug. They are usually of relatively short duration and focus on the effects of the drug on clinical and/or valid surrogate endpoints of therapeutic effectiveness. The principal goal of Phase 2 is to provide unequivocal evidence of the desired therapeutic effect. Hence, optimal experimental conditions are often employed, including use of relatively uncomplicated patients (little or no concomitant illness or disease), particularly close monitoring and attention to compliance, and attempts to use an unequivocally adequate dose by, e.g., titrating patients to the highest tolerated dose or blood concentration, use of a relatively short inter-dosing interval and use of a variety of therapeutic endpoints to gain an idea as to which is most satisfactory.

A second major goal is to gain information that will guide the additional clinical trials, generally larger and longer, carried out in Phase 3, such as the best dose range and titration scheme to use, the optimal dosing interval, needed adjustments of dose for people with organ dysfunction and concomitant medications, etc.

Often, a commercial sponsor does not want the Phase 2 (is the drug active in the disease?) to be prolonged and hence, the extra time needed to explore the full dose range and various dose intervals to obtain good dose and concentration response information may not be committed. Moreover, having established some effect at some dose, it is tempting to obtain the wider exposure in Phase 3 without ever defining these relationships, hoping that the efficacy will be evident in the further studies and that the adverse effects will be acceptable. Undoubtedly, this approach can be successful and it can be rapid. But on too many occasions failure to define dose-concentration-response relationships leads to unacceptable toxicity or adverse effect rates, marginal evidence of effectiveness (e.g., because the wrong dosing interval or dose was chosen), and a lack of information on how to individualize dosing. This is especially true when Phase 3 is designed with a series of concurrent studies, that allow no opportunity for the results of one trial to influence the design of subsequent trials.

Phase 3 studies overlap in intent and design with Phase 2 studies and include:

A. Additional controlled trials to establish effectiveness and dose-concentration-response.

B. Comparative trials with standard therapy.

C. Add-on or interaction studies, where the effect of the new agent is examined when added to other therapy.

D. Studies in special populations, e.g., patients with concomitant illness, varying severity of disease, specific demographic features (age, gender, race).

E. Longer-term studies, active-drug controlled or uncontrolled, to establish long term safety. These usually are only marginally (at best) useful for establishing effectiveness, but can be enhanced by employing randomized dose allocation (e.g. two or more doses of the test drug to gain dose-response information) or a randomized withdrawal phase.

F. Studies of long-term effectiveness or of clinical effects where only a surrogate end-point has been tested in Phase 2.

G. Studies of different regimens (q.d., where b.i.d. had been studied), titration schemes, or use of loading doses.

While there are no firm guidelines regarding how much of this information should be obtained in Phase 2 vs Phase 3, it seems obvious that there must be opportunity, for adaptive modification(s) whether this occurs after Phase 2 or during Phase 3. Moreover, the "unexpected" (toxicities, marginal (or lack of) efficacy, etc.) should be anticipated and possible means of understanding it and seeking it out should be utilized. This leads to two important principles.

1. Dose-concentration and concentration-response information, including an estimate of the lowest useful concentration, the concentration beyond which greater response is not seen (if toxicity does not preclude determination of this parameter), the highest concentration that is tolerated, and understanding of the concentration-effectiveness and concentration-toxicity curves, should be obtained as early in drug development as possible. Similarly, acceptable dose-interval(s) should be defined early.

2. Throughout Phases 2 and 3, systemic drug concentration data, apart from those related to concentration response trials should be routinely obtained on a survey basis to help explain unusual responses, to suggest the possibility for either the presence of or lack of drug-drug and drug-disease interactions, and to identify other unanticipated variability such as metabolic heterogeneity.

Specifically, applying these principles:

1. Ideally, the first or second Phase 2 controlled trial should be a concentration-response study, exploring the full tolerated range (found in Phase 1) of the drug. Concentration-response data may be derived retrospectively from randomized dose-response trials or more unambiguously from randomized concentration-controlled trials. While most experience to date is with parallel design trials, it is possible that titration-design trials, properly analyzed, can provide useful concentration-response and dose-concentration response data. Designs that expose a substantial fraction of the study group to more than one dose level are, however, the only designs that can provide information on the typical shape and distribution of individual dose-response curves. This information is important for dosage optimization, so that some such design (random sequence cross-over, dose titration, or other) should be used in at least some studies. Early concentration-response studies should be possible for drugs in a well-developed class, where the basic activity of the drug is easy to demonstrate and is highly probable based on clinical pharmacologic measures. Where the fundamental activity of the drug is not clear (first member of a new class) it may be reasonable to use maximum tolerated doses early, turning to

concentration-response later, but even here, the lack of prior information about toxicity argues that it is a desirable precaution to include one or more lower dose groups.

2. A well-designed Phase 3 will have an organized approach to establishing long-term safety, effectiveness and safety in relevant demographic and disease subgroups, clinical effectiveness where surrogates have been used, identifying the best dose-interval and dose adjustments needed in particular subsets (age, race, gender, patients with organ system dysfunction.)

Even a well-developed and carefully planned program cannot anticipate all possibilities. Moreover, specific studies of all possible subsets and interactions are costly, time consuming, and, probably unnecessary. The pharmacokinetic screen, (a small number of blood level measurements taken in some or all patients), coupled with the sorts of integrated overview analyses of effectiveness and safety data called for in FDA's Guideline to the Clinical and Statistical Sections of an NDA, or using more formal population models, can be used to identify and quantify important demographic and other subset differences. It will therefore be necessary to study formally only those interactions that require very precise definition or that would not be discerned in ordinary clinical studies because the correct measurements have not been taken.

IV. DRUG LABELING/INDIVIDUALIZATION OF DOSING USING PK/PD

It is the objective of labeling to advise the prescriber regarding the safe and effective method of use for a new drug in individual patients. Once the diagnosis has been made and the drug is chosen for use in treatment, then practical pharmacokinetic and pharmacodynamic information should be available in an organized and logical format to serve, when appropriate, as a basis for selection of dose and dosage interval. The known relationships between dose, plasma concentration and drug effects in typical patients may be used as a starting point in dosage individualization. The modifying effects of age, body weight, disease, and interacting drugs should be disclosed to practitioners, to help them adjust the dose or target exposure to suit the individual patient's needs and the practitioner's therapeutic goals. The entire clinical experience during Phases 1-3, in relationship to the derived exposure vs. effect relationships should be the basis of dosing recommendations for individualized treatment. The information derived therefore can be utilized in the following ways:

A. To guide practitioners when monitoring the desired and adverse effects of the drug, in relation to dose or plasma concentrations.

B. To assist practitioners in optimizing the use of the drug in a variety of patients, the algorithms for dosing particular subsets of patients are incorporated into the Dosing and Administration section. Ideally, labeling will include:

1. For systemic concentration monitoring (if indicated), the usual therapeutic concentration range, and suggested blood sampling times.

2. The methods that were used to assess drug response and drug toxicity so that therapeutic/toxic endpoints can be related to dose, exposure or systemic concentrations.

3. Alerts to the need for dose adjustments for concomitant use of interacting drugs, with attention to interactions that modify PK, PD or both.

4. The impact of variable compliance on therapeutic or toxic endpoints, if known, and, how this should affect dosing.

C. To help practitioners appreciate the existence of interpatient variability in response and its causes, and the way to avoid adverse drug experiences due to such variability.

Wording in the label should be developed to communicate to prescribers relevant kinetic and dynamic relationships, including some appreciation of intra- and inter-patient variability and its causes, so that they will be able to individualize treatment. In particular, variability can be expressed as ranges, standard deviations, coefficients of variation, etc. Information about intra-patient as well as inter-patient variability and their sources may be present in formulas, tables, or scattergrams.

V. CONCLUSIONS

The authors believe that a full understanding of the pharmacokinetics and pharmacodynamics of a new drug in preclinical animal species and humans, provides a scientific framework for efficient and rational drug development. Integration of the principles and practices outlined in this conference report into the drug development process should lead to identification of dosing regimens for individual patients that optimize therapeutic outcome.

DISCLAIMER: This report contains the personal opinions of the authors and does not necessarily represent the views or policies of the American Association of Pharmaceutical Scientists, U.S. Food and Drug Administration, or American Society for Clinical Pharmacology and Therapeutics. In particular, the report should not be construed as a guideline of the U.S. Food and Drug Administration.

REFERENCE

Skelly, J. P., G. L. Amidon, W. H. Barr, L. Z. Benet, J. E. Carter, J. R. Robinson, V. P. Shah and A. Yacobi (1990). In vitro and in vivo testing and correlation for oral controlled/modified release dosage forms. Pharm. Res. 7, 975-982 (1990).

GLOSSARY

AUC = Area Under Curve (plasma concentration time profile)
CL = Clearance
CLr = Renal Clearance
C_{max} = Maximum Concentration
C_{min} = Minimum Concentration
F = Fraction of Dose Available
V = Volume of Distribution

PUBLICATIONS

In order to reach wider circulation, and to have information available to scientists, by prior arrangement, this document was submitted and published in the following journals:

1. Pharmaceutical Research 9: 826-833 (1992)
2. Clinical Pharmacology and Therapeutics 51:465-473 (1992)
3. International Journal of Pharmaceutics 82: 9-19 (1992)
4. Journal of Pharmaceutical Sciences 81: 605-610 (1992)

AUTHOR INDEX

SUBJECT INDEX

Page numbers in **bold print** indicate that this subject is discussed on subsequent pages in the same chapter